CURRENT TOPICS IN ANEMIA

Edited by **Jesmine Khan**

Current Topics in Anemia
http://dx.doi.org/10.5772/66061
Edited by Jesmine Khan

Contributors

Yuriy Milovanov, Emmanuel Andres, Ana Isabel Lopes, Sara Valério Azevedo, Regilda Moreira-Araújo, Amanda Brandão, Elena Samohvalov, John Olaniyi, Greanious Alfred Mavondo, Mzingaye Maibongwe Louis Mzingwane, Ines Banjari I., Hong Yan, Lingxia Zeng, Leilei Pei, Chao Li, Ebru Dündar Yenilmez, Abdullah Tuli, Jelena Roganovic, Ksenija Starinac, Alina Solovyeva, Viola Gace, Cadiele Oliana Reichert, Filomena Marafon, Débora Levy, Luciana Morganti Ferreira Maselli, Margarete Dulce Bagatini, Solange Lúcia Blatt, Sérgio Bydlowski, Celso Spada

Published by InTech
Janeza Trdine 9, 51000 Rijeka, Croatia

Publishing Process Manager Dajana Pemac
Technical Editor SPi Global
Cover InTech Design team

First published February, 2018
Printed in Croatia
Legal deposit, Croatia: National and University Library in Zagreb

Additional hard copies can be obtained from orders@intechopen.com

Current Topics in Anemia, Edited by Jesmine Khan
p. cm.
Print ISBN 978-953-51-3774-0
Online ISBN 978-953-51-3775-7

For EU product safety concerns:
IN TECH d.o.o., Prolaz Marije Krucifikse Kozulić 3, 51000 Rijeka, Croatia,
info@intechopen.com or visit our website at intechopen.com.

Meet the editor

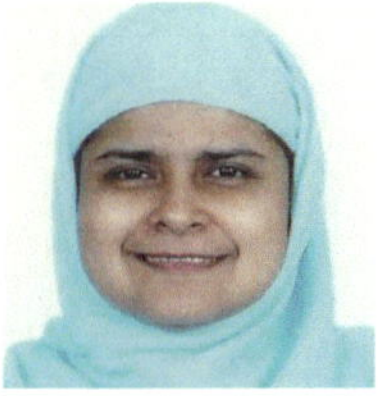

Jesmine Khan is affiliated with the Faculty of Medicine, Universiti Teknologi MARA (UiTM), Malaysia, as an associate professor. She obtained her MBBS degree from Mymensingh Medical College, Dhaka University, Bangladesh. She has special interest in nutrition and acquired her PhD degree in Surgical Nutrition from the Graduate School of Medicine, Osaka University, Osaka, Japan. She has vast experience in teaching at home and abroad. She is active in writings, has published numerous articles in scientific journals, works as an editorial board member and a reviewer of academic journals, and is involved in nutrition-related research and activities.

Contents

Preface

Anemia is a very common condition throughout the world. There are various causes of anemia. Anemia can develop from the disease itself either from chronic blood loss or from any other conditions, which cause malabsorption of nutrients required for the synthesis of red blood cells and hemoglobin. It might also result from the associated problems with the disease such as anorexia, nausea, and vomiting.

The objective of this book was to collect and compile the findings of reputable researchers from different countries of the world about common forms of anemia in some specific physiological conditions such as in children, elderly, and pregnant women and in pathological conditions such as inflammatory bowel disease, chronic kidney disease, systemic lupus erythematosus, and malaria. Different chapters of the book discuss the epidemiology, causes, pathophysiology, clinical features, laboratory diagnosis, and management of anemia in different diseases and conditions.

Chapters of this book might interest not only the physicians dealing with anemic patients but also other healthcare professionals and researchers involved in the care of anemic patients throughout the world. There are 13 chapters in this book, which gives an overall idea of the respective chapters of the authors' area of interest, where they shared their research and real-life experiences in managing their patients.

This book is divided into six sections. The first section includes two chapters, which discuss the common types of anemia: iron-deficiency anemia (IDA) and megaloblastic anemia. The first chapter of this section entitled "Iron-Deficiency Anemia" discusses the overall picture of iron-deficiency anemia. Iron-deficiency anemia is the most common anemia seen throughout the world. Before knowing about iron-deficiency anemia, it is very important to know iron metabolism. This chapter discusses the metabolism of iron, factors regulating iron metabolism, genetic variants and consequences of iron-deficiency anemia, standard diagnostic criteria, and treatment for iron-deficiency anemia. The second chapter of this book entitled "Megaloblastic Anemia" provides an overall idea of megaloblastic anemia including its causes, prevalence, clinical features, pathophysiology, laboratory diagnosis, differential diagnosis, and treatment.

The second section of the book includes chapters discussing anemia in different age groups such as in children, in women of reproductive age, in pregnant women, and in the elderly. The first chapter "Iron-Deficiency Anemia in Children" discusses the epidemiology, risk factors, causes, clinical presentations, screening, prevention, and treatment of iron-deficiency anemia in children in detail. The chapter "Iron-Deficiency Anemia and Pregnancy" discusses the prevalence of iron-deficiency anemia (IDA), bioavailability of iron during pregnancy, and intervention for IDA during pregnancy both from their own research and from others. This chapter also discusses the relationship between obesity and IDA in pregnancy. The third chapter of this section "Anemia in Women of Reproductive Age" discusses a common condition in women of childbearing age, leiomyoma, and abnormal and/or abundant uterine bleeding. This chapter also considers the main causes of bleeding and the therapy aimed at limiting the amount of blood loss, as well as preoperative treatment of iron deficiency in women with uterine leiomyomas, planning for pregnancy. The chapter "Nutritional Anemia in Elderly Patients" discusses the common nutrients responsible for causing anemia in elderly individuals of developed countries. It is thought that usually anemia is a problem of underdeveloped and developing countries. Very few people realize that it can be a problem of the developed countries as well. In this chapter, the author reviews the literatures by other researchers as well as by his own experience in this field.

The third section of the book includes several diseases as the cause of anemia such as inflammatory bowel disease, chronic kidney disease, severe malaria, and systemic lupus erythematosus. The first chapter of this section "Anemia and IBD: Current Status and Future Prospective" provides a detailed description of the prevalence, pathophysiology diagnostic criteria, and treatment of anemia in IBD patients to ensure better management and better quality of life. The second chapter of this section "Anemia in Chronic Kidney Disease (CKD) and after Kidney Allotransplantation" provides a literature summary concerning early diagnosis and treatment of anemia in CKD. As anemia in CKD has been recognized as a separate independent risk factor of cardiovascular events, this chapter might be useful for clinicians and contribute to decrease cardiovascular mortality. The third chapter of this section "The Pattern of Anemia in Lupus" discusses the pathophysiological mechanism of anemic syndrome in systemic lupus erythematosus (SLE) and the changes of the immune system, correlation between SLE and anemia of chronic disease, and different important methods to diagnose the pathological process of lupus as an immune disease. The fourth chapter of this section "Severe Malaria Anemia (SMA) Pathophysiology and the Use of Phytotherapeutics as Treatment Options" discusses postmalaria severe anemia that results in high malaria morbidity and mortality. The authors discuss the etiology, pathophysiology, and management of SMA by phytotherapeutics in reducing severe malaria anemia.

The fourth section "Hepcidin and Anemia" contains one chapter "Influence of Hepcidin in the Development of Anemia," which discusses the role of hepcidin, a peptide molecule that regulates iron homeostasis in the pathophysiology of anemia. Hepcidin contributes to the pathogenesis of iron-deficiency anemia, anemia of inflammation, and hemoglobinopathies, all of them are discussed in this chapter.

The fifth section "Laboratory Approach to Anemia" has one chapter that discusses and provides an overall idea of the use of algorithms as a tool in the determination of anemias in order to reduce the laboratory tests and accurately diagnose the underlying cause(s) in patients with anemia.

The sixth section "Management of Anemia by Novel Food Product" includes the chapter "Foods Produced with Cowpea Flour as a Strategy to Control Iron-Deficiency Anemia in Children" that discusses the usage of cowpea produced in Africa and Latin America, including Brazil, where the prevalence of anemia is high, to be used in the form of flour in the preparation of cookies for children for a new and promising strategy to reduce iron-deficiency anemia.

Jesmine Khan
Faculty of Medicine,
Universiti Teknologi MARA,
Malaysia

Section 1

Major Types of Anemia

Chapter 1

Iron Deficiency Anaemia

Lingxia Zeng, Leilei Pei, Chao Li and Hong Yan

Additional information is available at the end of the chapter

http://dx.doi.org/10.5772/intechopen.69048

Abstract

Iron deficiency anaemia as the most common nutrition disorder has only marginal reduction globally during recent decades, with the highest burden in pregnant women and young children. Insufficient iron storage and/or excessive loss of iron are common causes of iron deficiency anaemia. Therefore, understanding the complexity of the regulatory network required to maintain iron homeostasis and identifying the functional variants associated with iron metabolism should be fundamental and crucial to control and treat the iron deficiency anaemia. Sensitive and inexpensive measures to distinguish iron deficiency anaemia from the other kinds of anaemia should be developed for precise treatment. Original disease treatments combined with oral or intravenous iron therapy are key approaches in clinical practices. The integrated, multifactorial and multi-sectoral approach with food-based strategy and iron supplementation as the leading public health inventions is required to achieve iron deficiency anaemia control target. This chapter will focus on the advanced knowledge associated with iron metabolism, disease burden and health consequences of iron deficiency anaemia in different life course, newly parameters development in the diagnosis of iron deficiency anaemia, therapy choice in clinical practice and public health strategies to reduce iron deficiencies in high-burden areas.

Keywords: iron deficiency, iron deficiency anaemia, iron metabolism, hepcidin, iron supplementation, food fortification, ferritin, transferrin saturation

1. Introduction

As the most common nutrition disorder in both the developed and developing world, affecting more than two billion people, iron deficiency anaemia is recognized not only a clinical condition but also a serious public health issue, with pregnancy women and pre-school-age children at the highest risk [1–5]. The annual economic loss because of iron deficiency anaemia in 10 developing countries was estimated about 4% of gross domestic product [2]. Despite considerable economic and scientific advancement during recent decades, there has been only marginal reduction in the global prevalence of anaemia with more than 50% of cases caused by iron deficiency [2, 4].

This chapter will summarize the advanced knowledge associated with iron metabolism, health burden, newly parameters development in the diagnosis of iron deficiency anaemia, therapy choice and public health strategies to reduce iron deficiencies in high burden areas.

2. Iron metabolism and hepcidin, potential regulators associated with iron metabolism

2.1. Iron metabolism pathway

The absorption of dietary iron is a variable and dynamic process, depending on the two primary forms of haem and non-haem iron. Haem is a component of haemoglobin and myoglobin and haem iron is complexed as ferrous iron (Fe^{2+}) in the haem form, which is present in animal tissues such as meat, poultry, fish and shellfish [6]. Most of non-haem iron (Fe^{3+} or ferric iron) is provided by the vegetarian diet (black tea, cacao, cereals, dried fruit etc.). Although haem iron could represent ~40% of animal tissue iron and be better absorbed, it only accounts for less than 15% of total iron intake [7, 8]. In spite of the low absorption rate, the majority of the dietary iron is obtained from non-haem iron. Studies have confirmed that animal tissues (meat, poultry and fish) and vitamin C and organic acids could enhance iron absorption, while high intake of phytates, tannins, calcium and zinc may tend to inhibit the absorption of iron [9, 10].

It is currently well known that most of dietary iron is absorbed by enterocytes of the duodenal lining. The first step to absorb iron is that the insoluble ferric iron (Fe^{3+}) has to be converted into the ferrous form (Fe^{2+}) by a brush border ferric reductase (duodenal cytochrome B, DCYTB) in the duodenum and upper jejunum. The ferrous iron is then transferred across the enterocyte membrane into the cell by divalent metal transporter 1 (DMT1). Afterwards, the iron is stored in these intestinal lining cells as ferritin which is accomplished by Fe^{3+} binding to apoferritin, or could be released into the body via the only known iron exporter ferroportin. Cooperated with either of the ferroxidases hephaestin (enterocytes) or ceruloplasmin (other cell types) that facilitate iron extraction from the ferroportin channel, ferroportin at the basolateral membrane transports Fe^{2+} that is subsequently loaded onto plasma transferrin (Tf) [11].

In blood, plasma iron-loaded transferrin (Tf-Fe^{2+}) transports iron to all cells in a transferrin receptor-mediated endocytotic process [6]. Iron-loaded Tf binds to transferrin receptor 1 (TfR1), and their complex internalizes and enters into cells, wherein iron releases by pH-dependent mechanism. As it provides most of the iron required for various functions of an organism, plasma transferrin plays a crucial role in iron metabolism. TfR1 is highly expressed on haemoglobin-synthesizing erythroblasts. Most of plasma iron is used by bone marrow to synthesize haemoglobin in red blood precursors. Several other cell types, such as enterocytes, hepato-

http://dx.doi.org/10.5772/intechopen.69048

cytes and reticuloendothelial macrophages, are considered to be major iron storage sites. Iron release from or store in enterocytes, hepatocytes and macrophages depends on plasma iron levels, to meet the physiological demand. In a review published in Cell, Hentze et al. carefully discussed these mechanisms and summarized them in a single figure (**Figure 1**) [11].

2.2. Hepcidin and potential regulators associated with iron metabolism

In the human body, the iron homeostasis is tightly regulated to avoid both deficiency and excess. Hepcidin is a core regulator of the entry of iron into the circulation, which is a peptide hormone synthesized mainly in the liver, which was discovered in 2000. Previous studies have confirmed that hepcidin is not liver specific but also expressed in other tissues, such as the kidney, heart and lungs [12]. Hepcidin is first synthetized as an 84-amino acid (aa) prepropeptide, and then further processed into 60–64-aa prohepcidin. Finally, mature and biologically active 25-aa hepcidin is produced by truncating the proregion from prohormon convertase furin [13]. When the hepcidin level is abnormally high, serum iron falls due to iron trapping in macrophages and liver cells, and decreased gut iron absorption by reducing iron transport across the gut mucosa (enterocytes). In the instances, it is clear that anaemia will develop due

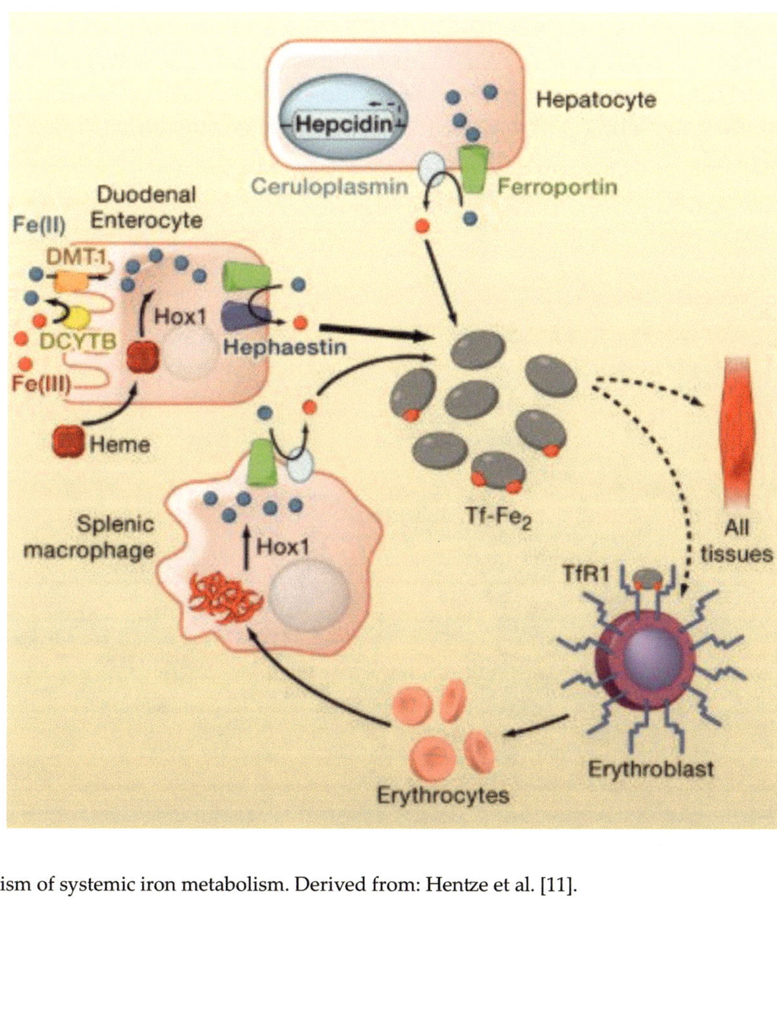

Figure 1. Mechanism of systemic iron metabolism. Derived from: Hentze et al. [11].

to lack of inadequate amount of serum iron being available for developing red cells. In the state in which the hepcidin level is abnormally low, on the contrary, iron overload occurs due to increased iron efflux from storage and gut iron absorption. Tandara et al. have discussed the mechanisms of hepcidin regulating iron homeostasis and summarized them in a single figure (**Figure 2**) [14].

So far, at least four major separate pathways in hepcidin regulation have been confirmed, such as regulation by iron status; dietary iron and iron stores; regulation by inflammation; regulation by hypoxia/anaemia and regulation by erythroid factors [15, 16]. These different regulatory inputs are integrated transcriptionally.

At the molecular level, it is not still completely clear that iron stores regulate hepcidin synthesis, but haemojuvelin (HJV), haemochromatosis protein (HFE) and transferrin receptor 2 (TfR2) have been proven to be upstream regulators of hepcidin. HFE acts as a bimodal switch between two sensors of the concentration of Tf-Fe^{2+}, TfR1 and TfR2, on the plasma membrane of hepatocytes [17]. HFE binds the ubiquitously expressed TfR1 at a site that overlaps the transferrin binding domain, and Tf-Fe^{2+} thus competes with HFE binding to TfR1. By contrast, TfR2 can bind both HFE and Tf-Fe^{2+} simultaneously [18]. Although HFE and TfR2 clearly contribute to hepcidin activation, the bone morphogenetic protein (BMP) signalling pathway is quantitatively the most critical. It has been proposed that HJV acts as co-receptor that binds to bone morphogenetic protein (BMP) ligands and BMP type I and type II receptors on the cell surface. This complex (HJV-BMP ligand-BMP receptors) consequently induces an intracellular BMP signalling pathway which in turn activates the SMAD4 signalling pathway.

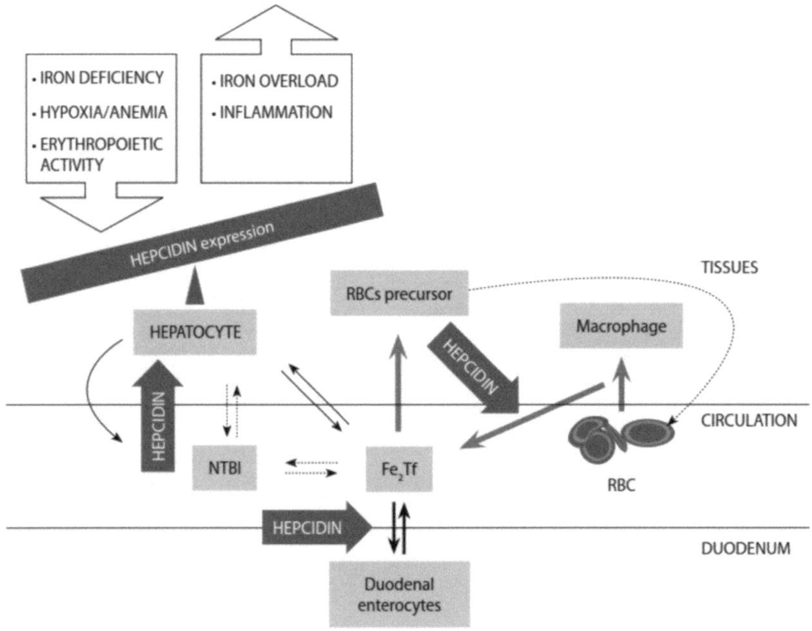

Figure 2. Maintenance of systemic iron homeostasis regulated by hepcidin. Derived from: Tandara and Salamunic [14].

The drosophila mothers against decapentaplegic (SMAD) complex translocate to nucleus and directly increases hepcidin gene transcription [19–21]. BMP/SMAD signalling cascade of HJV is important for basal regulation of hepcidin transcription [22]. Thus, HJV is central for hepcidin expression, and the point of convergence of multiple regulatory inputs. Transmembrane protease, serine 6 (encoded by the TMPRSS6 gene) has been identified as an inhibitor of hepcidin activation by cleaving membrane HJV under normal conditions [11, 23, 24]. If TMPRSS6 gene mutations occur, hepcidin levels increase and result in insufficient iron absorption [25].

Hepcidin synthesis is also dramatically induced by infection and inflammation. In particular, interleukin 6 (IL-6) is the central inducer of hepcidin synthesis during inflammation [14, 26, 27], which acts on hepatocytes and stimulates hepcidin production through signal transducer and activators of transcription (STAT3) signalling pathway [28]. Hepcidin mediated by IL-6 often results in cellular iron retention and hypoferremia, thus anaemia develops due to restricted iron availability in haemoglobin synthesis [14]. In the condition in which anaemia/hypoxia develops, hepcidin gene expression decreases along with the increase of erythropoietin expression. Tissue hypoxia increased erythropoiesis and further suppress hepcidin expression. Several bone marrow-derivated signal molecules that regulate the process of erythropoiesis mediating hepcidin have been found, including growth differentiation factor 15 (GDF15), twisted gastrulation protein homologue 1 (TWSG1), hypoxia inducible factors (HIF) and hormone erytropoetin [29–31]. Furthermore, iron responsive element (IRE)/iron responsive proteins (IRP) system also tightly regulates cellular iron uptake and storage and coordinatively keeps cell iron homeostasis.

Iron responsive proteins 1 (IRP1) and 2 (IRP2) in cytoplasmic can sense the level of iron in transit pool and bind specifically to RNA stem-loops (iron responsive element, IRE), and post-transcriptionally modify the expression of proteins involved in iron metabolism [14].

2.3. Genetic variants associated with iron deficiency anaemia from genome-wide association studies

The iron metabolism is tightly and precisely regulated by several interacting iron-binding factors. The development of genome-wide association studies (GWAS) has confirmed that the mutation of genes in iron metabolism, like transferrin, transferring receptors, matriptase-2, hepcidin, may determine the phenotypic variation in iron homeostasis between individuals [32]. Mutations in the gene (HAMP) encoding hepcidin can increase iron absorption and lead to juvenile haemochromatosis [33]. Due to the same regulatory pathway, mutations in these genes, including those encoding HJV, HFE and TfR2, clearly result in iron loading syndromes [32].

However, limited information is available about gene variants associated with iron deficiency anaemia. The inherited disorders of iron metabolism played an important role in iron deficiency anaemia. For example, in two association studies of iron metabolism disorders, the SNP rs235756 in BMP2 brings about the decrease of serum ferritin level [34, 35]. Mutations in the DMT1 gene occur in patients with microcytic anaemia, low serum ferritin and liver iron overload [36]. Studies also showed that mutations in the matriptase gene (TMPRSS6) cause iron-refractory iron deficiency anaemia [11]. It has been suggested that the mutation G277S of the TF gene alone does not affect iron absorption in iron deficient women and a combination of polymorphisms may be involved in iron metabolism [32, 37]. The recently determined mutation in the glutaredoxin 5 (GLRX5) gene leads to microcytic, hypochromic anaemia with iron overload and the presence of ringed sideroblasts in the bone marrow upon Perl's staining [38]. According to the European Network of Rare Congenital Anaemia, 62 rare anaemia subtypes are shown recently, including haemolytic anaemia and anaemia arising from mutations in genes that control duodenal iron absorption (e.g. SLC11A2), systemic iron homoeostasis (e.g. TMPRSS6) or erythroid iron absorption and utilization [8]. The genetic forms of sideroblastic anaemia such as mutations in glutaredoxin 5, aminolevulinic acid synthetase 2 and ABCB7 genes provide the updated information.

3. Disease burden and adverse health consequences of iron deficiency anaemia in different life courses

3.1. Disease burden

WHO estimated that the highest prevalence of anaemia was in the population of pre-school-aged children, pregnant and non-pregnant women, but lower for school-aged children, men and the elderly [8]. Data in 2010 showed more than 2.2 billion people were affected by anaemia and global prevalence of anaemia was 32.9%, and iron deficiency was reported as the most common cause of anaemia [4]. WHO estimates that 50% of cases are due to iron deficiency, and regional disparities exist [4, 39]. In detail, results from studies conducted in the United States reported the prevalence of iron deficiency ranges from 4.5 to 18.0%. But the proportion of anaemia caused by iron deficiency in central Asia, south Asia and Andean Latin America were 64.7, 54.8 and 62.3%, respectively [8, 40].

In 2010, global anaemia causing 68.36 million years lived with disability (8.8% of total for all conditions) [4]. The distribution of anaemia prevalence was unbalanced across regions, central and West Africa and south Asia were the highest anaemia prevalence regions in middle- and low-income areas, and high-income areas had lowest anaemia prevalence (**Table 1**). In addition, this trend was similar among the higher risk population of anaemia (children under 5 years, pregnant women from 15 to 49 years, non-pregnant women from 15 to 49 years) [5].

3.2. Consequences of iron deficiency anaemia

The population of pre-school-aged children, pregnant and non-pregnant women was the highest prevalence of anaemia [8], the consequences of iron deficiency anaemia among pre-school-aged children, pregnant and non-pregnant women should be emphasized.

The consequences of iron deficiency of pregnant women are multiple. First, iron deficiency during pregnancy was significantly associated with increasing perinatal mortality. Evidence from six observational studies showed a combined odds ratio of 0.75 (association between anaemia and maternal mortality) associated with a 10 g/L increase in haemoglobin [41, 42]. In addition, the combined OR was 0.72 for perinatal mortality associated with a 10 g/L increase in haemoglobin [41, 42]. Another study (RCT) conducted in China found prenatal supplementation with iron-folic acid was associated with a reduction in early neonatal mortality compared with

	Prevalence of anaemia (%)		
	Children (<5 years)	Non-pregnant women (15–49 years)	Pregnant women (15–49 years)
Middle- and low-income areas			
Central and west Africa	71	48	56
East Africa	55	28	36
South Africa	46	28	31
South Asia	58	47	52
East and southeast Asia	25	21	25
Central Asia, Middle East and north Africa	38	33	31
Oceania	43	28	36
Andean and central Latin America and Caribbean	33	19	27
Southern and tropical Latin America	23	18	31
Central and eastern Europe	26	22	24
High-income areas	11	16	22

Table 1. Distribution of anaemia prevalence in middle- and low-income areas by different population.

prenatal folic acid supplementation only [43]. Second, many studies have determinate the association between iron deficiency anaemia and pre-term and low birth weight [44–46]. Evidence from a retrospective population-based study showed maternal anaemia during pregnancy was risk factor for pre-term delivery (OR = 1.2) and low birth weight (OR = 1.1) [44]. Results from a meta-analysis reported that analysis of cohort studies showed a higher risk of pre-term birth (OR = 1.21) and low birth weight (OR = 1.29) with anaemia in the first or second trimester of pregnancy [45]. Significant association between prenatal iron deficiency anaemia and low birth weight was also found in low and middle-income counties [42]. Third, previous study reported that the fetal brain could be at risk when iron supply does not meet iron demand [47]. In addition, several observational studies reported the reverse effect of iron deficiency during pregnancy on intellectual development and motor development of children [48, 49]. One longitudinal study conducted in China found that prenatal iron deficiency anaemia in the third trimester is significantly associated with mental development of children [48]. Another prospective study conducted in Vietnam reported that prenatal iron deficiency anaemia hasadverse effects on child cognitive development [49].

Iron deficiency is more likely in women of reproductive age because of menstrual blood loss [50]. Results from some RCTs showed that iron improves cognitive ability, physical performance and mood in iron-depleted non-anaemia women [51–53]. In detail, a study found iron supplementation improved physical performance and mood of female soldiers [51]. One study conducted in the United States reported iron status was significantly associated with cognitive ability in women of reproductive age. The iron-sufficient women completed the cognitive tasks faster than women with iron deficiency anaemia, and got higher accuracy of cognitive function over a broad range of tasks [52]. Another study also reported the negative effect of maternal anaemia diagnosed postpartum on language comprehension of children [54].

Children under 5 years with iron deficiency anaemia test lower in social-emotional, cognitive and motor development than control group children [47, 55–59]. For motor development, an observational study conducted in African-America found poorer motor function in iron deficiency infants [56]. Another longitudinal study found lower motor scores in infants with chronic iron deficiency anaemia. In addition, long-term effect of chronic iron deficiency anaemia in infancy on motor development in early adolescence was exist, and even iron treatment at the age of 12–23 months did not prevent long-term effect of iron deficiency in infancy on motor development [57]. A study conducted in the United States showed positive effect of iron status of infants at 9 months on gross motor development and motor coordination/sequencing [58]. For cognitive development, a meta-analysis estimated that a 10 g/L haemoglobin increase was significantly associated with a 1.73 increase in IQ tests [41]. Another study found children with iron deficiency anaemia at 54–60 months age had lower score for verbal reasoning test compared to non-anaemia children [59].

Iron deficiency anaemia is prevalent in the elderly, particularly after the age of 80 [60]. Chronic blood loss, micronutrient-related anaemia and renal disease are important mechanisms for low haemoglobin level [61]. A cohort study conducted in Taiwan reported iron deficiency was significantly associated with cardiovascular disease and all-cause mortality in elderly [62]. A prospective study conducted in Korea found anaemia was associated with physical functioning impairment and instrumental activities of daily living in elderly [63]. A Norwegian prospective study reported the significant association between low iron status and increasing risk of death from ischaemic heart disease [64]. Result from a cross-sectional study conducted in England reported the significant relationship between iron status and symptoms of depression [65]. Many studies have extensively investigated the association between iron deficiency and productivity [42, 66], because the role of iron in oxygen transport to muscles and other tissues, and in other metabolic pathways by which iron deficiency can cause aerobic work capacity reduction [42]. Previous studies reported the positive effect of iron supplementation on work productivity of female cotton-mill workers in China, female tea-plantation workers in Sri Lanka and rubber plantation workers in Indonesia [66, 67]. Iron deficiency would cause work performance reduction and has substantial economic consequences accordingly in countries in which physical labour is prevalent [42, 67].

In summary, the consequences of iron deficiency anaemia in different populations were multiple. For pregnant women with iron deficiency anaemia, the effects were mainly on perinatal mortality, pre-term birth, low birth weight, offspring intellectual development and motor development. For non-pregnant women, the effects were mainly on cognitive ability, physical performance and mood. For infant, the effects were mainly focus on further social-emotional, cognitive and motor development. For elderly, the effects were mostly on cardiovascular disease, all-cause mortality, physical functioning impairment, instrumental activities of daily living, increasing risk of death from ischaemic heart disease and symptoms of depression. The effect of iron deficiency in adults on work productivity was also reported.

4. Standard diagnosis criteria of iron deficiency anaemia

At the population level, haemoglobin concentration is the most reliable indicator of anaemia. Meanwhile, measurement of haemoglobin concentration is frequently used as a proxy indicator of iron deficiency, because measurement of haemoglobin concentration is relatively inexpensive and easy. According to the criterion of World Health Organization, an adult man is considered as anaemic when the haemoglobin concentration is less than 130 g/L, whereas an adult woman is deemed anaemic when her haemoglobin concentration is less than 120 g/L, and this cut-off should be lowered to 110 g/L if the woman is in pregnancy. This cut-off threshold is 115 g/L between 5 and 11 years, and 110 g/L under 5 years (**Table 2**) [8, 68].

Patients with severe anaemia can be usually detected by clinical examination such as pallor of eyelids, tongue, palms and nail beds [8, 39, 69]. In poor areas where laboratory testing is not feasible, clinical examination should be regularly used to monitor women and children. As the frequency of conjunctivitis caused redness even in anaemia patients, palm pallor is preferred to eyelid pallor as a clinical sign for diagnosis of young children. But, clinical measures are more subjective and have more room for error accordingly compare to haemoglobin concentration [39].

Because of the complex diagnosis of iron deficiency, use of several indicators in combination could be better for us to assess iron deficiency [8]. First, red cell indices on full blood counts show a reduced mean cell volume, which corresponds to microcytosis, and a reduced mean cell haemoglobin, corresponding to hypochromia. But the thresholds are not commonly agreed [70]. Second, mean cell haemoglobin and volume are widely available, sensitive and inexpensive measures, but these indictors become abnormal only in longstanding iron deficiency. Moreover, mean cell volume could be normal if combined with nutrient deficiency [71].

Serum ferritin measurement is the most sensitive and specific test and widely used to identify iron deficiency [8, 39, 72], but it is spuriously elevate in malignancy, inflammatory conditions or liver disease. Serum ferritin below the cut-off of 15 μg/L in patients older than 5 years could be diagnosed as iron deficiency [72]. However, results from previous study indicated that if the cut-off of ferritin level increase to 30 μg/L, the diagnostic accuracy would be improved. The sensitivity would increase from 25 to 92% according, compared with the 12 μg/L (cut-off value), and specificity was unchanged (98%) [73]. For the patients with malignant disease, acute and chronic inflammatory disorders and liver disease, cut-off value equal or larger than 50 μg/L could still be iron deficient [4, 72]. Results from previous studies suggested cut-off of

Children (0–14 years)	Hb threshold (g/L)	Adult (≥15 years)	Hb threshold (g/L)
0.5–4 years	110	Non-pregnant women	120
5–11 years	115	Pregnant women	110
12–14 years	120	Men	130

Table 2. Haemoglobin threshold in different population.

100 μg/L for patients with chronic kidney disease [74], and suggested increasing cut-off to 200 μg/L in case of haemodialysis [75].

A low transferrin saturation level (less than 16%) also strongly indicates iron deficiency (iron supply insufficient to support normal erythropoiesis), but the threshold will increase to 20% in patients with inflammation. Because the serum iron will reduce with the increasing of total iron-binding capacity if the patients with iron deficiency, and finally result in reduction in transferrin saturation [8, 39].

Serum soluble transferrin receptor (sTfR) is another useful biomarker in diagnosis of iron deficiency, and is not influenced by inflammation. The synthesis of transferrin receptors will increase if patients with iron deficiency and lead to an increase in sTfR accordingly [73]. But there are some limitations when using sTfR to determine iron deficiency. One of the limitations is that if the patients with disorders associated with increased erythropoiesis (haemolytic anaemia, chronic lymphocytic leukaemia), concentrations of sTfR can be raised accordingly. Another limitation is that the guidelines are only published in the UK, but standardized cut-offs worldwide are still absent [75].

Recently, bone marrow aspiration is another option to assess iron stores, and thought of as the highly specific and not affected by inflammation for diagnosis of iron deficiency. But it is not used frequently only when other tests are conflicting or negative. As it is expensive and affected by recombinant human erythropoietin, it is uncomfortable for the patients [8, 39].

For diagnosis of iron deficiency anaemia, it is important to consider the whole picture rather than relying on single test results when determining the iron deficiency. The diagnosis of iron deficiency for the patients with inflammation is challenging and also cannot be determined on the basis of a single test result.

5. Therapy choice in clinical practices

The goals of treating iron deficiency anaemia are to treat its underlying cause and supply enough iron to normalize haemoglobin concentrations and replenish iron stores. Considering its cause and severity of iron deficiency anaemia, treatments may include dietary changes and supplements, medicines and surgery. Severe iron deficiency anaemia may require a blood transfusion, iron injections or intravenous (IV) iron therapy, which may need to be addressed in a hospital.

5.1. Oral iron therapy

Medical care starts with establishing the diagnosis and reason for the iron deficiency. Iron supplementation is used to prevent iron deficiency anaemia in at-risk populations, or to treat patients with proven disease. Treatment with oral iron supplements is simple, inexpensive and a relatively effective way of treating iron deficient conditions. WHO has recommended daily iron supplementation with 60 mg of elemental iron to prevent iron deficiency in menstruating adolescent girls and women, and 2 mg/kg daily in children aged 0–5 years and 30 mg daily in children aged 5–12 years [76–78]. In general, four common iron preparations are often adopted, i.e. ferrous sulphate, ferrous sulphate exsiccated, ferrous gluconate and ferrous fumarate. When side effects occur (dark stools, constipation, stomach irritation and heartburn), iron can be taken with meals, but doing so decreases absorption to 40% [8]. The best source of iron is red meat, especially beef and liver. The body tends to absorb iron from meat better than iron from non-meat foods. However, some non-meat foods can also help you raise your iron levels. Furthermore, Vitamin C helps the body absorb iron, whose good sources are vegetables and fruits, especially citrus fruits.

In most patients, the iron deficiency should be treated with oral iron therapy, and the underlying etiology should be corrected so the deficiency does not recur. However, there are cases that iron supplements are inappropriate to patients, for example, those who have a microcytic iron-overloading disorder (e.g. thalassemia and sideroblastic anaemia).Therefore, it may be necessary to identify the etiology of the anaemia, such as gene mutation related to iron metabolism, occult blood loss undetected with chemical testing of stool specimens; for identification of a source of bleeding that requires endoscopic examinations or angiography; or for treatment of an underlying major illness (e.g. neoplasia and ulcerative colitis).

5.2. Intravenous (IV) iron therapy

The British Society of Gastroenterology guidelines suggest that all patients require iron supplementation and that parenteral iron can be used if oral preparations are not well tolerated. For therapeutic iron supplementation, treatment with IV iron in some clinical situations could present some advantages over oral iron, such as faster and higher increases of haemoglobin (Hb) levels and body iron stores. Friedrisch et al. suggest the main clinical indications for IV iron treatment, which contains post-gastrectomy/bariatric surgery, anaemia of chronic kidney disease, intestinal malabsorption syndromes, anaemia associated to inflammatory diseases, inflammatory bowel diseases, anaemia of cancer, intolerance to oral iron or non-compliance to an oral regimen, iron-refractory iron deficiency anaemias and so on [79].

Recently, three new IV iron compounds (ferric carboxymaltose [FCM], iron isomaltoside 1000 [Monofer®] and Ferumoxytol [FeraHeme®]) have been released for clinical use in patients with Iron Deficiency Anaemia (IDA) [80–82]. Do not administer IV iron therapy to patients who should be treated with oral iron, as anaphylaxis may result. Uncommonly, post-menopausal women are unresponsive to iron supplementation, including parenteral iron, because they have primary defective iron reutilization due to androgen deficiency. This condition responds only to androgen replacement. Danazol is a reasonable choice for these patients, as it is less masculinizing.

6. Public health strategies to reduce iron deficiencies in high-burden areas

Although the global anaemia burden has been actually improved and age-standardized prevalence of anaemia was down from 33.3% in 1990 to 27% in 2013, according to the analysis based on 188 countries, 20 age groups, the total population with anaemia increased from 1.83 billion in

1990 to 1.93 billion in 2013 [2]. Developing countries account for more than 89% of the burden, with the greatest prevalence in central and western sub-Saharan African and greatest number of case in South Asia. Children with the highest burden of anaemia consistently have improved less than adults [2]. Iron deficiency anaemia is the dominant cause of anaemia globally and in most populations, accounting for 62.6% of the total of anaemia cases, and IDA was also the greatest causes of anaemia-related disability with 60% of total years lived with disability (YLD) [2, 83]. Monitoring and controlling IDA has been the crucial driver of reduced global anaemia burden since 1990 [2, 3]. Individual-level and population-level interventions targeted iron deficiency anaemia were implemented and the efficacy and effectiveness of these intervention strategies were also evaluated with a priority in high-risk, high-burden population such as preschool-children and pregnant women. Especially, further actions on iron deficiency anaemia prevention and treatment are highly required in order to reach the global nutrition targets of a 50% reduction of anaemia in women of reproductive age by 2025 [84].

The World Health Organization (WHO) has published a series of guidelines that support policies for the prevention and control of iron deficiency anaemia targeted on population in highest burden of IDA [78, 85–88]. The most common cause of iron deficiency anaemia in high-burden areas is prolonged negative iron balance, caused by inadequate dietary iron intake or absorption, increased needs for iron during pregnancy or growth periods, and increased iron losses as a result of menstruation and parasitic infections [84].

Public health strategies to prevent and control iron deficiency anaemia include improvements in dietary diversity; food fortification with iron, folic acid and other micronutrients; distribution of iron-containing supplements. The efficacy and effectiveness of different strategies were evaluated, based on the evidence from the community-based large-scale intervention studies.

6.1. Improvements in dietary diversity

Health education about food and nutrition such as dietary counselling is one of three recommended intervention strategies to decrease the IDA burden. Although dietary counselling commonly resulted in a better dietary intake profile in targeted subpopulation, such as breastfed for longer and had non-human milk introduced later among infant, consumed more meat and had diets with better iron bioavailability in relation to the children or pregnant women; however, this kind of interventions was not sufficient to prevent occurrence of anaemia, ID or IDA in population with high IDA burden [89–91].

6.2. Food fortification with iron

Food fortification as one of the leading public health interventions was recommended to prevent and control micronutrient deficiencies including iron deficiency and iron deficiency anaemia by adding the micronutrients containing iron to processed food vehicles, or home fortification. The choice of processed food vehicles varies widely by region and context, depending on the subpopulation targeted, food consumption and acceptability, food availability and sustainability, as well as the financial and technical concerns. The staple food is the most commonly used as vehicle of fortification, in addition, milk powder, beverages, biscuits, the most commonly used sauce, such as soy sauce, drink and water, can also be used as fortified foods [92–104].

More than 80 countries have mandated fortification of wheat and maize flour with at least iron and folic acid in 2015 [93]. A review of efficacy and effectiveness of flour fortification programmes on iron status and anaemia found that flour fortification is associated with consistent reductions in low ferritin prevalence in women, but not in children. Further, a reduction in anaemia prevalence was observed in only one-third of the subgroups of women and children studied [93].

A recently published review on the effect of multiple micro-nutrients (MMN) containing iron-fortified non-dairy beverages among school-aged children in low-middle-income counties showed a clear benefit of MMN fortified non-dairy beverages intervention from 8 weeks to 6 months on anaemia (42% reduction in prevalence), iron deficiency (66% reduction in prevalence) and iron deficiency anaemia (83% reduction in prevalence) compared to iso-caloric controls [99].

Biscuits have been identified to be an ideal vehicle for fortification for school-aged children due to its convenience with regard to storage, distribution and long shelf life. A nutrition intervention trial conducted in India showed that iron-fortified biscuits led to a significant enhancement in haemoglobin status of anaemic school children in rural areas [98]. Another study showed that maize porridge fortified with multi-micronutrient powder contained low dose, highly bioavailable iron can reduce the prevalence of IDA in pre-school children [102]. Home fortification with multi-micronutrient powder with low dosages of bioavailable iron may therefore be a promising strategy to improve iron status among children.

A study involved 3029 students of the boarding schools in the 27 provinces in China showed that iron-fortified soy sauce could be effective for the improvement of the haemoglobin level and reduce anaemia prevalence of boarding school students [97].

The beneficial of fortified complementary feeding supplement on the growth of young children aged 6–23 months have been confirmed by a large number of nutrition intervention programme conducted in population with low socio-economic status. Furthermore, the risk of anaemia among young children was significantly reduced after the daily fortified complementary feeding supplement introduced to infant diet in rural area, which implied that fortified complementary feeding supplement could be a best intervention strategy target on young children anaemia [105–112].

The successful implementation of food fortification programme commonly requires government-driven and multi-stakeholder participation, which has also become an obstacle to its sustainability.

6.3. Iron supplementation

Iron supplementation, provided in capsule, tablet or syrup form, is most suitable in contexts where certain subpopulation may not be reached, or when iron requirements may not be met by other intervention strategies.

A series of systematic reviews based on randomized control trial have been carried out to assess the effect of daily iron supplementation on haematologic and non-haematologic outcomes in high-burden subpopulations [113–119]. In children aged 4–23 months, daily iron supplementation effectively reduces anaemia by 39%, iron deficiency by 70% and iron deficiency anaemia by 86% [117]. In 2–5-year-old children, daily iron supplementation increases haemoglobin and ferritin; however, the evidence on the effect of iron supplementation on anaemia, iron deficiency and iron deficiency anaemia is limited [114]. In primary-school-aged children (5–12-year old), iron supplementation reduced the risk of anaemia by 50% and the risk of iron deficiency by 79% [116, 118].

The World Health Organization has published a series of iron supplementation guidelines, which provides global, evidence-based recommendations on the daily or intermittent use of iron supplements for high-burden subpopulation as a public health intervention to improve iron status and reduce the risk of iron deficiency anaemia in childhood, adolescence, pregnancy and lactation [85–88]. WHO suggested iron supplementation scheme targeted on variety of subpopulation was summarized in **Table 3**. In summary, the establishment of effective strategies, an integrated, multifactorial and multi-sectoral approach, is required to achieve IDA control target [84].

Target group	**Supplementation composition**	**Supplement form**	**Frequency**	**Duration**	**Settings**
Anaemic pregnant women	120 mg of elemental iron and 400 μg folic acid		Daily	Until women's Hb concentration rises to normal, then followed by the standard daily antenatal iron dose	Where prevalence of anaemia in pregnant women is 40% or higher
Non-anaemic pregnant women	30–60 mg of elemental iron and 400 μg folic acid		Daily	During pregnancy	Where prevalence of anaemia in pregnant women is 40% or higher
Non-anaemic pregnant women	120 mg of elemental iron and 2800 μg of folic acid		weekly	During pregnancy	Where anaemia prevalence among pregnant women is less than 20%
Postpartum women	iron supplementation, alone or combination with folic acid			6–12 weeks following delivery	Where gestational anaemia is of public health concern
Infants and young children aged 6–23 months	10–12.5 mg elemental iron	Drops/syrups	Daily	Three consecutive months in a year	Where the prevalence of anaemia in infants and young children is 40% or higher

Target group	Supplementation composition	Supplement form	Frequency	Duration	Settings
Pre-school-age children (24–59 months of age)	30 mg elemental iron	Drops/syrups/ tablets	Daily	Three consecutive months in a year	Where the prevalence of anaemia in infants and young children is 40% or higher
Pre-school-age children (24–59 months of age)	25 mg of elemental iron	Drops/syrups	Weekly	3 months of supplementation followed by 3 months of no supplementation after which the provision of supplements should restart	Where the prevalence of anaemia in pre-school or school-age children is 20% or higher
School-age children (5–12 years of age)	30–60 mg elemental iron	Tablets or capsules	Daily	Three consecutive months in a year	Where the prevalence of anaemia in infants and young children is 40% or higher
School-age children (5–12 years of age)	45 mg of elemental iron	Drops/syrups	Weekly	3 months of supplementation followed by 3 months of no supplementation after which the provision of supplements should restart	Where the prevalence of anaemia in pre-school or school-age children is 20% or higher
Menstruating adult women and adolescent girls (non-pregnant females in the reproductive age group)	30–60 mg elemental iron	Tablets	Daily	Three consecutive months in a year	Where the prevalence of anaemia in menstruating adult women and adolescent girls is 40% or higher

Table 3. WHO suggested scheme daily iron supplementation in different subpopulation.

7. Conclusion—key results

Considering the complexity of the regulatory network required to maintain iron homeostasis, future fine-mapping studies, including rare and uncommon variants, and functional studies should be undertaken to better characterize loci and to identify the functional variants directly influencing iron levels in iron deficiency anaemia.

New parameters which can give useful information about the iron availability for erythropoiesis and the erythropoietic activity of the bone marrow, and with stable to inflammatory conditions, should be developed for the early detection of iron deficiency, monitoring effect of iron supplementation and treatment, and discrimination the types of anaemia.

Intravenous iron formulation for rapid and high-dose replenishment of depleted iron stores with very low immunogenic potential is ideal alternative choice for the treatment of iron deficiency anaemia. Iron supplementation and fortification, as two key public health strategies in reducing the iron deficiency anaemia burden, should be selected in terms of the certain population subgroups targeted. The establishment of effective strategies, an integrated, multifactorial and multi-sectoral approach, is required to achieve IDA control target.

Author details

Lingxia Zeng*, Leilei Pei, Chao Li and Hong Yan

*Address all correspondence to: tjzlx@mail.xjtu.edu.cn

Xi'an Jiaotong University Health Science Center, Xi'an, PR China

References

[1] Khambalia AZ, Aimone AM, Zlotkin SH. Burden of anemia among indigenous populations. Nutrition Reviews. 2011;**69**(12):693-719. DOI: 10.1111/j.1753-4887.2011.00437.x

[2] Kassebaum NJ. The global burden of anemia. Hematology/Oncology Clinics of North America. 2016;**30**:247-308. DOI: 10.1016/j.hoc.2015.11.002

[3] Global Burden of Disease Pediatrics Collaboration. Global and national burden of diseases and injuries among children and adolescents between 1990 and 2013-findings from the global burden of disease 2013 study. JAMA Pediatrics. 2016;**170**(3):267-287. DOI: 10.1001/jamapediatrics.2015.4276

[4] Kassebaum NJ, Jasrasaria R, Naghavi M, Wulf SK, Johns N, Lozano R, et al. A systematic analysis of global anemia burden from 1990 to 2010. Blood. 2014;**123**:615-624

[5] Stevens GA, Finucane MM, De-Regil LM, Paciorek CJ, Flaxman SR, Branca F, et al. Global, regional, and national trends in haemoglobin concentration and prevalence of total and severe anaemia in children and pregnant and non-pregnant women for 1995-2011: A systematic analysis of population-representative data. The Lancet Global Health. 2013;**1**(1):e16-e25

[6] McDermid JM, Lönnerdal B. Iron. Advances in Nutrition. 2012;**3**(4):532-533. DOI: 10.3945/an.112.002261

[7] Hurrell R, Egli I. Iron bioavailability and dietary reference values. American Journal of Clinical Nutrition. 2010;**91**(5):1461S-1467S. DOI: 10.3945/ajcn.2010.28674F

[8] Lopez A, Cacoub P, Macdougall IC, Peyrin-Biroulet L. Iron deficiency anaemia. Lancet. 2016;**387**(10021):907-916. DOI: 10.1016/S0140-6736(15)60865-0

[9] Kibangou IB, Bouhallab S, Henry G, Bureau F, Allouche S, Blais A, et al. Milk proteins and iron absorption: Contrasting effects of different caseinophosphopeptides. Pediatric Research. 2005;**58**(4):731-734. DOI: 10.1203/01.PDR.0000180555.27710.46

[10] Zimmermann MB, Chaouki N, Hurrell RF. Iron deficiency due to consumption of a habitual diet low in bioavailable iron: A longitudinal cohort study in Moroccan children. American Journal of Clinical Nutrition. 2005;**81**(1):115-121

[11] Hentze MW, Muckenthaler MU, Galy B, Camaschella C. Two to tango: Regulation of mammalian iron metabolism. Cell. 2010;**142**(1):24-38. DOI: 10.1016/j.cell.2010.06.028

[12] Kulaksiz H, Gherke DG, Rost A, Janetzko D, Kallinowski T, Bruckner B, et al. Prohepcidin: Expression and cell specific localisation in the liver and its regulation in hereditary haemochromatosis, chronic renall insufficiency, and renal anemia. Gut 2004;**53**:735-743. DOI: 10.1136/gut.2003.022863

[13] Valore E, Ganz T. Posttranslational processing of hepcidin in human hepatocytes is mediated by the prohormon convertase furin. Blood Cells, Molecules and Diseases. 2008;**40**(1):132-138. DOI: 10.1016/j.bcmd.2007.07.009

[14] Tandara L, Salamunic I. Iron metabolism: Current facts and future directions. Biochemical Medicine (Zagreb). 2012;**22**(3):311-328

[15] Zhang AS, Enns CA. Molecular mechanisms of normal iron homeostasis. Hematology American Society of Hematology Education Program. 2009:207-214. doi: 10.1182/asheducation-2009.1.207.

[16] Kemna EH, Kartikasari AE, van Tits LJ, Pickkers P, Tjalsma H, Swinkels DW. Regulation of hepcidin: Insights from biochemical analyses on human serum samples. Blood Cells, Molecules and Diseases. 2008;**40**(3):339-346. DOI: 10.1016/j.bcmd.2007.10.002

[17] Goswami, T, and Andrews, NC. Hereditary hemochromatosis protein, HFE, interaction with transferrin receptor 2 suggests a molecular mechanism for mammalian iron sensing. Journal of Biological Chemistry. 2006;**281**(39):28494-28498. DOI: 10.1074/jbc.C600197200

[18] Gao J, Chen J, Kramer M, Tsukamoto H, Zhang AS, Enns CA. Interaction of the hereditary hemochromatosis protein HFE with transferrin receptor 2 is required for transferrin-induced hepcidin expression. Cell Metabolism. 2009;**9**(3):217-227. DOI: 10.1016/j.cmet.2009.01.010

[19] Anderson GJ, Frazer DM, McLaren GD. Iron absorption and metabolism. Current Opinion in Gastroenterology. 2009;**25**(2):129-135. DOI: 10.1097/MOG.0b013e32831ef1f7

[20] Babitt JL, Huang FW, Wrighting DM, Xia Y, Sidis Y, Samad TA, et al. Bone morphogenetic protein signaling by hemojuvelin regulates hepcidin expression. Nature Genetics. 2006;**38**(5):531-539. DOI: 10.1038/ng1777

[21] Wang RH, Li C, Xu X, Zheng Y, Xiao C, Zerfas P, et al. A role of SMAD4 in iron metabolism through the positive regulation of hepcidin expression. Cell Metabolism. 2005;**2**(6):399-409. DOI: 10.1016/j.cmet.2005.10.010

[22] Bartnikas TB, Fleming MD. Hemojuvelin is essential for transferrin-dependent and transferrin-independent hepcidin expression in mice. Haematologica. 2012;**97**(2):189-192. DOI: 10.3324/haematol.2011.054031

[23] Hooper JD, Campagnolo L, Goodarzi G, Truong TN, Stuhlmann H, Quigley JP. Mouse matriptase-2: Identification, characterization and comparative mRNA expression analysis with mouse hepsin in adult and embryonic tissues. Biochemical Journal 2003;**373**(Pt 3):689-702. DOI: 10.1042/BJ20030390

[24] Silvestri L, Pagani A, Nai A, De Domenico I, Kaplan J, Camaschella C. The serine protease matriptase-2 (TMPRSS6) inhibits hepcidin activation by cleaving membrane hemojuvelin. Cell Metabolism. 2008;**8**(6):502-511. DOI: 10.1016/j.cmet.2008.09.012

[25] Kloss-Brandstätter A, Erhart G, Lamina C, Meister B, Haun M, Coassin S, et al. Candidate gene sequencing of SLC11A2 and TMPRSS6 in a family with severe anaemia: Common SNPs, rare haplotypes, no causative mutation. PLoS One. 2012;**7**(4):e35015. DOI: 10.1371/journal.pone.0035015

[26] Lee P, Peng H, Gelbart T, Beutler E. The IL-6 and lipopolysaccharide-induced transcription of hepcidin in HFE, transferrin receptor 2 and beta-2-microglobulin-deficient hepatocytes. Proceedings of the National Academy of Sciences of the United States of America. 2004;**101**(25):9263-9265. DOI: 10.1073/pnas.0403108101

[27] Kemna EP, Nemeth E, van der Hoeven H, Pickkers, Swinkels D. Time course analysis of hepcidin, serum iron, and plasma cytokine levels in humans injected with LPS. Blood 2005;**106**(5):1864-1866. DOI: 10.1182/blood-2005-03-1159

[28] Wrighting D, Andrews NC. Interleukin-6 induces hepcidin expression through STAT3. Blood 2006;**108**(9):3204-3209. DOI: 10.1182/blood-2006-06-027631

[29] Pinto JP, Ribeiro S, Pontes H, Thowfeequ S, Tosh D, Carvalho F, et al. Erythropoietin mediates hepcidin expression in hepatocytes through EPOR signaling and regulation of C/EBPalpha. Blood. 2008;**111**(12):5727-5733. DOI: 10.1182/blood-2007-08-106195.

[30] Tanno T, Bhanu NV, Oneal PA, Goh SH, Staker P, Lee YT, et al. High levels of GDF15 in thalassemia suppress expression of the iron regulatory protein hepcidin. Natural Medicines. 2007;**13**:1096-1101. DOI: 10.1038/nm1629

[31] Tanno T, Porayette A, Orapan S, Noh SJ, Byrnes C, Bhupatiraju A, et al. Identification of TWSG1 as a second novel erythroid regulator of hepcidin expression in murine and human cells. Blood. 2009;**114**(1):181-186. DOI: 10.1182/blood-2008-12-195503

[32] Blanco-Rojo R, Baeza-Richer C, López-Parra AM, Pérez-Granados AM, Brichs A, Bertoncini S, et al. Four variants in transferrin and HFE genes as potential markers of iron deficiency anaemia risk: An association study in menstruating women. Nature Medicine (London). 2011;**8**:69. DOI: 10.1186/1743-7075-8-69

[33] Andreani M, Radio FC, Testi M, De Bernardo C, Troiano M, Majore S, et al. Association of hepcidin promoter c.-582 A>G variant and iron overload in thalassemia major. Haematologica. 2009;**94**(9):1293-1296. DOI: 10.3324/haematol.2009.006270

[34] Milet J, Dehais V, Bourgain C, Jouanolle AM, Mosser A, Perrin M, et al. Common variants in the BMP2, BMP4, and HJV genes of the hepcidin regulation pathway modulate HFE hemochromatosis penetrance. American Journal of Human Genetics. 2007;**81**(4):799-807. DOI: 10.1086/520001

[35] Milet J, Le Gac G, Scotet V, Gourlaouen I, Thèze C, Mosser J, et al. A common SNP near BMP2 is associated with severity of the iron burden in HFE p.C282Y homozygous patients: A follow-up study. Blood Cells, Molecules and Diseases. 2010;**44**(1):34-37. DOI: 10.1016/j.bcmd.2009.10.001

[36] Beaumont C, Delaunay J, Hetet G, Grandchamp B, de Montalembert M, Tchernia G. Two new human DMT1 gene mutations in a patient with microcytic anaemia, low ferritinemia, and liver iron overload. Blood. 2006;**107**:4168-4170. DOI: 10.1182/blood-2005-10-4269

[37] Sarria B, Navas-Carretero S, Lopez-Parra AM, Perez-Granados AM, Arroyo-Pardo E, Roe MA, et al. The G277S transferrin mutation does not affect iron absorption in iron deficient women. European Journal of Nutrition. 2007;**46**(1):57-60. DOI: 10.1007/s00394-006-0631-x

[38] Ye H, Jeong SY, Ghosh MC, Kovtunovych G, Silvestri L, Ortillo D, et al. Glutaredoxin 5 deficiency causes sideroblastic anemia by specifically impairing heme biosynthesis and depleting cytosolic iron in human erythroblasts. Journal of Clinical Investigation. 2010;**120**(5):1749-1761. DOI: 10.1172/JCI40372

[39] WHO. Iron Deficiency Anaemia Assessment, Prevention, and Control: A Guide for Programme Managers. Geneva: World Health Organization; 2001. Available from: http://apps.who.int/iris/bitstream/10665/66914/1/WHO_NHD_01.3.pdf. [Accessed: 15 March 2017]

[40] Petry N, Olofin I, Hurrell RF, Boy E, Wirth JP, Moursi M, et al. The proportion of anemia associated with iron deficiency in low, medium, and high human development index countries: A systematic analysis of national surveys. Nutrients. 2016;**8**(11):693. DOI: 10.3390/nu8110693

[41] Ezzati M, Lopez AD, Rodgers AA, Murray CJL. Comparative Quantification of Health Risks: Global and Regional Burden of Disease Attributable to Selected Major Risk Factors. Geneva, Switzerland: World Health Organization; 2004. Available from: http://citeseerx.ist.psu.edu/viewdoc/download?doi=10.1.1.378.1301&rep=rep1&type=pdf. [Accessed: 15 March 2017]

[42] Balarajan Y, Ramakrishnan U, Özaltin E, Shankar AH, Subramanian SV. Anaemia in low-income and middle-income countries. The Lancet. 2012;**378**(9809):2123-2135. DOI: http://dx.doi.org/10.1016/S0140-6736(10)62304-5

[43] Zeng L, Cheng Y, Dang S, Yan H, Dibley MJ, Chang S, et al. Impact of micronutrient supplementation during pregnancy on birth weight, duration of gestation, and perinatal mortality in rural western China: Double blind cluster randomised controlled trial. British Medical Journal. 2008;**337**:a2001. DOI: https://doi.org/10.1136/bmj.a2001

[44] Levy A, Fraser D, Katz M, Mazor M, Sheiner E. Maternal anemia during pregnancy is an independent risk factor for low birthweight and preterm delivery. European Journal of Obstetrics & Gynecology and Reproductive Biology. 2005;**122**(2):182-186. DOI: 10.1016/j.ejogrb.2005.02.015

[45] Haider BA, Olofin I, Wang M, Spiegelm an D, Ezzati M, Fawzi WW, et al. Anaemia, prenatal iron use, and risk of adverse pregnancy outcomes: Systematic review and meta-analysis. British Medical Journal. 2013;**346**:f3443. DOI: 10.1136/bmj.f3443

[46] Abu-Saad K, Fraser D. Maternal nutrition and birth outcomes. Epidemiologic Reviews. 2010;**32**:5-25. DOI: https://doi.org/10.1093/epirev/mxq001

[47] Lozoff B, Georgieff MK. Iron deficiency and brain development. Seminars in Pediatric Neurology. WB Saunders 2006;**13**(3):158-165. DOI: 10.1016/j.spen.2006.08.004

[48] Chang S, Zeng L, Brouwer ID, Kok FJ, Yan H. Effect of iron deficiency anemia in pregnancy on child mental development in rural China. Pediatrics. 2013;**131**(3):e755-e763. DOI: 10.1542/peds.2011-3513

[49] Tran TD, Biggs BA, Tran T, Simpson JA, Hanieh S, Dwyer T, et al. Impact on infants' cognitive development of antenatal exposure to iron deficiency disorder and common mental disorders. PLoS One. 2013;**8**(9):e74876. DOI: 10.1371/journal.pone.0074876

[50] Harvey LJ, Armah CN, Dainty JR, Foxall RJ, John Lewis D, Langford NJ, et al. Impact of menstrual blood loss and diet on iron deficiency among women in the UK. British Journal of Nutrition. 2005;**94**:557-564. DOI: https://doi.org/10.1079/BJN20051493

[51] McClung JP, Karl JP, Cable SJ, Williams KW, Nindl BC, Young AJ, et al. Randomized, double-blind, placebo-controlled trial of iron supplementation in female soldiers during military training: Effects on iron status, physical performance, and mood. American Journal of Clinical Nutrition. 2009;**90**(1):124-131. DOI: 10.3945/ajcn.2009.27774

[52] Murray-Kolb LE, Beard JL. Iron treatment normalizes cognitive functioning in young women. American Journal of Clinical Nutrition. 2007;**85**(3):778-787

[53] Pasricha SR, Drakesmith H, Black J, Hipgrave D, Biggs BA. Control of iron deficiency anemia in low-and middle-income countries. Blood. 2013;**121**(14):2607-2617. DOI: 10.1182/blood-2012-09-453522

[54] Hamadani JD, Tofail F, Hilaly A, Mehrin F, Shiraji S, Banu S, et al. Association of post-partum maternal morbidities with children's mental, psychomotor and language devel-opment in rural Bangladesh. Journal of Health, Population and Nutrition.2012 Jun;**30**(2):193-204

[55] Lozoff B. Iron deficiency and child development. Food and Nutrition Bulletin 2007; **28**(4_suppl4):S560-S571

[56] Shafir T, Angulo-Barroso R, Jing Y, Angelilli ML, Jacobson SW, Lozoff B. Iron deficiency and infant motor development. Early Human Development. 2008;**84**(7):479-485. DOI: 10.1016/j.earlhumdev.2007.12.009

[57] Shafir T, Angulo-Barroso R, Calatroni A, Jimenez E, Lozoff B. Effects of iron deficiency in infancy on patterns of motor development over time. Human Movement Science 2006;**25**(6):821-838. DOI: 10.1016/j.humov.2006.06.006

[58] Shafir Liberzon T, Angulo-Barroso R, Calatroni A, Angelilli ML, Jacobson SW, Lozoff B. Iron deficiency affects motor development in 9-month-old infants. Pediatric Research. 2005;**57**:1731

[59] Gashu D, Stoecker BJ, Bougma K, Adish A, Haki GD, Marquis GS. Stunting, selenium deficiency and anemia are associated with poor cognitive performance in preschool children from rural Ethiopia. Nutrition Journal. 2016;**15**(1):38. DOI: 10.1186/s12937-016-0155-z

[60] Fairweather-Tait SJ, Wawer AA, Gillings R, Jennings A, Myint PK. Iron status in the elderly. Mechanisms of Ageing and Development. 2014;**136**:22-28. DOI: 10.1016/j.mad.2013.11.005

[61] Santos IS, Scazufca M, Lotufo PA, Menezes PR, Benseñor IM. Causes of recurrent or persistent anemia in older people from the results of the São Paulo Ageing & Health Study. Geriatrics & Gerontology International. 2013;**13**(1):204-208. DOI: 10.1111/j.1447-0594.2012.00888.x

[62] Hsu HS, Li CI, Liu CS, Lin CC, Huang KC, Li TC, et al. Iron deficiency is associated with increased risk for cardiovascular disease and all-cause mortality in the elderly living in long-term care facilities. Nutrition. 2013;**29**(5):737-743. DOI: 10.1016/j.nut.2012.10.015

[63] Bang SM, Lee JO, Kim YJ, Lee KW, Lim S, Kim JH, et al. Anemia and activities of daily living in the Korean urban elderly population: Results from the Korean Longitudinal Study on Health and Aging (KLoSHA). Annals of Hematology. 2013;**92**(1):59-65. DOI: 10.1007/s00277-012-1563-6

[64] Mørkedal B, Laugsand LE, Romundstad PR, Vatten LJ. Mortality from ischaemic heart disease: Sex-specific effects of transferrin saturation, serum iron, and total iron binding capacity. The HUNT study. European Journal of Cardiovascular Prevention & Rehabilitation. 2011;**18**(5):687-694. DOI: 10.1177/1741826710390134

[65] Stewart R, Hirani V. Relationship between depressive symptoms, anemia, and iron status in older residents from a national survey population. Psychosomatic Medicine. 2012;**74**(2):208-213. DOI: 10.1097/PSY.0b013e3182414f7d

[66] Haas JD, Brownlie T 4th. Iron deficiency and reduced work capacity: A critical review of the research to determine a causal relationship. Journal of Nutrition. 2001;**131**(2S-2):676-688S; discussion 688-690S

[67] Horton S, Ross J. The economics of iron deficiency. Food Policy. 2003;**28**:51-75. DOI: https://doi.org/10.1016/S0306-9192(02)00070-2

[68] World Health Organization. Haemoglobin concentrations for the diagnosis of anaemia and assessment of severity [Internet]. 2011. Available from: http://www.who.int/nutrition/publications/micronutrients/indicators_haemoglobin/en/ [Accessed: 20 January 2017].

[69] Huch Sr R. Iron Deficiency and Iron Deficiency Anaemia. Stuttgart: Thieme; 2006

[70] Jolobe OM. Prevalence of hypochromia (without microcytosis) vs microcytosis (without hypochromia) in iron deficiency. Clinical and Laboratory Haematology. 2000;**22**:79-80. DOI: 10.1046/j.1365-2257.2000.00293.x

[71] Goddard AF, James MW, McIntyre AS, Scott BB, and the British Society of Gastroenterology. Guidelines for the management of iron deficiency anaemia. Gut. 2011;**60**: 1309-1316

[72] Guyatt GH, Oxman AD, Ali M, Willan A, McIlroy W, Patterson C. Laboratory diagnosis of iron-deficiency anemia: An overview. Journal of General Internal Medicine. 1992;**7**:145-153. DOI: 10.1007/BF02598003

[73] Mast AE, Blinder MA, Gronowski AM, Chumley C, Scott MG. Clinical utility of the soluble transferrin receptor and comparisonwith serum ferritin in several populations. Clinical Chemistry. 1998;**44**:45-51

[74] Locatelli F, Aljama P, Bárány P, Canaud B, Carrera F, Eckardt KU, et al, and the European Best Practice Guidelines Working Group. Revised European best practice guidelines for the management of anaemia in patients with chronic renal failure. Nephrology Dialysis Transplantation. 2004;**19**(suppl 2):ii1–ii47

[75] Thomas DW, Hinchliff e RF, Briggs C, Macdougall IC, Littlewood T, Cavill I, and British Committee for Standards in Haematology. Guideline for the laboratory diagnosis of functional iron deficiency. British Journal of Haematology. 2013;**161**(5):639-648. DOI: 10.1111/bjh.12311

[76] WHO. Guideline: Intermittent Iron and Folic Acid Supplementation in Menstruating Women. Geneva: World Health Organization; 2011. http://apps.who.int/iris/bitstream/10665/44649/1/9789241502023_eng.pdf

[77] Fernández-Gaxiola AC, De-Regil LM. Intermittent iron supplementation for reducing anaemia and its associated impairments in menstruating women. The Cochrane Database of Systematic Reviews. 2011 Dec 7;(12):CD009218. doi: 10.1002/14651858.CD009218.pub2

[78] WHO. Guideline: Intermittent Iron Supplementation for Preschool and School-age Children. Geneva: World Health Organization; 2011. https://www.ncbi.nlm.nih.gov/books/NBK179850/

[79] Friedrisch JR, Cançado RD. Intravenous ferric carboxymaltose for the treatment of iron deficiency anemia. Revista Brasileira de Hematologia e Hemoterapia. 2015;**37**(6):400-405. DOI: 10.1016/j.bjhh.2015.08.012

[80] Lyseng-Williamsom KA, Keating GM. Ferric carboxymaltose: A review of its use in iron-deficiency anaemia. Drugs. 2009;**69**(6):739-756. DOI: 10.2165/00003495-200969060-00007

[81] Jahn MR, Andreasen HB, Futterer S, Nawroth T, Schunemann V, Kolb U, et al. A comparative study of the physicochemical properties of iron isomaltoside 1000 (Monofer), a new intravenous iron preparation and its clinical implications. European Journal of Pharmaceutics and Biopharmaceutics. 2011;**78**(3):480-491. DOI: 10.1016/j.ejpb.2011.03.016

[82] Lu M, Cohen MH, Rieves D, Pazdur R. FDA review of ferumoxytol (Feraheme) for the treatment of iron deficiency anemia in adults with chronic kidney disease. American Journal of Hematology. 2010;**859**(5):315-319

[83] Vos T, Flaxman AD, Naghavi M, Lozano R, Michaud C, Ezzati M, et al. Years lived with disability (YLDs) for 1160 sequelae of 289 diseases and injuries 1990-2010: A systematic analysis for the Global Burden of Disease Study 2010. Lancet. 2012;**380**:2163-2196

[84] World Health Organization. Global Nutrition Targets 2025: Anaemia Policy Brief [Internet]. 2014. Available from: http://www.who.int/nutrition/publications/globaltargets2025_policybrief_anaemia/en/ [Accessed: 20 January 2017]

[85] World Health Organization. WHO Recommendations on Antenatal Care for a Positive Pregnancy Experience [Internet]. 2016. Available from: http://www.who.int/reproductivehealth/publications/maternal_perinatal_health/anc-positive-pregnancy-experience/en/ [Accessed: 20 January 2017]

[86] World Health Organization. Guideline: Daily Iron Supplementation in Postpartum Women [Internet]. 2016. Available from: http://www.who.int/nutrition/publications/micronutrients/guidelines/daily_iron_supp_postpartum_women/en/ [Accessed: 20 January 2017]

[87] World Health Organization. Guideline: Daily Iron Supplementation in Infants and Children [Internet]. 2016. Available from: http://www.who.int/nutrition/publications/micronutrients/guidelines/daily_iron_supp_childrens/en/ [Accessed: 20 January 2017]

[88] World Health Organization. Guideline: Daily Iron Supplementation in Adult Women and Adolescent Girls [Internet]. 2016. Available from: http://www.who.int/nutrition/publications/micronutrients/guidelines/daily_iron_supp_womenandgirls/en/ [Accessed: 20 January 2017]

[89] Bortolini GA, Vitolo MR. The impact of systematic dietary counseling during the first year of life on prevalence rates of anemia and iron deficiency at 12-16 months. Jornal de Pediatria (Rio de Janeiro). 2012;**88**(1):33-39. DOI: 10.2223/JPED.2156

[90] Imdad A, Yakoob MY, Bhutta ZA. Impact of maternal education about complementary feeding and provision of complementary foods on child growth in developing countries. BMC Public Health. 2011;**11**(Suppl.3):S25. DOI: 10.1186/1471-2458-11-S3-S25

[91] Mokori A, Hendriks SL, Oriskushaba P, Oelofse A. Changes in complementary feeding practices and nutrition status in returnee children aged 6-23 months in north Uganda. South African Journal of Clinical Nutrition. 2013;**26**(4):201-211

[92] Cardoso MA, Augusto RA, Bortolini GA, Oliveira CSM, Tietzman DC, Sequeira LAS, et al. Effect of providing multiple micronutrients in powder through primary healthcare on anemia in young Brazilian children: A multicentre pragmatic controlled trial. PLoS ONE. 2016;**11**(3):e0151097. DOI: 10.1371/journal.pone.0151097

[93] Pachon H, Spohrer R, Mei Z, and Serdula MK. Evidence of the effectiveness of flour fortification programs on iron status and anemia: A systematic review. Nutrition Reviews. 2015;**73**(11):780-795. DOI: 10.1093/nutrit/nuv037

[94] Best C, Neufingerl N, Del Rosso JM, Transler C, Van den Briel T, Osendarp S. Can multi-micronutrient food fortification improve the micronutrient status, growth, health, and cognition of school children? A systematic review. Nutrition Review. 2011;**69**:186-204

[95] De-Regil LM, Suchdev PS, Vist GE, Walleser S, Pena-Rosas JP. Home fortification of foods with multiple micronutrient powders for health and nutrition in children under two years of age (review). Evidence Based Child Health. 2013;**8**:112-201

[96] Yang Z, Huffman SL. Review of fortified food and beverage products for pregnant and lactating women and their impact on nutritional status. Maternal and Child Nutrition. 2011;**7**:19-43

[97] Chen D, Sun J, Huang J, Wang L, Piao W, Tang Y, et al. Effects of the iron fortified soy sauce on improving student's anemia in boarding schools. Journal of Hygiene Research. 2016;**45**(2):221-225

[98] Bal D, Nagesh K, Surendra HS, Chiradoni D, Gomathy G. Effect of Supplementation with iron fortified biscuits on the hemoglobin status of children in rural areas of Shimoga, Karnataka. Indian Journal of Pediatrics. 2015;**82**(3):253-259. DOI: 10.1007/s12098-014-1483-7

[99] Aaron GJ, Dror DK, Yang Z. Multiple-Micronutrient fortified Non-Dairy beverage interventions reduce the risk of anemia and iron deficiency in School-Aged children in Low-Middle income countries: A systematic review and Meta-Analysis. Nutrients. 2015;**7**:3847-3868. DOI: 10.3390/nu7053847

[100] Bilenko N, Fraser D, Vardy H, Belmaker I. Impact of multiple micronutrient supplementation ("Sprinkles") on iron deficiency anemia in bedouin Arab and Jewish infants. Israel Medicine Association Journal. 2014;**16**:434-438

[101] Almeida CA, De Mello ED, Ramos AP, Joao CA, Joao CR, Dutra-de-Oliveira JE. Assessment of drinking water fortification with iron plus ascorbic acid or ascorbic acid alone in daycare centers as a strategy to control Iron-Deficiency anemia and iron deficiency: A randomized blind clinical study. Journal of Tropical Pediatrics. 2014;**60**(1): 40-46. DOI: 10.1093/tropej/fmt071

[102] Macharia-Mutie CW, Moretti D, Van den Briel N, Omusundi AM, Mwangi AM, Kok FJ, et al. Maize porridge enriched with a micronutrient powder containing Low-Dose iron as NaFeEDTA but not amaranth grain flour reduces anemia and iron deficiency in Kenyan Preschool Children. Journal of Nutrition. 2012;**142**:1756-1763. DOI: 10.3945/in. 112.157578

[103] Thankachan P, Selvam S, Surendran D, Chellan S, Pauline M, Abrams SA, et al. Efficacy of a multi micronutrient-fortified drink in improving iron and micronutrient status among schoolchildren with low iron stores in India: A randomised, double-masked placebo-controlled trial. European Journal of Clinical Nutrition. 2013;**67**:36-41. DOI: 10.1038/ejcn.2012.188

[104] Bokhari F, Derbyshire EJ, Hickling D, Li W, Brennan CS. A randomized trial investigating an iron-rich bread as a prophylaxis against iron deficiency in pregnancy. International Journal of Food Sciences and Nutrition. 2012;**63**(4):461-467. DOI: 10.3109/09637486.2011.634790

[105] Lazzerini M, Rubert L, Pani P. Specially formulated foods for treating children with moderate acute malnutrition in low- and middle-income countries. Cochrane Database of Systematic Reviews. 2013(6). Art. No.: CD009584. DOI: 10.1002/14651858.CD009584.pub2

[106] Sun J, Dai Y, Zhang S, Huang J, Yang Z, Huo J, Chen,C. Implementation of a programme to market a complementary food supplement (Ying Yang Bao) and impacts on anaemia and feeding practices in Shanxi, China. Maternal & Child Nutrition. 2011;**7**(Suppl 3):96-111

[107] Phu PV, Hoan NV, Salvignol B, Trecge S, Wieringa FK, Dijkhuizen MA, et al. A six-month intervention with two different types of Micronutrient-Fortified complementary foods had distinct short- and long-term effects on linear and ponderal growth of Vietnamese infants. The Journal of Nutrition. 2012;**142**:1735-1740. DOI: 10.3945/jn.111.154211

[108] Campbell RK, Hurley KM, Shamim AA, Shaikh S, Chowdhury ZT, Mehra S, et al. Effect of complementary food supplementation on breastfeeding and home diet in rural Bangladeshi children. America Journal of Clinic Nutrition. 2016;**104**:1450-1458. DOI: 10.3945/ajcn.116.135509

[109] Christian P, Shaikh S, Shamim AA, Mehra S, Wu L, Mitra M, et al. Effect of fortified complementary food supplementation on child growth in rural Bangladesh: A cluster-randomized trial. International Journal of Epidemiology. 2015;**44**(6):1862-1876. DOI: 10.1093/ije/dyv155

[110] Wang YY, Chen CM, Wang FZ, Jia M, Wang KA. Effects of nutrient fortified complementary food supplements on anemia of infants and young children in poor rural of Gansu. Biomedical and Environmental Sciences. 2009;**22**:194-200

[111] Muslihah N, Khomsan A, Briawan D, Riyadi H. Complementary food supplementation with a small-quantity of lipid-based nutrient supplements prevents stunting in 6-12-month-old infants in rural West Madura Islan, Indonesia. Asia Pacific Journal of Clinical Nutrition. 2016;**25**(Suppl 1):S36-S42. DOI: 10.6133/apjcn.122016.s9

[112] Mangani C, Maleta K, Phuka J, Cheung YB, Thakalakwa C, Dewey K, et al. Effect of complementary feeding with lipid-based nutrient supplements and corn-soy blend on the incidence of stunting and linear growth among 6- to 18-month-old infants and children in rural Malawi. Maternal & Child Nutrition. 2015;**11**(Suppl. 4):132-143. DOI: 10.111/mcn.12068

[113] Gera T, Sachdev HPS, Nestel P, Sachdev SS. Effect of iron supplementation on haemoglobin response in children: Systematic review of randomised controlled trials. Journal of Pediatric Gastroenterology and Nutrition. 2007;**44**(4):468-486

[114] Thompson J, Biggs BA, Pasricha SR. Effects of daily iron supplementation in 2- to 5-Year-Old children: Systematic review and Meta-analysis. Pediatrics. 2013;**131**(4):739-753. DOI: 10.1542/peds.2012-2256

[115] Neuberger A, Okebe J, Yahav D, Paul M. Oral iron supplements for children in malaria-endemic areas (Review). Cochrane Database of Systematic Reviews. 2016;(2):CD006589. DOI: 10.1002/14651858.CD006589.pub4

[116] Low M, Farrell A, Biggs BA, Pasricha SR. Effects of daily iron supplementation in primary-school–aged children: Systematic review and meta-analysis of randomized controlled trials. Canadian Medical Association Journal. 2013;**185**(17):E791-E802. DOI: 10.1503/cmaj.130628

[117] Pasricha SR, Hayes E, Kalumba K, Biggs BA. Effect of daily iron supplementation on health in children aged 4-23 months: A systematic review and meta-analysis of randomised controlled trials. Lancet Global Health. 2013;**1**:e77-e86

[118] De-Regil LM, Jefferds M, Sylvetsky AC, Dowswell T. Intermittent iron supplementation for improving nutrition and development in children under 12 years of age. Cochrane Database of Systematic Reviews. 2011;(12):CD009085. DOI: 10.1002/14651858.CD009085.pub2

[119] Casey GJ, Montresor A, Cavalli-Sforza LT, Thu H, Phu LB, Tinh TT, et al. Elimination of iron deficiency anemia and soil transmitted helminth infection: Evidence from a Fifty-four month Iron-Folic acid and De-worming program. PLOS Neglected Tropical Diseases. 2013;7(4):e2146. DOI: 10.1371/journal.pntd.0002146

Chapter 2

Megaloblastic Anemia

Olaniyi John Ayodele

Additional information is available at the end of the chapter

http://dx.doi.org/10.5772/intechopen.70063

Abstract

Megaloblastic anemia is a multisystem disorder, which can easily be diagnosed with high index of suspicion and by correct application of its pathogenetic mechanisms. Any factor inhibiting deoxyribonucleic acid (DNA) synthesis, drugs (medications), infections like human immunodeficiency virus (HIV) and gas like nitrous oxide will cause megaloblastosis. However, poor diet, problems with absorption, transportation and metabolism of the vitamins, as well as factors that increase demand and ultimately exhaust the store of the vitamins like chronic hemolytic states, pregnancy, malignancies happen to be the commonest causes of megaloblastic anemia. A complete blood count, blood and marrow films review reflect the typical pathognomonic cytologic appearance of megaloblastic anemia. Logically selected biochemical tests help in establishing diagnosis through determination of serum levels of both folate and cobalamin and assessment of the metabolites, which are considered to be more sensitive and specific. Also, full endoscopic studies are required to confirm the presence of disorders of gastrointestinal tract responsible for impaired absorption. Clinical features are subtle and widely varied. It is highly amenable to therapy once the primary cause is established and managed. Appropriate replacement therapy of deficient nutrient, cobalamin or folate or both, easily corrects anemia. Pernicious anemia often requires lifelong therapy with parenteral cobalamin.

Keywords: anemia, megaloblast, blood and marrow smears review, neuropathies, replacement therapy

1. Introduction

Anemia, technically, describes a condition in which an individual's hemoglobin level (or hematocrit) falls two standard deviations below the average mean of normal for individuals of same age, sex, and altitude [1, 2]. The functional consequence of anemia decreased oxygen carrying capacity of the blood and general tissue hypoxia.

Megaloblastic anemia refers to a group of anemias that have in common a selective reduction in the rate of deoxyribonucleic acid (DNA) synthesis; however, transcription, translation, and protein synthesis proceed normally. Consequently, a resultant unbalanced cell growth ensues and the dichotomy between the rates of cytoplasmic and nuclear maturation widens with each division during erythropoiesis until eventually the cell either dies or omits terminal division making it to survive as oversized end stage cell (macrocytes) with a shortened lifespan. Therefore, the retarded DNA synthesis leads to accumulation of dead and dying megaloblasts in the marrow, creating a spurious appearance of marrow hyperplasia but with a gradual reduction in the number of matured cells being pushed out and eventually progressed to pancytopenia. The megaloblastic anemias are caused by vitamin B_{12} deficiency, folate deficiency, or by related conditions that caused impaired DNA synthesis.

1.1. History

Many researchers sequentially contributed to the discovery and identification of its etiology. Addison in 1849 was the first to characterize it as anemia, general languor, and debility [3]. In 1877, Osler and Gardnerin discovered its association with neuropathy and its association with myelopathy was documented 10 years later by Lichtheim. Megaloblasts were identified by Ehrlic in 1880 while the abnormalities in leukocytes were described in 1920. It was confirmed by Minot and Murphy that the disease is reversible by the intake of large amount of liver [4]. Castle, in 1929, discovered the presence of "intrinsic factor" in gastric acid that facilitates the absorption of the "extrinsic factor" [5]. The structure of vitamin B_{12} was later identified by Hodgkin and this earned him a Nobel Prize [6]. However, it was Herbert, in 1948, who discovered the structure of folic acid and described its link with the causation of megaloblastic anemia [7].

2. Epidemiology

Epidemiological studies on megaloblastic anemia in Nigeria and in Africa are sparse. However, the frequency of megaloblastosis is highest in countries in which malnutrition is rampant and routine vitamin supplementation for elderly individuals and pregnant woman is not available. Faulty preparations of foods and increased demand for folate during pregnancy are the most common causes of megaloblastic anemias.

About 1 in 7500 people develops pernicious anemia in the US per year but this has been modified by current fortification of foods and vitamin supplementations in elderly patients in the US. International statistics showed that pernicious anemia and folate deficiency usually occur in individuals older than 40 years and the prevalence increases with older populations. The incidence of pernicious anemia is reported to be higher in Sweden, Denmark, and United Kingdom than in other developed countries [8].

3. Physiology of cobalamin and folate

Vitamin B_{12} consists of a corrin ring with a cobalt atom in its center attached to a nucleotide portion and they are termed cobalamins. The biologically inactive pharmacologic preparations of vitamin B_{12} include cyanocobalamin and hydroxocobalamin whereas adenosylcobalamin and methylcobalamin that are generated through enzymatic synthesis are the biologically active forms, whereas adenosyl-cobalamin is the tissue form of vitamin B_{12}, methylcobalamin circulates in blood. Although a normal diet provides a large excess of vitamin B_{12}, the daily requirement is about 1–2 μg in adults. In the process of digestion, R-protein, either of salivary or parietal cells origin, binds to liberated cobalamin from complex dietary protein through the action of gastric secretion made up of pepsin and hydrochloric acid. The cobalamin-R protein complex is degraded pancreatic secretions in the duodenum to release free cobalamin that then binds to intrinsic factor that was secreted in the stomach. The cobalamin-intrinsic factor complex is now transported to the terminal ileum where absorption takes place. Failure of physiological activity at any of these points results in megaloblastic anemia. Following absorption, the released vitamin binds a transport protein called transcobalamin (TCII), which transports the vitamin to enterohepatic circulation. Vitamin B_{12} is stored primarily in the liver in an amount of 2–3 mg, which is 1000-fold in excess of daily requirement.

The physiologic role of vitamin B_{12} include:

a. Conversion of methyl-malonyl-coenzyme A (CoA) to succinyl CoA by adenosyl cobalamin.

b. Conversion of homocysteine to methionine.

c. Synthesis of S-adenosyl-methionine.

3.1. Physiology of folate (pteroyl glutamic acid)

Folic acid, a composite molecule consists of pteridine, p-amino benzoic acid, and glutamic acid. Folates are available as polyglutamates in many foods like the green leafy vegetables, yeast, and liver. However, overcooking easily destroys the folate. Folate is absorbed as monoglutamates in the upper jejunum. The daily requirement of folate is 150 μg and the body stores of folate are sufficient for 6 months. The major intracellular compounds are folate polyglutamates with attached additional glutamates. Folates are essential in many biochemical reactions like synthesis of purines, thymine, and deoxyribonucleic acid (DNA).

4. Etiology and pathogenesis

The principal causes of megaloblastic anemia in clinical practice are folate and cobalamin deficiency either directly or indirectly (see **Table 1**).

4.1. Major causes of cobalamin deficiency include

Dietary: Dietary cause of cobalamin deficiency is rare except in strict vegetarians who avoid taking meat, eggs, and dairy products.

Problems with cobalamin absorption: Atrophic gastritis and achlorhydria, which commonly occur in elderly people are the two conditions which are responsible for impaired release of cobalamins bound to food. Hence, cobalamin is not released from food for absorptive process.

I. Cobalamin deficiency	II. Folate deficiency	III. Drug-induced suppression of DNA synthesis	IV. Inborn errors
(i) Dietary deficiency (ii) Deficiency of gastric IF Pernicious anemia or gastrectomy (iii) Intestinal malabsorption Ileal resection or ileitis Familial selective cobalamin malabsorption Competitive parasites or infections Fish tapeworm Bacteria overgrowth in malformed small bowel (iv) Increased Requirement	(i) Dietary deficiency (ii) Impaired absorption Sprue Extensive small bowel disease or resection Intestinal short circuits Anticonvulsants and oral contraceptives (iii) Increased requirement Pregnancy Hemolytic anemia Myeloproliferative and other hyperproliferative disorders	(i) Folate antagonists (ii) Metabolic inhibitors of purine pyrimidine thymidylate synthesis Other inhibitors (iii) Alkylating agents D. Nitrous oxide (IV) Inborn errors **a.** Defective transport of cobalamin **b.** Defective cobalamin utilization **c.** Defective folate metabolism **d.** Hereditary orotic aciduria **e.** Lesch-Nyhan syndrome	(i) Defective transport of cobalamin (ii) Defective cobalamin utilization (iii) Defective folate metabolism (iv) Hereditary orotic aciduria E. Lesch-Nyhan syndrome

Table 1. Pathogenetic classification of megaloblastic anemia [9].

Also, autoimmune destruction of gastric parietal cells may lead to failure of intrinsic factor production. This condition is called pernicious anemia. Pernicious anemia is recognized as the best-known cause of cobalamin deficiency. It is diagnosed in 1% of people older than 60 years and the incidence is slightly higher in women than in men.

Inhibition of intrinsic factor production can also be caused by H_2 antagonists.

The release of cobalamin from R-proteins can also be inhibited by the alkaline environment in the small intestine emanating from pancreatic insufficiency.

On the contrary, the acidic environment seen in conditions like Zollinger Ellison syndrome, also prevents binding of cobalamin to intrinsic factor hence leading to diminished binding to intrinsic factor and ultimate interference with cobalamin absorption.

The disorders of the terminal ileum, site of uptake of cobalamin-intrinsic factor complex, can cause cobalamin deficiency. Disorders that can possibly affect the terminal ileum include tropical sprue, inflammatory bowel disease, lymphoma, as well as ileal resection. Autoimmune destruction of the ileal receptor, cubilin, as found in Imerslund Grasbeck syndrome equally distrupts the uptake of cobalamin bound to intrinsic factor.

Also, bacteria colonization can occur in intestines deformed by strictures, surgical blind loops, scleroderma, inflammatory bowel disease, or amyloidosis blind loop syndrome can result to

http://dx.doi.org/10.5772/intechopen.70063

cobalamin deficiency. In this condition, bacteria competes with the host for cobalamin for the uptake of cobalamin bound to intrinsic factor.

Fish tapeworm such as *Diphyllobothrium latum* infestation, which is common in places like Canada, Alaska, and the Baltic sea, feeds on cobalamin in the intestine thereby reducing the amount of cobalamin available for ingestion by the host.

Miscellaneous causes of cobalamin deficiency include exposure to nitrous oxide, which through oxidative inactivation of cobalamin causes megaloblastosis. Prolonged exposure to nitrous oxide can lead to severe mental and neurological disorders. Various medications like purine analogs (six mercaptopurine, six tioguanine), pyrimidine analogs (five fluorouracil and five azacytidine), and drugs that affect cobalamin metabolism like P-aminosalicylic acid, phenformin, and metformin that can cause cobalamin deficiency.

4.2. Major causes of folate deficiency

The main cause of loss of folate from food is poor food preparation through excessive dilution of food in water, through excessive heating, and subsequent inactivation of folate since folate is thermolabile. However, food fortification with folate and other vitamins are circumventing this problem in developed countries. This has to be aggressively promoted in many developing countries.

The storage of folate is for about 4 weeks after which folate deficiency sets in if folate intake is stopped. The daily requirement for adult is about 0.4 mg/day.

Folate deficiency occurs in situations where there is impaired absorption due to certain intestinal disorders like tropical sprue, nontropical sprue (celiac disease), amyloidosis, and inflammatory bowel disease.

Folate deficiency occurs in situations where there is increased physiologic demand for folate like chronic hemolytic states like sickle cell anemia, hereditary spherocytosis, and elliptocytosis; pregnancy, lactation, rapid growth, hyperalimentation, renal dialysis, where there is escalated loss of rapidly dividing cells like psoriasis and exfoliative dermatitis.

Also, medications such as phenytoin, metformin, phenobarbitone, dihydrofolate reductase, folate inhibitors like trimethoprim and pyrimethamine, methotrexate, sulphonamides, can cause folate deficiency.

Megaloblastic changes in human immunodeficiency virus (HIV) infection and myelodysplastic disorders are due to direct effect on deoxyribonucleic acid (DNA) in hemopoietic and other rapidly dividing cells.

4.3. Pathophysiology of megaloblastic anemia

The two vitamins, that is, folate and cobalamin act synergistically in generating the thymidylic acid used for DNA synthesis. Therefore, in cobalamin deficiency, the megaloblastic arrest is actually caused by a deficit in folate utilization. As shown in **Figure 1** (activated methyl cycle), methionine is generated by transfer of methylene group from N5-methyl tetrahydrofolate

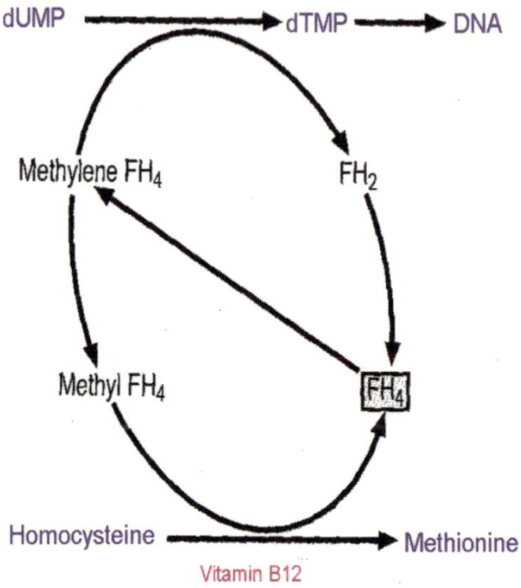

Figure 1. Activated methyl cycle.

(FH4) to homocysteine using the enzyme methyl transferase (Methionine synthase). In this biochemical process, methylcobalamin is the factor that assists in methyl transfer as coenzyme form of cobalamin. This is why the morphological abnormalities emanating from either cobalamin or folate deficiency appear exactly alike.

5. Clinical features

Megaloblastic anemias, irrespective of the cause, share certain general features. The anemia develops slowly with little or no symptoms until the hematocrit is severely depressed and at this point, symptoms like weakness, palpitation, fatigue, light headedness, and shortness of breath occur. Severe pallor and light jaundice combine to produce a telltale lemon yellow skin. Slight differences occur in clinical symptoms and signs of megaloblastic anemia depending on whether it is caused by folate deficiency or by vitamin B_{12} deficiency. In folate deficiency, main clinical features include anemic syndrome, pallor, icterus, hunter's syndrome, nail pigmentation, change of hair color (early graying), and splenomegaly in about 10–15% of patients. In addition to the above mentioned features, cobalamin deficiency manifests with neurological symptoms, which include loss of joint position sense in the second toes, loss of vibration sense in toes and fingers, paraesthesia, hypoesthesia, tingling sensation, gait abnormalities, loss of coordination, muscle weakness, spasticity, optic neuropathy, urinary and fecal incontinence, erectile dysfunction, dementia, memory loss. These neuropathies are symmetric and only affect lower extremities. Demonstrable signs include positive Romberg's sign, Babinsky reflex, thermittes's sign, spasticity, hyporeflexia, and clonus.

6. Laboratory features

The laboratory features of megaloblastic anemia revolve around the laboratory investigations and findings of vitamin B_{12} and folate deficiencies (see **Figure 2**).

6.1. Blood cells

All the blood cells are affected. Erythrocytes vary markedly in size and shape (anisopoikilocytosis), some are large (twice in volume of normal red cells) and oval (egg shaped) (macro-ovalocytes) and in severe cases erythrocytes show basophilic stiplings and contain nuclear remnants (Howell-Jolly bodies, cabot rings). The morphologic changes are directly proportional to the severity of anemia. Circulating megaloblasts (i.e., nucleated red cells that failed to mature appropriately) are visible in circulation with hematocrit less than 20%. Anemia is typically macrocytic with a mean corpuscular volume (MCV) of 100–150 FL or more. However, the macrocytic appearance may be masked by coexisting iron deficiency, thalassaemia trait, and inflammation. It is noteworthy that slight macrocytosis is the earliest sign of megaloblastic anemia. Also mingled with macrocytes are fragmented red cells and tear drop poikilocytes. Reticulocytopenia (a reticulocyte count of <1%) is a frequent finding. This occurs because of inordinate impairment of erythropoiesis culminating in intramedullary destruction of megaloblasts and resultant reticulocytopenia. This is referred to as ineffective erythropoiesis (see **Figure 3**).

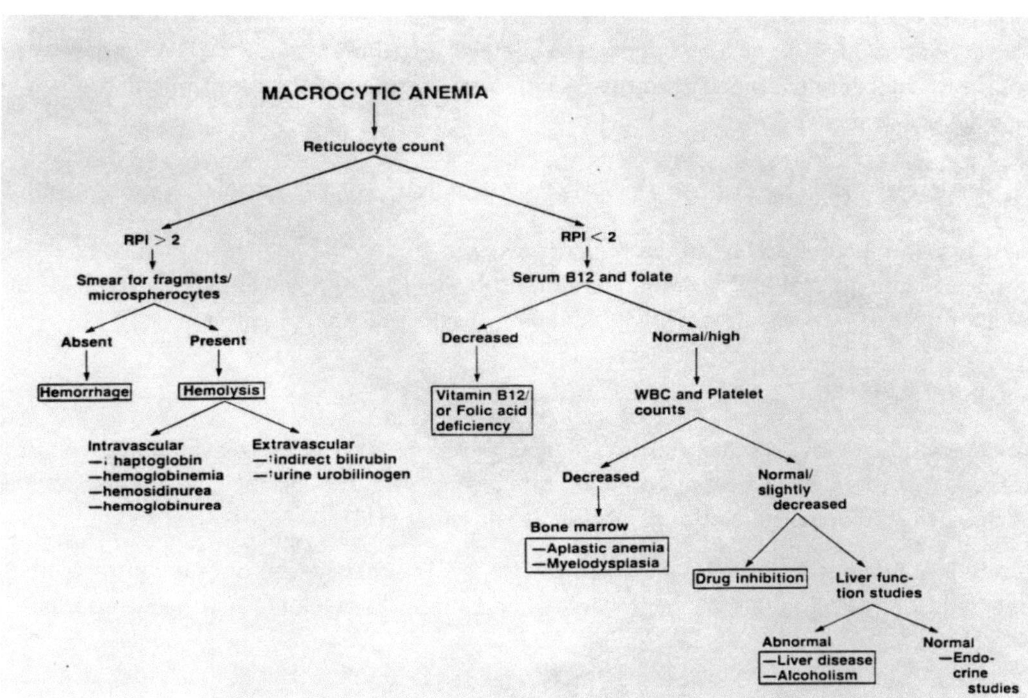

Figure 2. Algorithm for the investigation of macrocytic anemia.

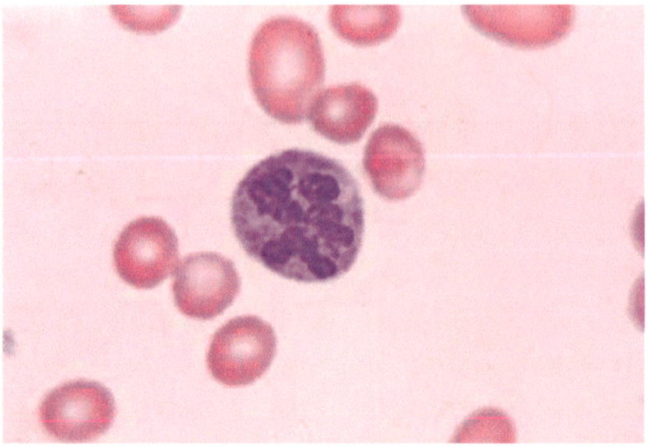

Figure 3. Cytologic abnormalities of megaloblastic anemia on blood smear.

As concerned about the leukocytes, there is a progressive reduction in white blood cells count but it rarely falls below 2000 cells/μL. Neutrophil hypersegmentation is another cardinal feature of megaloblastic anemia. In this case, neutrophil hypersegmentation is declared if neutrophils have more than the usual 3–5 nuclear segments/lobes. In other words, finding of a neutrophil having six or more nuclear segments or 5% of neutrophils have five or more lobes or in fact if most neutrophils have four or more lobes are strongly indicative of megaloblastic anemia. It is noteworthy that in nutritional megaloblastic anemias, hypersegmented neutrophils are an early sign of megaloblastosis.

Platelets vary widely in size and increased platelet distribution width (PDW) is the usual indicator. The complete blood count (CBC) often reveals anemia, leukopenia, and at times thrombocytopenia.

6.2. Serum vitamin B_{12} and folate

These tests are known to be limited by their low sensitivity and specificity, and it has been shown that the normal lower limits for vitamin B_{12} levels are not well defined [10]. Aside, these tests are expensive and not always available to the practicing clinician.

6.3. Serum B_{12} levels

Previous studies showed that vitamin B_{12} levels were found normal or elevated in myeloproliferative disorders, liver disease, congenital transcobalamin II deficiency, intestinal bacterial overgrowth, and antecedent administration of vitamin B_{12} [11]

Falsely low vitamin B_{12} levels with folate deficiency, pregnancy, use of oral contraceptives, congenital deficiency of serum haptocorrins, and multiple myeloma had been reported in Ref. [11].

6.4. Serum folate levels

Folic acid deficiency is rare where food fortification is the order of the day like in the US [12]. Although tissue stores may be normal, serum folate levels can decrease within a few days of dietary folate restriction [11]. Thus, patients should fast prior to testing for serum folate levels, as serum folate levels increase with feeding. Mild degree of hemolysis can falsely display elevated serum folate levels because of high concentration of folate within the red blood cell (RBC) [11].

Inspite of adequate tissue store of folate, certain conditions like pregnancy, use of certain anticonvulsant drugs and alcohol intake may also cause a decrease in serum levels of the vitamin. However, in vitamin B_{12} deficiency serum folate levels tend to increase, probably because of impairment of the methionine synthase pathway and trapping of methyltetrahydrofolate, which happens to be the principal form of folate in the serum [13, 14].

6.5. Red blood cell (RBC) folate

In RBC, folate level is regarded as a more reliable source of determining tissue stores of folate. Unlike serum folate which is affected by dietary intake, RBC folate levels remain constant throughout the lifespan of the cell. However, assays for measuring RBC folate levels have also been fraught with unreliability [14–16]. Vitamin B_{12} deficiency has been established to be a cause of low RBC folate levels [14, 17, 18]. It is estimated that approximately 60% of patients with pernicious anemia have low RBC folate levels, presumably because vitamin B_{12} is necessary for normal transfer of methyl tetrahydrofolate from plasma to RBCs [13, 16, 19–21].

6.6. Bone marrow examination

The aspirated marrow is often hypercellular with striking imbalance in nuclear-cytoplasmic maturation often referred to as nuclear-cytoplasmic asynchrony. This asynchrony occurs because of progressive impaired DNA synthesis and nuclear derangements that accumulate with each cell division thereby slowing down nuclear replication and causes cummulative retardation with each step of maturation division. Therefore, the imbalance in cell growth becomes most apparent in matured hematopoietic cells. Sideroblasts, red cell precursors containing increased number of iron granules, are increased in proportion. Also, because of erythroid hyperplasia, the ratio of myeloid to erythroid precursors (M/E ratio) is reversed and may fall to 1:1 or even lower.

In severe cases, numerous giant pronormoblasts (promegaloblasts) having an unusually large number of mitotic figures are present. Macrophage iron content is often increased. Even with the attempt of masking megaloblastic anemia by the coexistence of microcytic anemia, a megaloblastic anemia will usually show hypersegmented neutrophils in the blood and giant metamyelocytes and bands in the marrow.

Substantial disintegration of erythroblasts occurs within the marrow sinuses sequel to undue prolonged detention of the erythroblasts with uncondensed nuclei wherein products of their disintegration are scanphage by macrophages. This process is referred to as ineffective erythropoiesis.

It is noteworthy that a megaloblastic anemia may be misdiagnosed as acute leukemia when megaloblastic anemia is very severe. In this case, the typical megaloblasts are obviously absent, and rather most cells available are bizarre megaloblastic pronormoblasts that dominate the marrow because of lack of maturation of the erythroid series and hence raising the possibility of erythroleukemia. On the contrary, a patient with just macrocytosis, no anemia, and without any cellular abnormality on the peripheral blood film may not require bone marrow examination.

The granulocytes and megakaryocytes are equally affected by the imbalance of cell growth in megaloblastic anemia. Myeloid cells are generally oversized but it is the presence of giant metamyelocytes and giant bound forms that are actually pathognomonic of megaloblastic anemia. There is also complex lobular hypersegmentation (pseudo hyperdiploidy) of megakaryocytes. There may be megakaryocyte fragments and giant platelets in circulation.

6.7. Serum concentrations of methylmalonic acid (MMA) and homocysteine

Several important metabolic pathways require the functions of cobalamin and folate as co-factors. The generation of methionine from homocysteine requires the co-factors of vitamin B_{12} and folate. However, the production of succinyl CoA from L-methylmalonyl CoA requires only vitamin B_{12}. The generated succinyl CoA is involved in oxidative phosphorylation reactions within the cells. Therefore, early information regarding the cellular state of vitamin B_{12} and folate are provided by these metabolites. The serum levels of these metabolites are helpful in distinguishing folate from vitamin B_{12} deficiency [22, 23], whereas most patients with only folate deficiency have normal methylmalonic acid (MMA) or mildly elevated levels, patient with just vitamin B_{12} deficiency do have significantly elevated level. It is noteworthy that almost 50% of patients with elevation of these metabolites do have normal serum vitamin B_{12} levels. Hence, emphasizing the low sensitivity of serum vitamin B_{12} levels, especially when there are implicating signs and symptoms.

Overall, measuring serum MMA and homocysteine levels are well established way of differentiating cobalamin deficiency from folate deficiency, whereas in cobalamin deficiency, both metabolites are elevated but anemic cobalamin deficient patient show more marked elevations [22, 24].

Nonanemia cobalamin deficient patients are better identified using MMA, which is far more sensitive than homocysteine, whereas in folate deficient patients there is marked elevation of homocysteine levels while serum levels of MMA are not elevated [22, 24].

Hence, measurement of serum level of these two metabolites provides a means of distinguishing cobalamin from folate deficiency as well as providing a reliable degree of accuracy in diagnosing these deficiency states [22, 24].

However, the sensitivity of identifying patients with cobalamin deficiency is masked by renal dysfunction leading to a falsely elevated serum MMA [24, 25]. Also, hereditary hyperhomocysteinemia, where elevated homocysteine may cause confusion in diagnosing folate deficiency. It is recommended that measurement of MMA should be undertaken only if the initial levels of vitamin B_{12} and or homocysteine are abnormal.

6.8. Holotranscobalamin II (holoTC II)

When there is a discordance between vitamin B_{12} levels and its metabolites, or even before measuring vitamin B_{12}, MMA, and/or homocysteine serum levels; holotranscobalamin II (holoTCII) is becoming an emerging marker that may be useful in establishing a diagnosis of

http://dx.doi.org/10.5772/intechopen.70063

early vitamin B_{12} deficiency. It is also a very useful marker in cases of renal failure or myeloproliferative diseases in which vitamin B_{12} concentrations may be falsely elevated B_{12} [24, 25]. Cobalamin is transported to cell membrane receptors by holotranscobalamin II and its serum concentration indirectly measures the amount of available vitamin B_{12}. It has been validated that holoTcII has greater sensitivity and specificity than serum level of vitamin although its routine use has not been recommended [23, 26].

Overall, the gold standard for the diagnosis of vitamin B_{12} deficiency is yet to be established. Meanwhile, it is recommended that with low initial vitamin B_{12} level (i.e., <150 ng/L) and in the setting of high clinical index of suspicion of vitamin B_{12} deficiency, a repeat of serum level of the vitamin is suggested preferably along with MMA and homocysteine serum levels [27, 28]. However, in a case of unexplained macrocytic anemia, a complete diagnostic testing following a specific algorithm is necessary (**Table 2**) [29].

Laboratory studies and diagnostic ranges	Situations affecting results
Serum folate <2 ng/mL is diagnostic	Falsely low: Pregnancy, alcohol consumption, anti-seizure >4 ng/mL rules out deficiency drugs, temporarily (a few days) deficient diet (with normal)
Serum folate 2–4 ng/mL Falsely elevated	Requires quantification of methylmalonic acid, homocysteine and intra-erythrocyte folate. Single intake of folate-rich food.
Methyl-tetrahydrofolate [MTHF] and formyl-tetrahydrofolate (FTHF) <100–160 mg/L [Indicates deficiency]	Falsely low: Pregnancy, alcohol consumption, anti-seizure temporarily (a few days) deficient diet (with normal intra-erythrocyte folate). Compared with serum folate, less likely to alter due to transient variations such as dietary changes. Falsely elevated: Single intake of folate-rich food.
Serum cobalamin <200 pg/mL [diagnostic of deficiency] >300 pg/mL [rules out deficiency in 95% of cases]	Falsely low: Pregnancy, folate deficiency, HIV/Aids, anti-seizure drugs, multiply myeloma, hairy cell leukemia
200–300 pg/mL [indicates need to quantify methylmalonic acid and homocysteine]	Aplastic anemia, myelodysplastic syndromes, paroxysmal nocturnal hemoglobinuria, Gaucher's disease, oral contraceptives, Intra-individual variation: up to 23%, idiopathic origin, laboratory error.
Methylmalonic acid (MMA) Normal: 70–270 mmol/L	Falsely elevated: Kidney failure, methylmalonic acidemia. Intra-individual variation: up to 23%. Falsely low: Use of antibiotics. Usually elevated with comorbid cobalamin deficiency
Homocysteine Normal: 5–14 mmol/L	Falsely elevated: Hereditary hyperhomocysteinemia: Intra-individual variation: 17% changes in methyl-THFR, cystathionine beta-synthase, betaine usually elevated with comorbid cobalamin and folate synthesis. deficiency.
Elevated MMA and homocysteine:	Cobalamin deficiency (sensitivity: 94%, specificity: 99%). Normal MMA and homocysteine: rules out deficiency of both vitamins. Normal MMA and elevated homocysteine: folate deficiency (sensitivity: 86%, specificity: 99%).

Table 2. Specific laboratory investigations in suspected case of folate and cobalamin deficiency.

7. Differential diagnosis

Macrocytosis with MCV (not exceeding 110 FL) occurs in alcoholism, liver disease, hypothyroidism, aplastic anemia, myelodysplasia, pregnancy, and in certain disease states associated with a reticulocytosis (e.g., autoimmune hemolytic anemia).

8. Pernicious anemia (PA)

In pernicious anemia, the gastric parietal cells are destroyed by autoantibody and this results in failure or impaired production of intrinsic factor [30]. Frequently, both parietal cells and intrinsic factors are attacked by autoantibodies. The identification of parietal cell autoantibodies is more sensitive whereas the identification of intrinsic factor autoantibody is more specific.

Studies had shown that about 70% of patients with pernicious anemia will produce detectable levels of such autoantibodies. The clinical symptoms of pernicious anemia developed slowly as B_{12} stores are sufficient for about 5 years before deficiency lead to the onset of clinical symptoms. Therefore, the full clinical picture of severe intramedullary hemolysis culminating in progressively severe chronic anemia, along with severe neurological symptoms with demyelinisation leading to weakness and paraplegia occurs only rarely. Treatment with parenteral vitamin B_{12} will lead to a rapid increase of reticulocytes (within 48–72 h) and subsequent correction of anemia.

It is more common in males than in females and has an age peak around 60 year. In pernicious anemia, the gastric mucosa is atrophic and the secretion of intrinsic factor is defective. Inflammatory infiltrate of the gastric submucosa is the earliest gastric lesion in patients with PA. A type A gastritis involving the fundus and sparing the antrum is the typical finding in a patient with autoimmune pernicious anemia. The autoantibodies both to parietal cells and intrinsic factor are detectable both in the serum and gastric secretions. These autoantibodies particularly target the H^+/K^+-ATPase in the parietal cell resulting to gastric atrophy and achlorhydria. Studies had shown that parietal cell autoantibody is detectable in 90% of patients with pernicious anemia and also in 30% of first degree relatives who do not have pernicious anemia, and only about 2–8% of the normal population have low titer of these autoantibodies [31]. There are two types of anti-intrinsic factor autoantibodies. The type I autoantibodies blocks the binding of vitamin B_{12} to intrinsic factor and type II auto antibody, seen in 35–40% of patients binds to different epitope of intrinsic factor [32].

A selective malabsorption of vitamin B_{12} underlies the pathogenesis of autoimmune pernicious anemia. The eventual deficiency of vitamin B_{12} resulted to megaloblastic anemia and ineffective erythropoiesis.

9. Treatment of cobalamin deficiency

To treat a case of megaloblastic anemia, all efforts should be applied to exclude the underlying cause. Drug-related causes, MDS, and others should be clearly excluded. Since

http://dx.doi.org/10.5772/intechopen.70063

anemia of megaloblastosis insidiously develops, patients progressively adjust to the low hemoglobin and hence blood transfusion is not an option except only in patients with severe uncompensated and life threatening anemia.

Megaloblastic anemia with established cobalamin deficiency should be given intramuscular cobalamin of 1000 μg daily for 2 weeks or alternatively thrice weekly for 2 weeks for six doses and then weekly for another six doses until hematocrit returns to normal. It is given monthly for life in certain cases like pernicious anemia and in partial or total gastrectomy. Patients with neurological and mental impairment resulting from cobalamin deficiency deserve a very aggressive approach.

Oral cobalamin can be adopted when there is enough evidence that the absorptive capacity for cobalamin is intact. It is administered at 1000–2000 μg but a wide range of doses and schedules have been recommended. It is important to monitor closely for desired response since absorption can be variable and may be inadequate in some patients. Although intramuscular cobalamin is often preferable since it has the potential to bypass all abnormalities of cobalamin absorption. However, oral cobalamin is less expensive, better tolerated by patients, and preferable in patients with bleeding disorders like hemophilic patients in whom intramuscular injection should be avoided.

There is a need to apply multidisciplinary approach to the management of megaloblastic anemia. The hematologist hold a crucial position in making diagnosis and in management while the neurologists should be at hand to diagnose and manage potential neurological complications. The gastroenterologists are involved in ruling out the gastroenterological causes of the disease by doing both upper and lower endoscopy searching for diseases like atrophic gastritis, carcinoma of the stomach, and terminal ileitis. Also, pediatricians are needed in diagnosing and managing children with inborn errors and having megaloblastosis.

9.1. Folate therapy

In folate deficiency, a full hematologic response to physiologic doses of folate at 200 μg daily distinguishes it from cobalamin deficiency pharmacologic doses of folate at 5 mg daily is required to achieve full hematologic response [30]. This should not be recommended as a diagnostic test because neurologic problems may develop in cobalamin deficient patients treated with cobalamin alone. However, cobalamin may cause a partial response in folate deficiency [31].

Oral administration of folate is always the case except in difficult situation when parenteral administration may be indicated. At times folate rich diet may suffice. The dose of folate ranges between 1 and 5 mg daily but a higher dose is indicated in hemolytic conditions like sickle cell disease, hereditary elliptocytosis, hereditary spherocytosis, and in hyper-homocysteinemia. Food fortification with folate and supplementation are recommended to reduce the risk of pancreatic, cervical and colonic cancers, end stage renal disease and in elderly persons [32].

It is however noteworthy that administration of folate to individuals with Cobalamin deficiency increases the risk and frequency of cobalamin-induced neurological and neuropsychiatry disorders. Therefore, folate should not be instituted in patients with megaloblastic anemia when cobalamin deficiency has not been ruled out [33, 34].

The response to therapy should be closely monitored using complete blood count (CBC), reticulocyte count, lactate dehydrogenase (LDH) levels, indirect bilirubin, hemoglobin level, serum potassium and serum ferritin. It is expected that LDH and indirect bilirubin should fall rapidly with treatment while there is evident reticulocytosis within 3–5 days and it peaks between 4 and 10 days. The hemoglobin is expected to rise by 1 g/dL per week and should rise to normal level within 2 months. It is very important to closely monitor the serum potassium which falls with treatment and may result to death. Potassium supplementation should be given in case of hypokalemia using oral potassium supplement (slow K) Iron deficiency can occur because of escalated erythropoiesis and this may impede the rate of response. Iron therapy is equally necessary [33, 34].

A diagnostic therapeutic trial is allowed when the results of laboratory evaluation become ambiguous, a clinical trial of cobalamin therapy may be given. This is done only when cobalamin deficiency has been ruled out.

Particular attention should be placed on the followings:

Hypokalemia, that is, low serum potassium, can occur in a severe megaloblastic anemia on treatment because of ongoing rapid restoration of erythropoiesis in the bone marrow.

Only about 1% of ingested cobalamin is absorbed through the ileal mucosa when intrinsic factor is deficient. Therefore, a maintenance daily dose of 1 mg may be sufficient to maintain steady levels in patients not willing to receive regular injections.

It is also noteworthy that neurological symptoms may be irreversible or may respond slowly if folic acid was given without cobalamin in combined deficiency or while dealing with very severe and long standing cobalamin deficiency.

Author details

Olaniyi John Ayodele

Address all correspondence to: ayodeleolaniyi8@gmail.com

Department of Haematology, College of Medicine, University College Hospital, University of Ibadan, Ibadan, Nigeria

References

[1] Glader B. Anemia: General aspects. In: Greer JP, Foerster J, Lukens JN, et al, editors. Wintrobe's Clinical Hematology. 11th ed. Baltimore, Md: Williams & Wilkins; 2004. pp. 947-978

[2] Hoffbrand V, Provan D. ABC of clinical haematology: Macrocytic anaemias. British Medical Journal. 1997;**314**:430-433

[3] Addison T. Anaemia-disease of the supra-renal capsules. London Medical Gazette. 1849;**43**:517-518

[4] Minot GR, Murphy WP. Treatment of pernicious anemia by a special diet. Blood. 1948;**3**:8-21

[5] Castle WB. The effect of the administration to patients with pernicious anemia of the contents of the normal human stomach recovered after the ingestion of beef muscle. American Journal of the Medical Sciences. 1929;**87**:470-476

[6] Hodgkin DC, Kamper J, Mackey M, et al. Structure of vitamin B_{12}. Nature. 1956;**178**:64-66

[7] Alpers DH. What is new in vitamin B(12)? Current Opinion in Gastroenterology. 2005;**21**:183-186

[8] Chanarin I. The Megaloblastic Anaemias. 2nd ed. Oxford, England: Blackwell Scientific Publishers; 1979

[9] Castellanos-Sinco HB, Ramos-Penafiel CO, Santoyo-Sanchez A, Callazo-Jaloma J, et al. Megaloblastic anaemia: Folic acid and vitamin B_{12} metabolism. REVISTA MEDICAL DEL Hospital General DE MEXICO. Document descargado de http://www.elsevier.es el

[10] Ward PC. Modern approaches to the investigation of vitamin B_{12} deficiency. Clinics in Laboratory Medicine. 2002;**22**:435-445

[11] Snow CF. Laboratory diagnosis of vitamin B_{12} and folate deficiency: A guide for the primary care physician. Archives of Internal Medicine. 1999;**159**:1289-1298

[12] Ashraf MJ, Goyal M, Hinchey K, Cook JR. Clinical utility of folic acid testing for anemia and dementia screen. Journal of General Internal Medicine. 2004;**19**(s1):130

[13] Chanarin I. The Megaloblastic Anaemias. 2nd ed. Oxford, England: Blackwell Scientific Publishers; 1979

[14] Handin RI, Lux SE, Stossel TP. Blood: Principles and Practice of Hematology. 1st ed. Philadelphia, PA: Lippincott Williams & Wilkins; 1995. p. 1421

[15] Davidson RJ, Hamilton PJ. High mean red cell volume: Its incidence and significance in routine haematology. Journal of Clinical Pathology. 1978;**31**:493-498

[16] Lindenbaum J, Allen RH. Clinical spectrum and diagnosis of folate deficiency. In: Bailey LB, editor. Folate in Health and Disease. New York, NY: Marcel Dekker; 1995. pp. 43-73

[17] Handin RI, Lux SE, Stossel TP. Blood: Principles and Practice of Hematology. 1st ed. Philadelphia, PA: Lippincott Williams & Wilkins; 1995. p. 1421

[18] Tisman G, Herbert V. B12 dependence of cell uptake of serum folate: An explanation for high serum folate and cell folate depletion in B12 deficiency. Blood. 1973;**41**:465-469

[19] Antony AC. Megaloblastic anemias. In: Hoffman R, Benz EJ Jr, Shattil SJ, Furie B, Cohen HJ, Silberstein LE, McGlave P, editors. Hematology: Basic Principles and Practice. 3rd ed. New York, NY: Churchill Livingston; 2000. pp. 446-485

[20] Jaffe JP, Schilling RF. Erythrocyte folate levels: A clinical study. American Journal of Hematology. 1991;**36**:116-121

[21] Stabler SP, Marcell PD, Podell ER, Allen RH, Savage DG, Lindenbaum J. Elevation of total homocysteine in the serum of patients with cobalamin or folate deficiency detected by capillary gas chromatography-mass spectrometry. Journal of Clinical Investigation. 1988;**81**:466-474

[22] Savage DG, Lindenbaum J, Stabler SP, Allen RH. Sensitivity ofserum methylmalonic acid and total homocysteine determinations for diagnosing cobalamin and folate deficiencies. American Journal of Medicine. 1994;**96**:239-246

[23] Solomon LR. Cobalamin-responsive disorders in the ambulatory care setting: Unreliability of cobalamin, methylmalonic acid, and homocysteine testing. Blood. 2005;**105**: 978-985

[24] Alpers DH. What is new in vitamin B_{12}? Current Opinion in Gastroenterology. 2005;**21**: 183-186

[25] Lloyd-Wright Z, Hvas A, Moller J, Sanders TA, Nexo E. Holo-transcobalamin as an indicator of dietary vitamin B12 deficiency. Clinical Chemistry. 2003;**49**:2076-2078

[26] Nilsson K, Isaksson A, Gustafson L, Hultberg B. Clinical utility of serum holo-transcobalamin as a marker of cobalamin status in elderly patients with neuropsychiatric symptoms. Clinical Chemistry and Laboratory Medicine. 2004;**42**:637-643

[27] Robinson AR, Mladenovic J. Lack of clinical utility of folate levels in the evaluation of macrocytosis or anemia. American Journal of Medicine. 2001;**110**:88-90

[28] Andres E, Fothergill H, Mecili M. Efficacy of oral cobalamin (vitamin B12) therapy. Expert Opinion on Pharmacotherapy. 2010 Feb;**11**(2):249-256. [Medline]

[29] Robinson AR, Mladenovic J. Lack of clinical utility of folate levels in the evaluation of macrocytosis or anemia. American Journal of Medicine. 2001;**110**:88-90

[30] Antony AC. Megaloblastic Anemias. In: Hoffman R, Benz EJ Jr, Silberstein LE, Heslop HE, Weitz JI, Anastasi J. Hematology: Basic Principles and Practice. 6th ed. Philadelphia, PA: Elsevier; 2013. pp. 473-504

[31] Wang YH, Yan F, Zhang WB, et al. An investigation of vitamin B12 deficiency in elderly inpatients in neurology department. Neuroscience Bulletin. 2009 Aug;**25**(4):209-215. [Medline]

[32] Hoffbrand AV. Megaloblastic anemias. In: Kasper DL, Fauci AS, Hauser SL, Longo DL, Jameson JL, Loscalzo J, editors. Harrison's Principles of Internal Medicine. 19th ed. New York, NY: McGraw-Hill Education; 2015

[33] Bunn HF. Vitamin B12 and pernicious anaemia-The dawn of molecular medicine. The New England Journal of Medicine. 2014;**370**:773-776. DOI: 10.1056/NEJM,Mcibr 1315544

[34] Schick P, Talaesera F, Sacher RA, Besa E, et al. Megaloblastic Anaemia in Medscape update 2017 (Jan). emedicine.medscape.com/article/204066-overview

Section 2

Anemia in Different Age Groups

Chapter 3

Iron Deficiency Anemia in Children

Jelena Roganović and Ksenija Starinac

Additional information is available at the end of the chapter

http://dx.doi.org/10.5772/intechopen.69774

Abstract

Iron deficiency and iron deficiency anemia remain a major and global public health problem that affects particularly infants, young children, and women of childbearing age in developing countries. The prevalence of iron deficiency anemia is still common in industrialized countries despite efforts to improve public awareness and strengthen programs for the prevention and control of iron deficiency. The most common risk factors for iron deficiency in early childhood are rapid growth, perinatal risk factors, poor dietary intake, and gastrointestinal blood loss due to excessive consumption of cow's milk. Iron deficiency and iron deficiency anemia cause a wide variety of symptoms and changes in many different tissues. The most concerning consequences of iron deficiency in children are the alterations of cognitive, motor, and behavioral performance. Persistent neurocognitive changes despite iron repletion have increased the importance of prevention and early detection of iron deficiency. The main principles of treatment include investigation and elimination of the underlying cause, iron supplementation, improvement of nutrition, and education of the patient and family. Oral iron supplements are desirable as first-line therapy. Follow-up is very important to confirm the diagnosis and to ensure that anemia is adequately treated.

Keywords: iron deficiency, anemia, child, prevention, iron supplementation

1. Introduction

Iron deficiency is the most common micronutrient deficiency worldwide and one of the most important public health problems, affecting approximately 25% of the world's population according to the World Health Organization (WHO). Iron deficiency is the most common in preschool children and women of childbearing age, particularly in regions of Asia and Africa with poor access to iron-rich foods [1, 2]. There are lower rates of iron deficiency in developed countries such as the United States and other industrialized regions with healthy food rich in nutrients. However, the problem still exists and can have a great impact on mental and physical development, health maintenance, and the quality of life of affected children.

2. Epidemiology

Approximately 8% of toddlers in the United States have iron deficiency, and 2–3% have iron deficiency anemia (IDA) [3]. As age increases, prevalence decreases until adolescence. Sixteen percent of adolescent girls have iron deficiency, and 3% have IDA [4]. Among American females aged 12–15 years, the incidence of iron deficiency was 9% and the incidence of IDA was 2%; in the age group 16–19 years, the incidence was 11 and 3%, respectively [5]. Less than 1% of adolescent males had iron deficiency. Higher incidence of iron deficiency was found in both male and female adolescents in some other countries [6, 7]. The rate of iron deficiency did not decline much during the last 40 years, but there were significant improvements in some subgroups of young children. For example, in children aged 12–24 months, iron deficiency rates declined from 23 to 11% between two study periods [3].

The prevalence of iron deficiency in the United States is higher in children who live in poverty, in low-income families, and in immigrant groups. The highest prevalence was shown in children with African-American and Hispanic origin [3, 8]. Other risk factors associated with higher prevalence of IDA are low birth weight, prematurity, and childhood obesity [3, 8, 9]. These high-risk pediatric subgroups should undergo screening.

Pinhas-Hamiel and co-workers showed that the prevalence of iron deficiency was significantly associated with increased body mass index (BMI) [10]. Obesity was a risk factor in both males and females, but it was about three times higher in girls [10, 11]. It is unclear why obesity is linked to iron deficiency and IDA, but low-quality foods and increased needs comparing to body weight may be connected.

Adolescent athletes, vegetarians, adolescents with chronic illnesses, heavy menstrual blood loss (>80 ml/month), or children who are underweighted or malnourished are at higher risk for iron deficiency and IDA, and they should also have laboratory screening for anemia [12, 13].

In developing countries, where diets do not contain sufficient red meat, IDA is approximately seven times more frequent than in Europe or North America. Despite the fact that there is enough dietary iron in some cases, this is the case because heme iron is absorbed better than nonheme iron. IDA was found in 2/3 of children and adolescents in Nepal and in Sudan [14], and in 48.5% of Egyptian children in 2005 [15]. Parasites like hookworm can worsen iron deficiency due to profound gastrointestinal blood loss.

Neonates have total body iron of 250 mg (80 mg/kg), obtained from maternal sources. In the first 6 months of life, during the period when the infant gets iron-deficient milk diet, this amount decreases to 60 mg/kg. Infants fed with cow's milk are at greater risk to develop serious IDA because calcium from cow's milk is competing with iron for absorption. Children should get 0.5 mg more iron than is lost daily in order to maintain a normal body iron of 60 mg/kg.

The prevalence of iron deficiency exceeds 50% in countries with limited food and nutrient sources, such as most countries in Africa, Southeast Asia, and Latin America [16]. The prevalence of anemia ranges from 45 to 65% in children, 20 to 60% in women, and 10 to 35% in men [1]. Half of these cases are presumed to be caused by iron deficiency.

The prevalence of IDA is still high in infancy and preschool children, despite improvements in public health awareness, increased breastfeeding rate, and the presence of iron-fortified foods in diet [17, 18]. All these facts emphasize the importance of constant surveillance and early detection, prevention, and intervention toward iron deficiency in childhood, particularly in high-risk groups. Special attention should be paid to discover and treat iron deficiency during pregnancy and the earliest periods of life, because severe iron deficiency can have a great impact on child's growth, development, and learning skills.

3. Definitions

Iron deficiency is a condition when the body lacks sufficient iron to maintain normal physiological functions. It is defined as decreased total body iron or, in some cases, by serum ferritin level <12 mg/l in children up to 5 years and <15 mg/l in children 5 years and older. Although the serum ferritin level is useful in defining iron deficiency, this definition can be considered only if other conditions that can affect ferritin levels (i.e., inflammation or liver disease) are absent. For children less than 5 years of age with concurrent infection, serum ferritin concentrations <30 mg/l are reflective of depleted iron stores [19].

Anemia is defined as a hemoglobin concentration more than 2 standard deviations below the mean reference value for age- and sex-matched healthy population. WHO hemoglobin thresholds used to define anemia in different age groups are [2]:

- children 6 months to 5 years: 11 g/dl;
- children 5–12 years: 11.5 g/dl;
- children 12–15 years: 12 g/dl;
- nonpregnant women: 12 g/dl;
- pregnant women: 11 g/dl; and
- men ≥15 years: 13 g/dl.

IDA develops when body iron is too low to maintain normal red blood cell (RBC) production. IDA in young children (up to 5 years) is defined as the presence of ferritin level <12 mg/l and hemoglobin level <11 g/dl, in the absence of other conditions that can affect these findings [20].

The terms "iron deficiency" and "IDA" are often used in the same context. However, iron deficiency without anemia is three times as common as IDA. If iron requirements are below iron intake, total body iron reduces gradually. Hemoglobin levels are initially normal, reflecting the stage when iron deficiency exists in the absence of anemia. At that point, ferritin level and transferrin saturation are reduced. As total body iron decreases and iron stores are exhausted, hemoglobin levels drop below normal values. Thus, iron deficiency is defined as reduced body iron but hemoglobin levels are still above the cut-off value for anemia. Worsening of that condition leads to iron-deficient erythropoiesis and finally to development of IDA.

4. Pathophysiology

Iron is an essential micronutrient in the human body. It plays an important role in many metabolic processes, such as oxygen transport, electron transport, and DNA synthesis. Iron is a component of many cellular proteins and enzymes. Heme proteins, hemoglobin and myoglobin, contain about 3/4 of total body iron. The rest of body iron is stored in ferritin and hemosiderin, and about 3% is part of enzyme systems, such as catalase and cytochromes [21]. Iron is mostly recycled from senescent RBCs by macrophages. Only a small proportion of total body iron enters and leaves the body on a daily basis. Consequently, mechanisms that affect intestinal absorption and intercellular iron transport have great impact on iron balance. The serum iron concentration is regulated by absorptive cells in the proximal small intestine, which can regulate iron absorption to compensate for iron body loss. There are three different pathways of iron uptake in the small intestine: the heme pathway and two specific pathways for ferric and ferrous iron, respectively.

Enterocytes absorb heme iron and nonheme iron noncompetitively. Dietary iron contains both chemical forms of iron. Heme iron is mainly found as ferrous iron (Fe^{2+}), while the most part of nonheme dietary iron is ferric iron (Fe^{3+}). When heme enters the enterocyte, it is degraded by heme oxygenase with release of iron. It passes the basolateral membrane of the enterocyte and competes with nonheme iron to bind transferrin in the plasma. The way of nonheme iron transport in the body is still not known. The concentration of iron in the enterocytes depends on the body's needs for iron. Individuals who are iron-deficient have a small amount of iron in enterocytes, while those who have sufficient body iron have higher amounts of iron in the absorptive intestinal cells. Iron in the enterocyte regulates absorption by either up-regulation of receptors or saturation of an iron-binding protein, or both. Iron that is delivered to other nonintestinal cells in the body is bound to transferrin. There are two pathways through which transferrin iron can be delivered into nonintestinal cells: classical transferrin receptor pathway and the pathway independent of the transferrin receptor.

In adults, only 5% of total body iron requirements is from different food sources. This amount is the same as iron loss, which is mainly from the gastrointestinal tract. The majority (95%) of iron comes from the breakdown of old RBCs. In children, approximately 30% of iron comes from diet, probably due to fast growth in pediatric age [21, 22].

There are three major factors that can influence intestinal iron absorption: iron stores in ferritin and transferrin, erythropoietic rate, and bioavailability of iron in foods. When iron stores decrease, receptors in the intestinal mucosa increase in order to raise iron uptake. Iron absorption also increases when there is increased or ineffective erythropoiesis.

5. Risk factors

5.1. Perinatal risk factors

During the intrauterine period, the only source of iron is the iron that is crossing through the placenta. The majority of healthy infants have iron stores of about 80 mg/kg, and 2/3 of total iron is bound in hemoglobin molecules. Normal hemoglobin concentration is 15–17 g/dl. Healthy infants have enough body iron for the first 5–6 months of life [22, 23]. There are some conditions that can reduce iron stores at birth or can act through other mechanisms, thus increasing the risk for developing IDA during the first months of life. These conditions are maternal iron deficiency, prematurity, administration of erythropoietin for anemia of prematurity, fetal-maternal hemorrhage, twin-twin transfusion syndrome, other perinatal hemorrhagic events, and insufficient intake of dietary iron during early infancy. Delayed clamping of the umbilical cord (approximately 120–180 seconds after delivery) can improve the amount of iron and significantly reduce the risk of IDA [24].

Deficiency of iron during pregnancy increases the risk of iron deficiency in the infancy. A study of Kumar et al. showed that iron in the cord blood sample was in correlation with mother's hemoglobin and ferritin levels [25]. The content of iron in breast milk was reduced in mothers with severe anemia, but it was normal in mothers with mild or moderate anemia. It is recommended to implement iron supplementation during pregnancy in the populations with high prevalence of maternal IDA. It is also important to provide different kinds of iron-fortified foods for pregnant women who are at risk to develop IDA [26].

Prematurity is one of the risk factors for IDA because premature infants have smaller total blood volume at birth compared to healthy term infants, decreased ferritin concentrations, poor gastrointestinal absorption, and increased blood loss through phlebotomies [27]. Iron is mostly accumulated during the third trimester of gestation that is shorter in preterm infants. There is also increased risk for iron deficiency after use of erythropoietin for the prevention and the treatment of the anemia of prematurity [23].

Chronic fetal-maternal hemorrhage and twin-twin transfusion syndrome (TTTS) can reduce iron stores and cause anemia in term or premature infants. A small amount of fetal blood (<0.1 ml) is commonly found in maternal circulation. Causes of increased loss of fetal blood into the maternal circulation are seen as a result of trauma, placental abruption, or may be spontaneous and idiopathic. Manifestations of fetal-maternal hemorrhage depend on the amount and the rapidity of blood loss [28]. TTTS is a rare complication of monochorionic twins (or higher multiple gestations). It is the result of blood transfusion from one twin (donor) to another twin (recipient) through placental vascular anastomoses. The donor twin is smaller and often anemic, and the recipient twin is often plethoric with hemoglobin differences greater than 5 g/dl. Advanced stages of TTTS have 60–100% mortality rate, and fetuses who survive are at risk of severe cardiac, neurologic, and developmental disorders [29].

5.2. Dietary factors

Feeding and all dietary aspects are very important in early infancy and childhood because they can greatly impact development of IDA. There are many dietary factors that can affect iron metabolism. The most common factors are poor iron intake, decreased iron absorption, consumption of unmodified cow's milk before 12 months of age, and occult intestinal blood loss due to cow's milk protein-induced colitis [30].

Poor iron intake in infancy usually occurs when babies are fed with infant formulas or transitional foods which are not fortified with iron. In the study from Chile, the prevalence of IDA was higher in infants fed with the formula without iron (20%), much lower in those fed with iron-fortified formula (0.6%), and medium in infants fed with human milk (15%) [31]. In another study, an increased prevalence of IDA in infancy was observed in infants fed with nonformula cow's milk > 600 ml or more daily or > 6 breast feeds per day [32]. The amount of iron in human milk is highest during the first month of life, but gradually decreases in the following period. This amount varies among individuals. Maternal diet does not affect iron amount in the human milk.

Intestinal iron absorption depends on the form of iron in the foods. Dietary sources of heme iron, such as fish, meat, and poultry, have higher bioavailability of iron compared to nonheme sources of iron, such as fruits, vegetables, and grains. There are also various components of food that influence intestinal iron absorption. Vitamin C increases iron absorption from bread, cereals, fruits, and vegetables (nonheme iron) but has little effect on the absorption of heme iron. IDA is a common problem in children who follow a vegetarian diet. Intestinal absorption of ferrous and ferric iron is inhibited by tannins in different kinds of teas, foods rich in phosphates, oxalates, carbonates, and phytates (seeds and grains). Purified heme is absorbed poorly because heme polymerizes into macromolecules. Globin prevents the formation of insoluble heme polymers so that it remains available for absorption. Peptides from the degraded globin bind to iron and prevent iron polymerization and precipitation. Different forms of iron can be absorbed better when given together (i.e., spinach with meat).

One of the most important risk factors for IDA is early introduction of unmodified (nonformula) cow's milk. It increases the risk for intestinal blood loss in infants compared with the formula or breast feeding, mainly due to colitis [33]. Daily intake of 720 ml or more of cow's milk in preschool children is associated with increased risk for iron deficiency. The reasons are low concentration of iron in cow's milk, low bioavailability of iron, and possibly increased intestinal blood loss [34]. Sutcliffe et al. reported increased risk for iron deficiency in children with continued bottle-feeding compared with children with cup-feeding in the age of 2–3 years, mainly due to the greater volumes of cow's milk in bottle-feeding [35].

5.3. Gastrointestinal disease

Dietary iron is absorbed mainly throughout duodenum. Gastrointestinal malabsorption of iron occurs in diseases that affect this portion of the intestine, including celiac disease, Crohn disease, giardiasis, and resection of the proximal small intestine. In children, anemia secondary to iron, folic acid, and vitamin B12 malabsorption is a common complication of celiac disease, and further screening with tissue transglutaminase antibodies has been strongly recommended [36]. Conditions that cause gastrointestinal blood loss are also associated with iron deficiency. These include cow's milk protein-induced colitis, inflammatory bowel disease (IBD), duodenal/gastric ulcers, and chronic use of nonsteroidal anti-inflammatory drugs or aspirin. Iron deficiency occurs in about 60–80% of patients with IBD. Anemia of chronic disease, vitamin B12 deficiency, folic acid deficiency, and hemolysis contribute to the development of anemia in patients with IBD [37, 38].

6. Screening recommendations

Routine screening for IDA should be obtained in children 6–24 months of age. Screening consists of reviewing risk factors during any possible occasion or visit (risk assessment), and laboratory testing (laboratory screening) at least once during the mentioned period. Screening is recommended at all times for all infants and children who have any risk factor (malnutrition, low birth weight, prematurity, signs and symptoms of IDA, or living in the area with high prevalence of iron deficiency).

6.1. Risk assessment

Review of risk factors in all children is recommended at 4, 15, 18, 24, and 30 months, at 3 years, and once yearly afterward. This is currently the most important and valuable screening tool, more useful than laboratory testing of hemoglobin. Risk assessment consists of focused dietary history. The most vulnerable groups are children with the history of prematurity or low birth weight, infants using low-iron formula, nonformula cow's milk, soy milk or goat's milk before 12 months of age, infants having less than two iron-rich meals daily after 6 months of age, preschool children drinking more than 600 ml milk per day, or having less than three iron-rich meals daily.

6.2. Laboratory screening

American Academy of Pediatrics (AAP) suggests laboratory testing as the screening tool for iron deficiency at 1 year of age [30]. Universal laboratory screening is recommended for all children 9–12 months of age. Additional laboratory screening is recommended for children with risk factors for iron deficiency and IDA. There are two groups of children that should undertake additional laboratory screening:

- children with high risk for iron deficiency—repeated laboratory testing at 15–18 months of age or when some risk is identified; and
- children with special health needs (chronic diseases, inflammatory disorders, restricted diets)—repeated laboratory testing in the period of early childhood (2–5 years of age).

Laboratory screening in most cases includes complete blood count, which includes hemoglobin, hematocrit, mean corpuscular volume (MCV), and red blood cell distribution width (RDW). The minimum laboratory screening is measurement of hemoglobin with the normal value greater than 11 g/dl.

Laboratory testing of serum ferritin at the time of the first screening is the major diagnostic tool in children with risk factors for iron deficiency and IDA [30]. Ferritin levels should be always evaluated carefully because ferritin is nonspecifically elevated in a wide variety of inflammatory conditions. A C-reactive protein can help to validate the results of serum ferritin levels. Other screening measurements that can be taken into account as a different approach for iron deficiency include reticulocyte hemoglobin concentration and combination of soluble transferrin receptor and hemoglobin [39].

It is recommended by AAP to perform risk assessment once a year during the period of adolescence. Adolescents with risk factors (those with a history of IDA, low-iron diet, or girls with heavy menstrual bleeding) should have laboratory testing for anemia [40]. Considering different opinions on screening recommendations in adolescents, each physician should personally decide about the screening process based on the risk factors. Laboratory testing should be done every 5 years starting from age 13 in girls, and at least once during the rapid growth period in boys. Children with any risk factor (increased physical activity, special diets, obesity, malnutrition, chronic illnesses, and heavy menstrual bleeding in girls) should be monitored more frequently [12].

There is some controversy on routine screening for iron deficiency in areas with low rates of iron deficiency and IDA (i.e., United States). Studies provide little evidence that routine screening or iron treatment improves child's growth and neurodevelopmental outcome. On the other hand, routine screening is recommended because of the important health benefits. Besides, a physician should not decide about screening program only based on symptoms and risk factors in a child. Those who favor screening for iron deficiency in the adolescent period list high prevalence of anemia in that population and adverse consequences of iron deficiency [41]. The screening tests are generally minimally invasive (blood sample), and therapy for IDA is safe.

7. Prevention

Many recommendations for prevention of iron deficiency and IDA have been published, and the most commonly used are those provided by WHO and AAP. Widely used approaches include iron-fortified foods in a diet, iron-rich formulas, introduction of cow's milk in a diet from 12 months of age, screening for iron deficiency, and iron prophylaxis in infants [30].

It is important to emphasize that only a fraction of dietary iron is absorbed from food, depending on bioavailability (dietary iron absorption). Human milk contains only 0.3–1.0 mg/l of iron, but the bioavailability of iron is 50%, while milk formulas contain 12 mg/l of iron with bioavailability of iron 4–6% only [42]. As mentioned above, dietary iron has two main forms: heme and nonheme iron. Plants and iron-fortified foods contain nonheme iron only, whereas meat, seafood, and poultry contain both heme and nonheme iron. Heme iron has higher bioavailability than nonheme iron. The bioavailability of iron is approximately 14–18% from mixed diets, and 5–12% from vegetarian diets. Daily iron requirements vary depending on age and gender. Requirements for iron are 0.6 mg/day in healthy infants and 0.8 mg/day in preadolescent children. Adult males need 1 mg/day of iron, and adult females need 1.5 mg/day [43]. The recommended dietary iron for healthy full-term infants (from birth to 12 months of age) is 1 mg/kg/day (maximum 15 mg); for premature infants 2–4 mg/kg/day (maximum 15 mg); for toddlers 1–3 years of age 7 mg/day; for children aged 4–8 years 10 mg/day; for children aged 9–13 years 8 mg/day; for adolescent boys aged 14–18 years 11 mg/day, and for adolescent girls aged 14–18 years 15 mg/day [43]. Boys have increased requirements during pubertal growth because of expanding blood volume and increase in hemoglobin concentration. Increased requirements in girls during puberty are mostly due to menstrual blood loss, although the loss differs in various individuals. Besides, adolescent girls more often have a tendency to eat food that contains less iron and to avoid high iron-containing foods, contributing to iron deficiency [44].

7.1. Recommendations for supplementation

Infants who are not breastfed, obtain sufficient amount of iron from iron-fortified formula. Breastfed infants should receive an additional source of iron (as iron supplement or complementary food) in these doses:

- Full-term breastfed infants should receive an iron supplement from the age of 4 months (1 mg/kg/day, maximum 15 mg) until the infant has sufficient iron-rich complementary foods in a diet.
- Premature breastfed infants should receive an iron supplement starting from the age of 2 weeks (2–4 mg/kg/day, maximum 15 mg) throughout the first year of life (as supplements or iron-fortified formula).

Supplementation of iron is necessary to meet requirements in infants from populations with high rates of iron deficiency and IDA. In a prospective randomized trial of early versus late iron supplementation in low-birth-weight infants, infants who received early iron supplementation (started when feedings reached 100 ml/kg/day) had lower risk of infection and lower number of blood transfusions compared to infants who received late supplementation (started at 61 days of age) [45]. In a study from India that included breastfed infants at the age of 4–6 months, oral iron supplementation resulted in better growth, especially in infants who had anemia or were otherwise nutritionally deficient [46].

Prevention of iron deficiency and IDA varies by geographical region, age group, and other conditions. In countries with high prevalence of IDA, comprehensive strategies and interventions for high-risk groups are implemented, in particular for young children, adolescent girls, women in reproductive age, and pregnant and breastfeeding women. In some regions, food fortification with iron, control of helminth infection, and control of malaria are effective approaches to prevent IDA [17].

7.2. Dietary recommendations

The optimal way to reach iron requirements is an improvement of food quality. In countries with low prevalence of iron deficiency, recommended dietary intake should assure expected iron requirements. Exclusive breastfeeding is recommended for the first 4–6 months of life. Preterm breastfed infants should receive an iron supplement from 2 weeks of age. Additional source of iron should be given to infants starting at 4 months of age, first as an iron supplement, followed by iron-fortified foods (two or more meals/day meet the expected requirements for iron). Partially breastfed and nonbreastfed infants should consume exclusively iron-fortified formulas [47].

Starting from the age of 6 months, infants should receive one feeding rich in vitamin C (green vegetables, fruits, and juices) daily. After 6 months of age, meat should be introduced in a diet. Heme iron (meat and fish) is more bioavailable than nonheme iron (vegetables and cereals). Combining heme foods with nonheme foods also increases the absorption of iron [48]. Moreover, consumption of meat meets many requirements besides iron.

Infants should not be given nonformula cow's milk until the age of 12 months. The higher concentration of calcium in cow's milk inhibits absorption of iron. Children aged 1–5 years should drink less than 600 ml of milk daily. Besides, they should take enough iron-containing foods to fulfill daily iron requirements. Children, who do not eat at least 2 or 3 iron-rich foods every day, may have inadequate iron intake and may need iron supplementation [49].

8. Signs and symptoms

IDA is the final stage of iron deficiency, and the first one that can recover with iron supplementation. Iron deficiency without anemia may also be associated with some clinical signs and symptoms, such as fatigue, cognitive dysfunction, or decreased energy.

The most common presentation of IDA in an asymptomatic infant or a child, who is well-nourished and otherwise healthy, is mild-to-moderate microcytic and hypochromic anemia. Slowly progressive paleness may sometimes be missed, but anemia also produces nonspecific pallor of the mucous membranes. Signs of epithelial tissues that may be associated with IDA are koilonychia, glossitis, and angular stomatitis. Severe form of IDA is much rare and is presented with poor feeding, irritability, lethargy, tachypnea, and cardiomegaly. Growth is impaired in children with severe IDA, and splenomegaly may be present.

Symptoms of IDA are presented by many body systems and functions of the affected child: impaired psychomotor and/or mental development, effects on immunity and susceptibility to infection, decreased exercise capacity, weakness, pica and/or pagophagia, headache, irritability, beeturia, and restless leg syndrome in older children. Some of these symptoms may lead to long-term consequences. Iron deficiency significantly contributes to thrombotic risk. In cases of severe IDA, some children may experience acute life-threatening conditions, including hypotension, tachycardia, tachypnea, respiratory distress, and congestive heart failure. The presence of one or more of these findings requires immediate hospital admission and prompt treatment. Severe IDA may rarely be associated with increased intracranial pressure, clinical signs of pseudotumor cerebri, or papilledema. All these symptoms resolve with iron supplementation [50].

8.1. Neurodevelopmental signs and symptoms

Impaired psychomotor and/or mental development is common in infants with iron deficiency, and neurocognitive impairment in adolescents with IDA [51–53]. Negative impact on social and emotional behavior may appear and can lead to the development of attention deficit hyperactivity disorder (ADHD) [54]. Mood swings are frequent. Children with iron deficiency get tired easier and faster, and play less compared to healthy children. Numerous randomized trials performed on different pediatric age groups showed that iron supplementation prevented or corrected neurodevelopmental delay. These studies were mostly performed in low- or middle-income countries [55–57]. In the study from Costa Rica, iron deficiency and IDA were more frequent in infants fed with nonfortified- iron formula. In these infants, psychomotor development declined at the age 9 and 12 months. There were not any significant changes in mental development and behavior [58]. Some other studies demonstrated that psychomotor impairment might not completely recover after treatment of moderate-to-severe IDA [56, 59–62]. Children who had iron deficiency at the inclusion in the study continued to have lower cognitive scores when tested at school age and in adolescence compared to children with good iron balance and no iron deficiency [59]. Children who were treated for iron deficiency during infancy had lower scores on electrophysiological tests on recognition memory at 10 years of age, comparing with children without iron deficiency during infancy. Behavioral tests showed similar results in these two groups [61].

The biologic basis of neurodevelopmental disorders is not fully understood. Iron deficiency decreases expression of dopamine receptors, disrupts function of several enzymes in the nervous system with subsequent alterations in brain energy, and decreases myelin formation. Myelination disruption or impairment can be associated with constant changes in transmission through auditory and visual systems. In a study from Chile, auditory brainstem responses (ABR) and visual evoked potentials (VEP) were measured in two groups of 4-year-old children: children who were treated for IDA in infancy and non-anemic children who also received iron supplementation [63]. Subtle auditory and visual dysfunction was demonstrated with longer VEP and ABR latencies in children who had IDA in infancy compared with control group.

The relationship between IDA and febrile seizures (FS) has been examined in several studies with conflicting results. Studies that suggest positive correlation between iron deficiency and FS aim that the possible mechanism is iron-dependent metabolism of some neurotransmitters [64, 65]. Other studies found no association between iron deficiency and FS [66]. Zehetner et al. showed that iron supplementation for 16 weeks in dosage 5 mg/kg/day reduced the severity and frequency of breath-holding spells in children with IDA [67].

8.2. Immunity and infection

Iron deficiency and IDA have numerous effects on immune system and susceptibility to infection. Iron deficiency in children can induce defective functions of leukocytes and lymphocytes, and defective production of interleukin (IL)-2 and IL-6 [68, 69]. On the contrary, iron overload can increase the risk of infections with specific types of bacteria. Accumulation of iron in immune cells interferes with their antibacterial activity, and some bacteria grow well in an iron-rich environment. Besides, iron-binding proteins transferrin and lactoferrin have bacteriostatic effects, and these effects are lost when these proteins are saturated with iron [70].

Since both iron deficiency and iron excess can compromise cellular function, the levels of iron that cells are exposed to should be regulated precisely. In populations with high prevalence of iron deficiency and IDA, iron supplementation has different effects on susceptibility to infection and immunity. Low iron status may protect against malaria infection, but malaria in turn is linked with anemia, and changes in iron metabolism during a malaria infection may modulate susceptibility to co-infections [71]. Recent study of Zlotkin and coworkers showed that iron supplementation did not increase the risk of malaria infection [72].

8.3. Exercise capacity

Iron is an essential cofactor in aerobic metabolism. In IDA muscles are forced to depend on anaerobic metabolism more than they do in healthy nonanemic individuals. Iron deficiency leads to decreased exercise capacity in children, especially adolescent athletes. IDA is associated with decreased work capacity [73, 74].

8.4. Pica and pagophagia

Pica refers to unusual appetite for substances that are not food. In children, pica is often associated with iron deficiency and IDA [75]. The most common form of pica is starch or clay ingestion. Both substances decrease absorption of dietary iron. Pagophagia is a particular form of pica characterized by repetitive and compulsive ingestion of ice, freezer frost, or iced drinks. Some children prefer cold vegetables instead of ice. Pagophagia is very common in iron deficiency without anemia and is present in a half of patients with IDA. It responds to iron supplementation very fast, earlier than hemoglobin recovery [76]. The mechanism through which iron deficiency causes pagophagia is unclear. Biochemical processes involving the central nervous system might elucidate the underlying mechanism. Pica is not specific for iron deficiency. It can be found in children with developmental disabilities, such as intellectual disability or autism. It is also described in children after brain injury [77].

8.5. Thrombosis

Both iron deficiency and overload have been associated with an increased thrombotic risk in experimental and clinical studies. It has been reported that IDA is associated with cerebral vein thrombosis [78]. In Canadian study, children with arterial or venous stroke who were previously healthy, had ten times more chance to have IDA than children without stroke [79]. The mechanism of this association is complex. It may be related to reactive thrombocytosis that is often finding in IDA. Iron deficiency may contribute to a hypercoagulable state by affecting blood flow patterns. Besides, IDA with hypoxia could precipitate situations of increased metabolic stress (i.e., infections) in particularly vulnerable areas of the brain supplied by end arteries [80].

8.6. Beeturia

Beeturia is defined as pink or red urine after the ingestion of beets. It is most common in individuals with iron deficiency [81]. This manifestation is caused by increased intestinal absorption and increased excretion of the red pigment betalaine (betanin). The pigment is decolorized by ferric ions, and urine excretion of betalaine is increased in iron deficiency.

8.7. Restless leg syndrome

This syndrome is a common sleep-related movement disorder characterized with uncomfortable urge to move legs. It occurs usually in the evenings, during periods of inactivity and rest, and is occasionally relieved by movement. Restless leg syndrome is associated with iron deficiency and is often improved by iron supplementation. The brain iron insufficiency has been documented by independently replicated cerebrospinal fluid and brain imaging studies for individuals without IDA [82].

9. Diagnosis

Detailed history and physical examination are essential in diagnosis of any disease. Detailed history from the parents is very important in diagnosing iron deficiency and anemia, especially about prenatal period and dietary habits including time of introducing solid foods.

Presumptive diagnosis of IDA is made by a combination of risk assessment and laboratory testing of hemoglobin level (<11 g/dl). In infants younger than 6 months, lower values of hemoglobin are observed because of physiological anemia, but hemoglobin values under 9 g/dl demand further evaluation in order to investigate if there is any accompanying factor. Other findings like low mean corpuscular volume (MCV) or high red cell distribution width (RDW) help to determine diagnosis. For a definite confirmation, additional steps are needed:

- Estimate risk factors for lead poisoning and measure blood lead level if it is indicated [30, 83].
- If there is no evidence of lead toxicity, and the most likely is dietary deficiency, apply empirical trial of oral iron supplementation*
  - For infants and toddlers less than 24 months of age with anemia—move directly to empirical trial because IDA is the most probable cause of anemia in this age group.
  - For children 24 months of age and older—besides hemoglobin, hematocrit, MCV, and RDW, evaluate reticulocyte count, peripheral blood smear, and stool for occult blood before starting empirical trial.
- In children with severe anemia, complicated medical history, and with signs and symptoms atypical for IDA, additional testing should be performed before starting treatment.

These additional steps are necessary because anemia is not sensitive or specific for iron deficiency. Two-thirds of children with iron deficiency in the United States are not anemic, namely 9% have iron deficiency and 3% are anemic. The prevalence of anemia is much higher in countries with higher rates of iron deficiency. On the other hand, two-thirds of anemic toddlers have some other cause of anemia apart from iron deficiency [30]. Evaluation for iron deficiency in adolescence should also include serum ferritin levels. IDA in adolescent is identified by hemoglobin concentration below 11 g/dl combined with low serum ferritin (<12 ng/ml).

9.1. Presumptive diagnosis and empirical trial

In infants and toddlers up to 24 months of age who have mild microcytic anemia with presumptive diagnosis of IDA based on screening results, the strategy of choice is therapeutic trial of iron [51]. The recommended dosage is 3 mg/kg of elemental iron, once or twice daily, best between meals (daily dosage 3–6 mg/kg). Ferrous sulfate is the convenient and most commonly used form of iron. If there is increase of hemoglobin concentration greater than 1 g/dl after 4 weeks of treatment, the diagnosis of iron deficiency is confirmed. In this case, iron supplementation and monitoring of the child with laboratory tests should be continued for at least several months, after hemoglobin levels reach normal range according to age.

IDA is less common in older children than in infants. Additional evaluation, besides complete blood count, MCV, and RDW, is suggested in children older than 2 years before starting iron treatment. This evaluation includes reticulocyte count, peripheral blood smear, and stool for occult blood. If results support the diagnosis of IDA, iron supplementation should be started. Additional evaluation is required only if there is no response to the treatment.

9.2. Laboratory testing

Basic laboratory testing in diagnosing IDA is complete blood count, including hemoglobin, hematocrit, MCV, and RDW. More detailed evaluation is needed for children with complicated medical histories, severe forms of anemia (hemoglobin <7 g/dl) or presence of features that are not typical for IDA. In these cases, several other tests should be performed: serum iron, serum ferritin, total iron-binding capacity (TIBC), transferrin saturation, and stools for the presence of occult blood. These tests, although nonspecific for IDA, can support the diagnosis of IDA in majority of cases. Low serum iron and ferritin levels with an elevated TIBC are diagnostic for iron deficiency.

Complete blood count shows the severity of anemia. Increased RDW is the first laboratory sign of iron deficiency [51, 84]. RDW is high in IDA because there is a wide variation in RBC size. MCV and mean corpuscular hemoglobin concentration (MCHC) are low. Platelet count is often elevated, and it normalizes after iron treatment. Peripheral blood smear is an important workup in patients with anemia. The first finding of IDA on peripheral smear is anisocytosis. Besides, RBCs are hypochromic and microcytic.

In infants and small children, iron deficiency is usually identified by a serum ferritin concentration <12 ng/ml. Diagnosis of IDA is based on the combination of hemoglobin concentration below 11 g/dl and serum ferritin levels below 12 ng/ml. However, when examining the results, it must be taken into consideration that ferritin is an acute-phase reactant. Elevated serum ferritin levels have been associated with a wide range of conditions including inflammation, infection, chronic disease, and malignancy [85].

Free erythrocyte protoporphyrin (FEP), soluble transferrin receptor (sTfR), and reticulocyte hemoglobin content (CHr) are very useful and reliable laboratory tests to support the diagnosis of iron deficiency. FEP is a precursor of heme that normally occurs in very low concentration in RBCs. Elevated FEP values thus indicate early impairment of iron status and provide information about gradual changes in the iron supply. The sTfR refers to the cleaved extracellular portion of the transferrin receptor 1 that is released into serum. Iron deficiency causes overexpression of transferrin receptor and sTfR levels. The sTfR is regarded as a more stable marker of iron levels in an inflammatory state. CHr is a measure of early iron-deficient erythropoiesis. Reticulocyte hemoglobin content decreases earlier than hemoglobin content of RBC because normal life span of RBC is 120 days [86]. It has been shown that CHr measurement is more reliable and accurate laboratory test for the diagnosis of iron deficiency than hemoglobin level <11 g/dl, resulting in detection of greater number of patients with iron deficiency comparing to hemoglobin. On the other hand, greater number of falsely identified patients with iron deficiency was detected also by CHr, which is, although more sensitive, less specific than hemoglobin [87]. Serum transferrin receptor is found on reticulocytes and increased number of transferrin receptors is observed in IDA.

Some other types of anemia and other conditions that can be confused with IDA are mild hereditary anemias (alpha or beta thalassemia traits), mild anemia after recent infection or immunization, anemia of chronic disease, and combined nutritional anemias (malabsorption with vitamin B12 or folate deficiency). If the child does not respond to iron supplementation nor has some predisposing factor, other conditions should be considered.

10. Treatment

10.1. Oral iron therapy

For the successful treatment of IDA in infants and children, it is necessary to determine the appropriate dose and scheduling of oral iron therapy, apply dietary modifications together with iron supplementation, and follow-up the response to treatment.

Suggested dose for oral supplementation for infants and children with IDA is 3–6 mg/kg/day of elemental iron. Ferrous sulfate is generally recommended in a dose of 3 mg/kg of iron once or twice daily (maximum total daily dose, 150 mg of elemental iron). Elemental iron constitutes 20% of ferrous sulfate. Ferrous fumarate and ferrous gluconate are other forms of oral iron salts with different content of elemental iron. The iron supplement should be given between meals and preferably with juice because absorption of ferrous sulfate is increased when it is given with juice rather than with milk or other fluids. For maximum absorption of iron, administration 30–45 minutes before meal or 2 hours after meal is highly recommended.

The same doses of oral iron supplementation are recommended as a therapeutic trial for infants and young children with mild microcytic anemia and presumptive diagnosis of IDA [51]. Treatment should result in an increase of hemoglobin concentration greater than 1 g/dl within 4 weeks [30].

Side effects of oral iron preparations are gastrointestinal intolerance in higher doses, gray staining of teeth and gums (especially when given as a liquid preparation), effects on immune system, and susceptibility to infection.

10.2. Dietary changes

Dietary changes are necessary not only to prevent iron deficiency but also to add oral iron therapy. Following dietary changes are recommended for infants and children with proven or suspected IDA:

1. Infants should not be fed with unmodified cow's milk or low-iron formula. If infants are not breastfed or are partially breastfed, they should be fed with iron-fortified formula. Infants fed with cow's milk may have iron deficiency as a result of intestinal blood loss due to cow's milk protein-induced colitis. Lack of iron fortification in unmodified cow's milk contributes to iron deficiency state.

2. When iron deficiency is detected or suspected in a child older than 12 months, intake of cow's milk should be limited to 600 ml/day. Higher intake of cow's milk has been associated with higher risk for iron deficiency in several studies [34, 88]. Discontinuing bottle-feeding is also recommended because it generally helps in limiting milk intake [89]. If IDA is persistent and stool is positive for blood, all milk products should be stopped. In these cases, child should receive appropriate amount of calcium in a diet (calcium-rich foods).

3. Parents should be advised to modify child's diet in order to increase iron consumption. Infants 6 months and older should have appropriate intake of iron from complementary foods. Diet should contain cereals fortified with iron, food rich in vitamin C, and pureed meat.

10.3. Response assessment

Follow-up assessment is necessary to confirm that anemia has been caused by iron deficiency and the treatment was administered at correct dosage and timing. After 4 weeks of therapy, complete blood count should be done. It is recommended to perform evaluation when child is healthy and without viral infection that may cause acute decrease in hemoglobin.

If hemoglobin has increased at least by 1 g/dl after 4 weeks of oral iron supplementation, therapy should be continued, and hemoglobin re-evaluated every 2–3 months until hemoglobin reaches the normal value. Iron therapy should be continued additional 2–3 months to replace iron storage pools. Discontinuation of the treatment can lead to the recurrence of IDA.

If the appropriate response is missing after 4 weeks of treatment, additional evaluation of anemia is recommended. Possible causes of persistent or recurrent IDA are ineffective treatment, blood loss, malabsorption, or incorrect diagnosis. Parents should be asked whether the iron preparation has been given at the appropriate dosage and timing, whether suggested dietary modifications have been done, and if there were any intercurrent illnesses that could transiently decrease hemoglobin level. If the patient had no intercurrent illness and has been taking iron supplement in an appropriate dosage and timing, it is suggested to proceed with the following evaluation:

1. Evaluation for the type of anemia—Measuring of serum ferritin level, hemoglobin electrophoresis, vitamin B12, and folate can rule out the thalassemia trait, chronic disease anemia, and mixed nutritional deficiency. These conditions may imitate or complicate IDA. Very rare genetic mutations may interfere with iron transport and cause anemia similar to IDA, but without response to iron supplementation [90].

2. Evaluation for gastrointestinal blood loss—Stool should be tested for occult blood in a few separate samples. If the results are positive, it is recommended to assess further investigation for common causes of gastrointestinal blood loss, including cow's milk protein-induced colitis, celiac disease, and inflammatory bowel disease.

10.4. Parenteral iron therapy

Parenteral iron therapy is reserved for patients with severe forms of anemia who are intolerant to oral preparations, have poor response to oral supplementation, poor compliance, or malabsorption. Children with chronic gastrointestinal diseases as inflammatory bowel disease may require parenteral iron therapy because they often do not tolerate oral supplementation.

Most commonly used form of iron for parenteral use in children is low molecular weight iron dextran. It produces mild infusion reactions in less than 1% of patients and serious adverse effects are very rare [91]. Recently, ferric carboxymaltose administered as a short intravenous infusion without a test dose proved to be safe and highly effective in children and adolescents with IDA refractory to oral iron therapy [92]. Evaluation of treatment is usually performed at 4–12 weeks after the initial infusion.

10.5. Blood transfusion

Blood transfusion is rarely required in children with IDA. Transfusions are not considered necessary even with hemoglobin levels 4–5 g/dl, if the child is otherwise well. Blood transfusion should be administered only when there is an urgent need to restore oxygen-carrying capacity, i.e., in severe decompensated anemia. IDA develops gradually and over periods long enough to allow compensatory mechanisms to maintain intravascular volume. Consequently, there is a real risk of fluid overload with transfusion, and these patients should receive transfusion with caution. Standard of practice recommends slow transfusion of packed RBC volume of 5 ml/kg over 4 hours to avoid complications [93].

11. Conclusion

Iron deficiency is the most common nutritional deficiency in the world, affecting more than a quarter of the global population. Iron plays an essential role in many physiological functions, including oxygen binding and transport, cell growth and differentiation, gene regulation, enzyme reactions, and neurotransmitter synthesis. Iron deficiency develops in stages. In the first stage, iron requirement exceeds intake, causing depletion of bone marrow iron stores. As stores decrease, absorption of dietary iron increases compensatory. During later stages, deficiency impairs erythropoiesis, ultimately causing anemia.

Iron deficiency and IDA have many systemic effects, and the most concerning are diminished mental, motor, and behavioral functioning that might not be completely reversible after treatment with iron. Therefore, intervention should focus on primary prevention, which includes breastfeeding, fortification of foods with iron, use of iron-rich formulas when breastmilk is insufficient, and avoiding cow's milk before 1 year of age. Routine laboratory screening is recommended for all children 9–12 months of age. Risk assessment, consisting of focused dietary history, presents the most valuable screening tool, and additional laboratory screening is recommended for children with risk factors for iron deficiency and IDA.

Treatment starts with establishing the diagnosis. The main therapeutic principles are detection of the condition that causes iron deficiency, correction of underlying etiology, iron supplementation, dietary modifications, and education of families. Oral iron is the first-line therapy, giving in appropriate dose and scheduling. Adequate follow-up assessment for response is also important. If the appropriate response is missing, further evaluation should be obtained to rule out conditions that might simulate or complicate IDA.

Abbreviations

WHO	World Health Organization
IDA	Iron deficiency anemia
BMI	Body mass index
RBC	Red blood cells
TTTS	Twin-twin transfusion syndrome
IBD	Inflammatory bowel disease
AAP	American Academy of Pediatrics
MCV	Mean corpuscular volume
RDW	Red blood cell distribution width
ADHD	Attention deficit hyperactivity disorder

ABR	Auditory brainstem response
VEP	Visual evoked potential
FS	Febrile seizures
IL	Interleukin
TIBC	Total iron-binding capacity
MCHC	Mean corpuscular hemoglobin concentration
FEP	Free erythrocyte protoporphyrin
sTfR	Soluble transferrin receptor
CHr	Reticulocyte hemoglobin content

Author details

Jelena Roganović[1,2]* and Ksenija Starinac[3]

*Address all correspondence to: roganovic.kbcri@gmail.com

1 Clinical Hospital Center Rijeka and School of Medicine, University of Rijeka, Rijeka, Croatia

2 School of Medicine, University of Rijeka, Rijeka, Croatia

3 Service for Healthcare for Children and Adolescents, Kruševac, Serbia

References

[1] Stoltzfus RJ. Iron deficiency: Global prevalence and consequences. Food and Nutrition Bulletin. 2003;**24**:S99-S103

[2] DeBenoist B, McLean E, Egli I, et al. Worldwide Prevalence of Anemia 1993-2005: WHO Global Database on Anemia. Geneva: World Health Organization; 2008

[3] Brotanek JM, Gosz J, Weitzman M, Flores G. Secular trends in the prevalence of iron deficiency among US toddlers, 1976-2002. Archives of Pediatrics & Adolescent Medicine. 2008;**162**:374-381

[4] Centers for Disease Control and Prevention (CDC). Iron deficiency—United States, 1999-2000. MMWR. Morbidity and Mortality Weekly Report. 2002;**51**:897-899

[5] Looker AC, Dallman PR, Carroll MD, et al. Prevalence of iron deficiency in the United States. JAMA. 1997;**277**:973-976

[6] Ghasemi A, Keikhaei B. Effects of nutritional variables in children with iron deficiency anemia. International Journal of Pediatrics. 2014;**2**:183-187

[7] Foo LH, Khor GL, Tee ES. Iron status and dietary iron intake of adolescents from a rural community in Sabah, Malaysia. Asia Pacific Journal of Clinical Nutrition. 2004;**13**:48-55

[8] Cusick SE, Mei Z, Cogswell ME. Continuing anemia prevention strategies are needed throughout early childhood in low-income preschool children. The Journal of Pediatrics. 2007;**150**:422-428

[9] Brotanek JM, Gosz J, Weitzman M, Flores G. Iron deficiency in early childhood in the United States: Risk factors and racial/ethnic disparities. Pediatrics. 2007;**120**:568-575

[10] Pinhas-Hamiel O, Newfield RS, Koren I, et al. Greater prevalence of iron deficiency in overweight and obese children and adolescents. International Journal of Obesity and Related Metabolic Disorders. 2003;**27**:416-418

[11] Nead KG, Halterman JS, Kaczorowski JM, et al. Overweight children and adolescents: A risk group for iron deficiency. Pediatrics. 2004;**114**:104-108

[12] Hagan JF, Shaw JS, Duncan PM. Bright Futures Guidelines for Health Supervision of Infants, Children, and Adolescents. 3rd ed. Elk Grove Village, IL: American Academy of Pediatrics; 2008

[13] Committee on Practice and Ambulatory Medicine and Bright Futures Periodicity Schedule Workgroup. 2016 recommendations for preventive pediatric health care. Pediatrics. 2016;**137**:1-3

[14] Eltayeb MS, Elsaeed AE, Mohamedani AA, Assayed AA. Prevalence of anaemia among Quranic school (Khalawi) students (Heiran) in Wad El Magboul village, rural Rufaa, Gezira State, Central Sudan: A cross sectional study. The Pan African Medical Journal. 2016;**24**:244-253

[15] El-Zanaty F, Way A. Egypt Demographic and Health Survey 2005. Cairo, Egypt: Ministry of Health and Population, National Population Council, El-Zanaty and Associates and ORC Macro; 2006

[16] DuBois S, Kearney DJ. Iron-deficiency anemia and *Helicobacter pylori* infection: A review of the evidence. The American Journal of Gastroenterology. 2005;**100**:453-459

[17] World Health Organization. Iron Deficiency Anaemia: Assessment, Prevention and Control: A Guide for Programme Managers. Geneva: World Health Organization; 2001

[18] Zlotkin SH, Christofides AL, Hyder SM, et al. Controlling iron deficiency anemia through the use of home-fortified complementary foods. Indian Journal of Pediatrics. 2004;**71**:1015-1019

[19] World Health Organization. Serum ferritin concentrations for the assessment of iron status and iron deficiency in populations. Vitamin and Mineral Nutrition Information System. Geneva: World Health Organization; 2011

[20] McDonagh MS, Blazina I, Dana T, et al. Screening and routine supplementation for iron deficiency anemia: A systematic review. Pediatrics. 2015;**135**:723-733

[21] Bhattacharya PT, Misra SR, Hussain M. Nutritional aspects of essential trace elements in oral health and disease: An extensive review. Scientifica (Cairo). 2016;**2016**:1-12. DOI: 10.1155/2016/5464373

[22] Lönnerdal B, Georgieff MK, Hernell O. Developmental physiology of iron absorption, homeostasis and metabolism in the healthy term infant. The Journal of Pediatrics. 2015;**167**:S8-S14

[23] Özdemir N. Iron deficiency anemia from diagnosis to treatment in children. Turk Pediatri Arsivi. 2015;**50**:11-19

[24] van Rheenen P. Less iron deficiency anaemia after delayed cord-clamping. Paediatrics and International Child Health. 2013;**33**:57-58

[25] Kumar A, Rai AK, Basu S, et al. Cord blood and breast milk iron status in maternal anemia. Pediatrics. 2008;**121**:e673-e677

[26] Rahimy MC, Fanou L, Somasse YE, et al. When to start supplementary iron to prevent iron deficiency in early childhood in sub-Saharan Africa setting. Pediatric Blood & Cancer. 2007;**48**:544-549

[27] Collard KJ. Iron homeostasis in the neonate. Pediatrics. 2009;**123**:1208-1216

[28] Stroustrup A, Plafkin C. A pilot prospective study of fetomaternal hemorrhage identified by anemia in asymptomatic neonates. Journal of Perinatology. 2016;**36**:366-369

[29] Wagner S, Repke JT, Ural SH. Overview and long-term outcomes of patients born with Twin-to-Twin Transfusion Syndrome. Reviews in Obstetrics & Gynecology. 2013;**6**:149-154

[30] Baker RD, Greer FR, Committee on Nutrition American Academy of Pediatrics. Diagnosis and prevention of iron deficiency and iron-deficiency anemia in infants and young children (0-3 years of age). Pediatrics. 2010;**126**:1040-1050

[31] Pizzaro F, Yip R, Dallman PR, et al. Iron status with different infant feeding regimens: Relevance to screening and prevention of iron deficiency. The Journal of Pediatrics. 1991; **118**:687-692

[32] Hopkins D, Emmett P, Steer C, et al. Infant feeding in the second 6 months of life related to iron status: An observational study. Archives of Disease in Childhood. 2007;**92**:850-854

[33] Morino GS, Cinelli G, Di Pietro I, Papa V, Spreghini N, Manco M. NutricheQ Questionnaire assesses the risk of dietary imbalances in toddlers from 1 through 3 years of age. Food & Nutrition Research. 2015;**59**:10.3402/fnr.v59.29686. DOI: 10.3402/fnr.v59.29686

[34] Gupta PM, Perrine CG, Mei Z, Scanlon KS. Iron, anemia, and iron deficiency anemia among young children in the United States. Nutrients. 2016;**8**:330. DOI: 10.3390/nu8060330

[35] Sutcliffe TL, Khambalia A, Westergard S, et al. Iron depletion is associated with daytime bottle-feeding in the second and third years of life. Archives of Pediatrics & Adolescent Medicine. 2006;**160**:1114-1120

[36] Halfdanarson TR, Litzow MR, Murray JA. Hematologic manifestations of celiac disease. Blood. 2007;**109**:412-421

[37] Stein J, Hartmann F, Dignass AU. Diagnosis and management of iron deficiency anemia in patients with IBD. Nat Rev Gastroenterol Hepatol. 2010;**7**:599-610

[38] Goldberg ND. Iron deficiency anemia in patients with inflammatory bowel disease. Clinical and Experimental Gastroenterology. 2013;**6**:61-70

[39] American Academy of Pediatrics. Iron. In: Kleinman RE, Greer FR, editors. Pediatric Nutrition. 7th ed. Elk Grove Village, IL: American Academy of Pediatrics; 2011. pp. 449-466

[40] Duncan PM, Duncan ED, Swanson J. Bright Futures: The screening table recommendations. Pediatric Annals. 2008;**37**:152-158

[41] Sekhar DL, Murray-Kolb LE, Wang L, Kunselman, Paul IM. Adolescent anemia screening during ambulatory pediatric visits in the United States. Journal of Community Health. 2015;**40**:331-338

[42] Pizarro F, Olivares M, Maciero E, Krasnoff G, Cócaro N, Gaitan D. Iron absorption from two milk formulas fortified with iron sulfate stabilized with maltodextrin and citric acid. Nutrients. 2015;**7**:8952-8959

[43] Institute of Medicine, Food and Nutrition Board. Dietary Reference Intakes for Vitamin A, Vitamin K, Arsenic, Boron, Chromium, Copper, Iodine, Iron, Manganese, Molybdenum, Nickel, Silicon, Vanadium, and Zinc. Washington DC: National Academy Press; 2000. pp. 339-344

[44] Hund L, Northrop-Clewes CA, Nazario R, et al. A novel approach to evaluating the iron and folate status of women of reproductive age in Uzbekistan after 3 years of flour fortification with micronutrients. PLoS One. 2013;**8**(11):e79726. DOI: 10.1371/journal.pone.0079726

[45] Franz AR, Mihatsch WA, Sander S, et al. Prospective randomized trial of early versus late enteral iron supplementation in infants with a birth weight of less than 1301 grams. Pediatrics. 2000;**106**:700-706

[46] Abdelrazik N, Al-Haggar M, Al-Marsafawy H, et al. Impact of long-term oral iron supplementation in breast-fed infants. Indian Journal of Pediatrics. 2007;**74**:739-745

[47] Prell C, Koletzko B. Breastfeeding and complementary feeding. Deutsches Ärzteblatt International. 2016;**113**:435-444

[48] West AR, Oates PS. Mechanisms of heme iron absorption: Current questions and controversies. World Journal of Gastroenterology. 2008;**14**:4101-4110

[49] National Institutes of Health, Office of Dietary Supplements. Dietary Supplement Fact Sheet: Iron. Available from: http://ods.od.nih.gov/factsheets/iron.asp [Accessed: 2017-03-21]

[50] Biousse V, Rucker JC, Viqnal C, Crassard I, Katz BJ, Newman NJ. Anemia and papilledema. American Journal of Ophthalmology. 2003;**135**:437-446

[51] Jáuregui-Lobera I. Iron deficiency and cognitive functions. Neuropsychiatric Disease and Treatment. 2014;**10**:2087-2095. DOI: 10.2147/NDT.S72491

[52] Halterman JS, Kaczorowski JM, Aligne CA, et al. Iron deficiency and cognitive achievement among school-aged children and adolescents in the United States. Pediatrics. 2001;**107**:1381-1386

[53] Carter RC, Jacobson JL, Burden MJ, et al. Iron deficiency anemia and cognitive function in infancy. Pediatrics. 2010;**126**:e427-e434

[54] Lozoff B, Clark KM, Jing Y, et al. Dose-response relationships between iron deficiency with or without anemia and infant social-emotional behavior. The Journal of Pediatrics. 2008;**152**:696-702

[55] Doom JR, Georgieff MK. Striking while the iron is hot: Understanding the biological and neurodevelopmental effects of iron deficiency to optimize intervention in early childhood. Current Pediatrics Reports. 2014;**2**:291-298

[56] Doom JR, Gunnar MR, Georgieff MK, et al. Beyond stimulus deprivation: Iron deficiency and cognitive deficits in post-institutionalized children. Child Development. 2014;**85**:1805-1812

[57] Lozoff B, Castillo M, Clark KM, Smith JB, Sturza J. Iron supplementation in infancy contributes to more adaptive behavior at 10 years of age. The Journal of Nutrition. 2014;**144**:838-845

[58] Lozoff B, Wolf AW, Jimenez E. Iron-deficiency anemia and infant development: Effects of extended oral iron therapy. The Journal of Pediatrics. 1996;**129**:382-389

[59] Lozoff B, Jimenez E, Smith JB. Double burden of iron deficiency in infancy and low socioeconomic status: A longitudinal analysis of cognitive test scores to age 19 years. Archives of Pediatrics & Adolescent Medicine. 2006;**160**:1108-1113

[60] Lukowski AF, Koss M, Burden MJ, et al. Iron deficiency in infancy and neurocognitive functioning at 19 years: Evidence of long-term deficits in executive function and recognition memory. Nutritional Neuroscience. 2010;**13**:54-70

[61] Congdon EL, Westerlund A, Algarin CR, et al. Iron deficiency in infancy is associated with altered neural correlates of recognition memory at 10 years. The Journal of Pediatrics. 2012;**160**:1027-1033

[62] Lozoff B, Smith JB, Kaciroti N, et al. Functional significance of early-life iron deficiency: Outcomes at 25 years. The Journal of Pediatrics. 2013;**163**:1260-1266

[63] Algarin C, Peirano P, Garrido M, et al. Iron deficiency anemia in infancy: Long-lasting effects on auditory and visual system functioning. Pediatric Research. 2003;**53**:217-223

[64] Hartfield DS, Tan J, Yager JY, et al. The association between iron deficiency and febrile seizures in childhood. Clinical Pediatrics (Philadelphia). 2009;**48**:420-426

[65] Sharif MR, Kheirkhah D, Madani M, Kashani HH. The relationship between iron deficiency and febrile convulsion: A case-control study. Global Journal of Health Science. 2015;**8**:185-189

[66] Bidabadi E, Mashouf M. Association between iron deficiency anemia and first febrile convulsion: A case-control study. Seizure. 2009;**18**:347-351

[67] Zehetner AA, Orr N, Buckmaster A, et al. Iron supplementation for breath-holding attacks in children. The Cochrane Database of Systematic Reviews. 2010;**5**:CD008132. DOI: 10.1002/14651858

[68] Ekiz C, Agaoglu L, Karakas Z, et al. The effect of iron deficiency anemia on the function of the immune system. The Hematology Journal. 2005;**5**:579-583

[69] Kumar V, Choundhry VP. Iron deficiency and infection. Indian Journal of Pediatrics. 2010;**77**:789-793

[70] Sandrini SM, Shergill R, Woodward J, et al. Elucidation of the mechanism by which catecholamine stress hormones liberate iron from the innate immune defense proteins transferrin and lactoferrin. Journal of Bacteriology. 2010;**192**:587-594

[71] Spottiswoode N, Duffy PE, Drakesmith H. Iron, anemia and hepcidin in malaria. Frontiers in Pharmacology. 2014;**5**:125. DOI: 10.3389/fphar.2014.00125

[72] Zlotkin S, Newton S, Aimone AM, et al. Effect of iron fortification on malaria incidence in infants and young children in Ghana: A randomized trial. JAMA. 2013;**310**:938-947

[73] Clark SF. Iron deficiency anemia. Nutrition in Clinical Practice. 2008;**23**:128-141

[74] Peeling P, Sim M, Badenhorst CE, et al. Iron status and the acute postexercise hepcidin response in athletes. PLoS One. 2014;**9**(3):e93002

[75] Yadav D, Chandra J. Iron deficiency: Beyond anemia. Indian Journal of Pediatrics. 2011;**78**:65-72

[76] Osman YM, Wali JA, Osman OM. Craving for ice and iron-deficiency anemia: A case series from Oman. Pediatric Hematology and Oncology. 2005;**22**:127-131

[77] Hagopian LP, Rooker GW, Rolider NU. Identifying empirically supported treatments for pica in individuals with intellectual disabilities. Research in Developmental Disabilities. 2011;**32**:2114-2120

[78] Benedict SL, Bonkowsky JL, Thompson JA, et al. Cerebral sinovenous thrombosis in children: Another reason to treat iron deficiency anemia. Journal of Child Neurology. 2004;**19**:526-531

[79] Maguire JL, deVeber G, Parkin PC. Association between iron-deficiency anemia and stroke in young children. Pediatrics. 2007;**120**:1053-1057

[80] Franchini M, Targher G, Montagnana M, Lippi G. Iron and thrombosis. Annals of Hematology. 2008;**87**:167-173

[81] Zaater MK. Iron deficiency anemia and thyroid dysfunction by RIA. Med J Cairo Univ. 2012;**80**:307-312

[82] Allen RP, Earley CJ. The role of iron in restless leg syndrome. Movement Disorders. 2007;**22**(S18):S440-S448

[83] Wright RO, Tsaih SW, Schwartz J, et al. Association between iron deficiency and blood lead level in a longitudinal analysis of children followed in an urban primary care clinic. The Journal of Pediatrics. 2003;**142**:9-14

[84] Sazawal S, Dhingra U, Dhingra P, et al. Efficiency of red cell distribution width in identification of children aged 1-3 years with iron deficiency anemia against traditional hematological markers. BMC Pediatrics. 2014;**14**:8-13

[85] Moore Jr C, Ormseth M, Fuch H. Causes and significance of markedly elevated serum ferritin levels in an academic medical center. Journal of Clinical Rheumatology. 2013;**19**:324-328

[86] Mast AE, Blinder MA, Dietzen DJ. Reticulocyte hemoglobin content. American Journal of Hematology. 2007;**83**:307-309

[87] Ullrich C, Wu A, Armsby C, et al. Screening healthy infants for iron deficiency using reticulocyte hemoglobin content. JAMA. 2005;**294**:924-930

[88] Soh P, Ferguson EL, McKenzie JE, et al. Iron deficiency and risk factors for lower iron stores in 6-24-month-old New Zealanders. European Journal of Clinical Nutrition. 2004;**58**:71-79

[89] Brotanek JM, Halterman JS, Auinger P, et al. Iron deficiency, prolonged bottle-feeding, and racial/ethnic disparities in young children. Archives of Pediatrics & Adolescent Medicine. 2005;**159**:1038-1042

[90] Finberg KE. Iron-refractory iron deficiency anemia. Seminars in Hematology. 2009;**46**: 378-386

[91] Plummer ES, Crary SE, McCavit TL, Buchanan GR. Intravenous low molecular weight iron dextran in children with iron deficiency anemia unresponsive to oral iron. Pediatric Blood & Cancer. 2013;**60**:1747-1752

[92] Mantadakis E, Roganovic J. Safety and efficacy of ferric carboxymaltose in children and adolescents with iron deficiency anemia. The Journal of Pediatrics. 2017;**184**:241. DOI: 10.1016/j.jpeds.2017.01.041

[93] Sharma S, Sharma P, Tyler LN. Transfusion of blood and blood products: Indications and complications. American Family Physician. 2011;**83**:719-724

Chapter 4

Iron Deficiency Anemia and Pregnancy

Ines Banjari

Additional information is available at the end of the chapter

http://dx.doi.org/10.5772/intechopen.69114

Abstract

Iron deficiency is the most common nutritional deficiency in the world with immense public health consequences. It has a complex etiology and prolonged imbalance between dietary intake, absorption, and body needs which leads to iron deficiency anemia. If developed during pregnancy, it significantly alters pregnancy outcomes. Low birth weight is one of the main features, and those infants are at increased risk of developing anemia later in life. Along with widely recommended and practiced supplementation during pregnancy, proper combination of foods remain the best way for an optimal absorption of iron. Dietary iron is directly related to the total dietary energy intake, but depending on the type of its dietary source, maximum absorption is up to 40% of the total intake. Plant foods, the basis of everyday diet, contain significant number of dietary factors that inhibit iron absorption in the gut. Therefore, planning a well-balanced diet in order to achieve maximum absorption of iron from foods can be challenging. Pregnancy, especially its earliest period, is considered as the *critical window* in fetal programing, an ideal time frame to reduce risk factors for a number of health conditions in a newborn. Healthy pregnancy should be observed as a prerequisite for a healthier society.

Keywords: iron deficiency, iron deficiency anemia, iron bioavailability, pregnancy outcomes, fetal programing

1. Introduction

Iron is usually discussed from the aspect of undeveloped or developing countries that often experience food insecurity, or even famine. Deficiency of iron is the most common nutritional deficit around the globe, therefore the issue of iron is global [1, 2].

This is a multiple stage metabolic process and its main feature is gradual progression of iron deficiency (ID) toward severely depleted stores of iron in the body when iron deficiency anemia (IDA) develops. The etiology of IDA (**Figure 1**) is very complex and includes iron stores, food

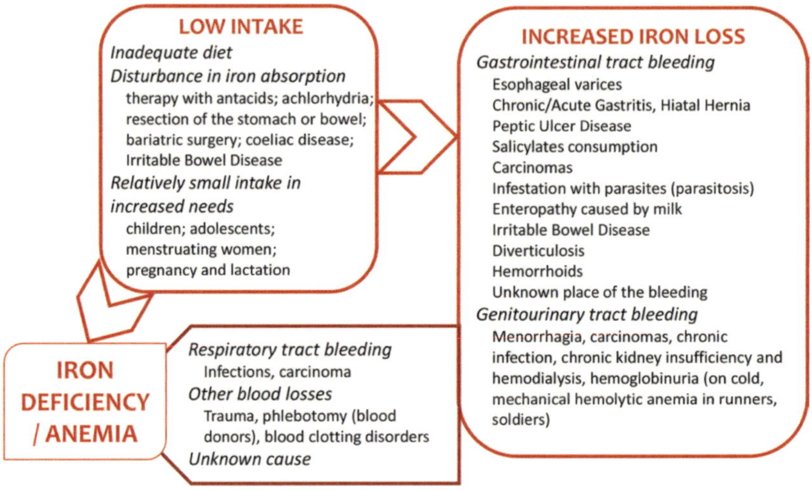

Figure 1. The etiology of iron deficiency and iron deficiency anemia (prepared according to Refs. [3, 6, 27]).

digestion, iron content, and bioavailability in foods, and iron distribution in the body through different stages in the life cycle (e.g., adolescence and pregnancy) [3–6]. In developed countries, the most common causes of IDA include genitourinary tract bleeding, fad dieting, and low consumption of iron-rich foods or foods that contain highly bioavailable iron. Additional component is economic poverty that significantly alters the quality of a person's diet [7].

However, even ID may cause loss of strength and tiredness, impaired immune response, poorer cognitive functioning, and behavior problems (social/emotional) [3, 8–13].

Pregnancy represents the *critical window* in child's development [14–18]. Therefore, pregnancy is considered an ideal time frame for all preventive interventions with focus put on not only iron status, but also obesity, diabetes, and other conditions.

Child's iron status reflects mother's iron status during pregnancy, and even before pregnancy. In terms of fetal programing, early pregnancy is considered extremely important [16, 19–22]. However, pregnancy outcomes, that is, fetal programing depends on numerous factors related to mother, from maternal age (the risk of adverse pregnancy outcomes increases at the age of 35 years, especially in the case of the first pregnancy), maternal state of nourishment (overweight and obesity significantly alters pregnancy outcomes), diabetes or gestational diabetes, and maternal weight gain during gestation [14]. Proper and specifically timed nutritional intervention could significantly reduce the risk of adverse pregnancy outcomes [19, 20].

From the aspect of iron status, it is important to note that a significant proportion of women start pregnancy with depleted iron stores [2, 23, 24]. In the United States, more than one-third of women of reproductive age have deprived iron stores [3]. Additionally, all women having ID are at the risk of developing IDA early in the course of gestation [1, 21, 25]. Requirements for iron increase significantly during pregnancy, so if not recognized and treated may cause adverse pregnancy outcomes, especially for a newborn. Adverse pregnancy outcomes include low birth weight infants, preterm delivery, labor complications, and higher rates of cesarean section [23, 24, 26–30]. The risk increases with the more severe stages of ID [21, 23, 24, 26, 27, 29]. A newborn enters an infinite loop of ID and its related health problems [31].

All stated additionally highlights the importance of proper food combination during pregnancy [32]. Timed recognition and proper treatment of ID could significantly alter health indicators, not only on an individual level but also on a population level. The more recent findings shed a new light on ID which favors the proposed idea; obesity has been linked to low iron stores, confirmed in both pregnant women and children [20, 33–37].

2. Definitions and prevalence

Prevalence around the world varies widely. According to the World Health Organization (WHO), the frequency of ID in developing countries is about 2.5 times that of anemia [1]. However, Croatia ID is 3.8 times more frequent among pregnant women at early pregnancy [25], which backs up the theory of depleted iron stores before pregnancy [3]. The incidence is high especially during pregnancy and lactation in both, industrialized and developing countries [2, 38]. Estimated prevalence of anemia is 43% in nonpregnant women in developing countries and 12% in wealthier regions [1]. On the other hand, estimates from the WHO report indicate that anywhere between 35 and 75% (56% on average) of pregnant women in developing countries and 18% of pregnant women from industrialized countries are ID, with half of them having IDA [1].

During pregnancy, maternal iron stores should be sufficient to maintain homeostasis of iron for the normal growth and development of fetus. Still, as pregnancy progresses physiologic anemia in later phases can be expected, due to hemodilution, a process of nonsimultaneous and disproportional increase in the total plasma volume (the total increase of around 50%, caused by aldosterone and estrogen) and the number of erythrocytes (the total increase of around 33%; erythropoiesis) [3–6, 21]. Moreover, physiology of pregnancy requires additional 800 mg of circulating iron during gestation [3, 6, 39, 40]. Therefore, ID and IDA often develop during the later stages of pregnancy even in women who enter pregnancy with relatively adequate iron stores [21, 23].

The WHO defines anemia as hemoglobin level below 110 g/l for pregnant women, or hematocrit level below 0.330 l/l [1, 41]. This criterion has been widely argued for its low sensitivity toward less severe stages of IDA [25, 30, 40, 42]. Therefore, clinical interpretation is useless unless iron-binding capacity values, that is, transferrin saturation percentage, are available at the same time [40, 42]. In IDA unsaturated-iron binding capacity (UIBC) and total iron-binding capacity (TIBC) are increased while usually transferrin saturation, which normally ranges between 20 and 50%, drops below 15.0%. So, for screening purpose and clinical decision, the WHO besides hemoglobin and hematocrit recommends either serum ferritin or transferrin saturation [1, 41, 42].

In Croatia, based on the WHO criteria, 17.7% (on hemoglobin basis) and 18.5% (on hematocrit basis) of pregnant women in early pregnancy had either ID or IDA. Clinical criteria showed that even 32.8% of pregnant women in early pregnancy had either ID or IDA (transferrin saturation <20.0%) [25]. The data support the global significance of proper iron stores among women and ID problem in developed countries.

3. Iron bioavailability

Various food sources have different amounts of bioavailable iron, that is, the amount of iron that can readily be absorbed in duodenum [6]. Still, a significant number of diet-related factors affect the final amount of iron available for the absorption.

For the iron absorption acidity in the stomach is very important (**Figure 2**). Absorption of nonheme iron is limited to duodenum [6]. Nonheme iron is presented in one of the two forms: ferric (Fe^{3+}) or ferrous (Fe^{2+}) form. The ferric form tends to form complex salts with anions and asks for a very low pH in the stomach (below 3). On the other hand, ferrous iron is soluble up to pH 8 [6, 43].

Iron in foods is present as heme and nonheme, deferring by solubility, sources, and absorption level [6]. Foods that are part of the usual, everyday meals have low iron content and low bioavailability. So, only 10–20% of the total iron intake is absorbed, but the absorption percentage is higher if IDA is present [1, 2, 44, 45]. The reason for low absorption lies in numerous inhibitors of iron absorption, such as phytic and oxalic acid, starch, polyphenols (i.e., tannins

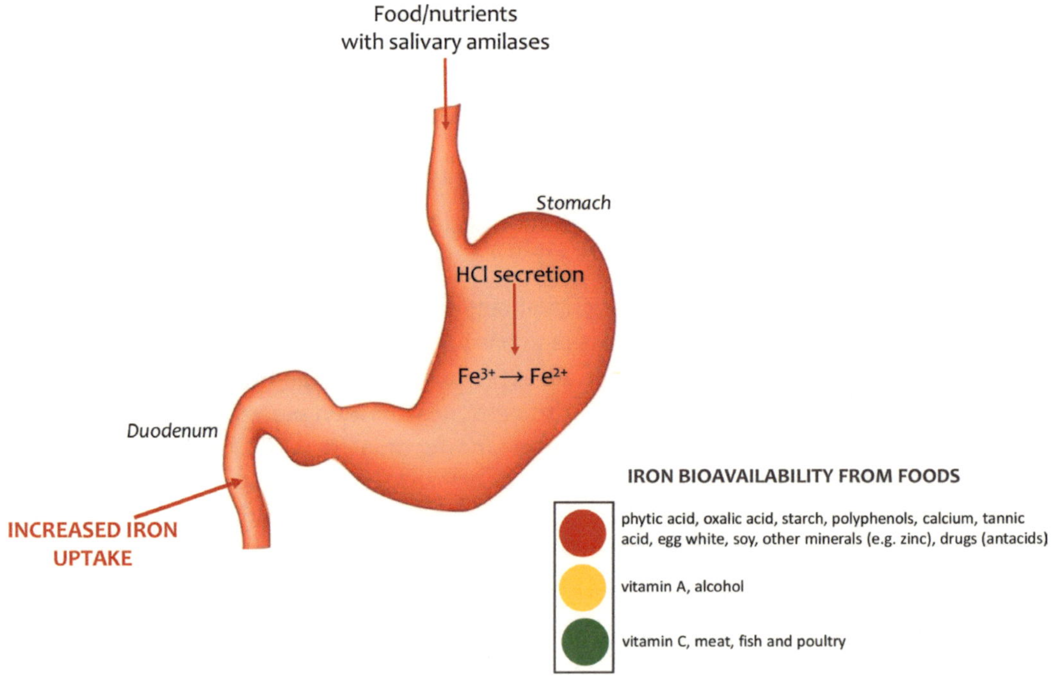

Figure 2. Parts of the gastrointestinal system important for the digestion and absorption of iron from foods and supplements.

from coffee and tea), egg white, calcium, other minerals (e.g., zinc), and numerous medicaments that diminish gastric secretion (e.g., antacids) [2, 32, 46–49].

Dietary intake of iron directly correlates with energy intake (on every 4184 kJ comes about 6 mg of iron) [3, 6, 39, 40]. Recommended intake (presented as dietary reference intakes (DRI) [50]) for pregnant women along with percentage increase from nonpregnant women recommendations is given in **Table 1**. Out of all micronutrients, iron and folic acid requirements increase by 50.0% in comparison to nonpregnant women. Folic acid role in pregnancy extends the scope of this chapter. For further details please refer to, for example, Banjari et al. [15].

Generally speaking, a well-balanced diet goes hand-in-hand with iron-rich foods. But, despite general belief of positive shifts in diet quality during pregnancy [51, 52], pregnant women do not change it significantly through pregnancy [4, 32]. However, changes in lifestyle habits are reflected in smoking cessation and supplement use, but not in diet quality [4, 32]. Educative programs for pregnant women could significantly alter their behavior, especially in terms of diet and not only during pregnancy but on a long-term basis [53–56].

Dietary intervention has shown to improve the iron status of pregnant women gradually and provides better results long-term [53, 55, 56]. Patterson et al. [56] conducted a 12-week intervention, with a follow-up 6 months after the intervention on ID and IDA pregnant women with either iron supplement or iron-rich diet. The supplement group took one tablet containing 350 mg of slow-release ferrous sulfate tablet per day, which was equivalent to 105 mg inorganic iron. On the other hand, the iron-rich diet group followed a diet planned to provide approximately 2.25 mg of absorbed iron per day. Both groups showed significant improvement in serum ferritin levels after the intervention and at follow-up. However, the increase was smaller in the diet group which continually improved iron

Nutrient	DRI	% increase	Nutrient	DRI	% increase
CHO (g/d)	175	34.6	Folate (μg/d)	600	50.0
Total fiber (g/d)	28	12.0	B_{12} (μg/d)	2.6	8.3
Protein (g/d)	71	54.0	Pantothenic acid (mg/d)	6	20.0
Vitamin A (μg/d)	770	10.0	Biotin (μg/d)	30	0.0
Vitamin C (mg/d)	85	13.3	Sodium (g/d)	2.3	0.0
Vitamin D (μg/d)	5	0.0	Ca (mg/d)	1000	0.0
Vitamin E (mg/d)	15	0.0	Cu (μg/d)	1000	11.1
Vitamin K (μg/d)	90	0.0	Fe (mg/d)	27	50.0
B_1 (mg/d)	1.4	27.3	Mg (mg/d)	350–360	10.9
B_2 (mg/d)	1.4	27.3	Mn (mg/d)	2.0	11.1
Niacin (mg/d)	18	28.6	Se (μg/d)	60	9.1
B_6 (mg/d)	1.9	46.2	Zn (mg/d)	11	37.5

Table 1. Dietary reference intakes (DRIs) for pregnant women (prepared according to IOM [50]).

status during 6 months follow-up [56]. These results clearly show the potential of properly balanced iron-rich diet as a mean for the improvement in iron status, and if timed properly present the best way to prevent ID and IDA in pregnancy.

The total dietary intake of iron increases significantly through gestation [28, 32, 38, 47, 52], reaching the highest peak at the third trimester [32]. Still, this amount is significantly under the recommended intake [50] and as reported by Banjari et al. [32], the total daily dietary intake of iron in pregnant women satisfies 35.2% in the first trimester, 37.4% in the second trimester, and increasing to 41.5% in the third trimester of the recommended DRI of iron. Shobeiri et al. [28] reported the intake of iron in Indian pregnant women to around 60% of DRI. On the other hand, even with relatively low total dietary intake of iron proper combination of foods may significantly improve the amount of iron absorbed [32, 56].

The presence of ID or IDA increases the amount of dietary iron which will be readily absorbed in the gut [2, 3, 6]. Barett et al. [57] have shown that the iron absorption increases through pregnancy, which is foreseeable as a normal physiologic process in pregnancy. Therefore, the iron absorption reaches its maximum by the end of gestation. In other words, the absorption of the total dietary iron starts with 7% absorbed in the first trimester, 36% in the second, and increases to 66% of absorbed iron in the third trimester, falling again postpartum to starting level (of around 11%) [57]. Banjari et al. [32] also confirmed that the amount of absorbed iron follows rising trend toward the end of pregnancy, being the highest in the third trimester being 1.33 mg of absorbed iron (out of 11.2 mg of total dietary iron intake) [32].

Banjari et al. [32] explained this low level of absorbed iron by the fact that plant foods present the main source of dietary iron for pregnant women, contributing more than 80% to the total dietary intake of iron [32]. Plant foods have been confirmed by numerous studies [2, 47–49, 56, 58, 59] to represent the main dietary source of iron for pregnant women.

Another possible reason includes low intake of meat; Banjari et al. [32] reported daily intake of meat to around 90 g a day. Therefore, the contribution of heme iron to the total dietary intake of iron is low, varying from 15.8, 16.4, and 16.6%, respectively, through gestation [32]. One of the main reasons is high consumption of chicken meat [32], which does not contain heme iron [60]. In the past two decades, consumption of poultry increased by 50% while simultaneously beef consumption fell by 40%; therefore, the amount of heme iron consumption is significantly lower [59]. Still, the so-called *meat factor* effect as well as amino acids with sulfur show positive influence on iron absorption [46, 61].

Consumption of cereals is very important part of a well-balanced diet. However, due to high content of phytates, one of the most potent inhibiting factors for iron bioavailability [46, 62] must be considered with special care, especially in countries with high consumption of cereals and cereal products [63–65]. According to Johnston et al. [59], cereals present the most important contributing source to overall intake of nonheme iron. These foods are the main source of the most potent inhibiting absorption factor, phytates [46, 62], which have been shown to correlate significantly with hemoglobin values of pregnant women, only in the first trimester of pregnancy [4]. This correlation points out that physiology of pregnancy diminishes the effect of inhibition by phytates as pregnancy progresses. Cereals and their products may be used as highly valuable foods by which an individual could increase the total daily dietary iron intake [48, 63] and have been used as functional foods, that is, foods enriched with iron either by a biofortification method or addition of different iron compounds (e.g., electrolytic iron, ferrous fumarate, ferrous pyrophosphate, ferrous lactate, etc.) [48]. Interventions based on iron fortification resulted in a significant drop of ID and IDA prevalence in countries, such as China, Brazil, Venezuela, Morocco, and others [48]. In addition, potential adverse effects of high intake of iron must be considered [6], but never the less, functional cereal products enriched with iron could serve as a good basis to improve the total dietary intake of iron of not only pregnant women, but also menstruating women and children, that is, population groups at the risk of insufficient intake of iron [63, 66].

Consumption of coffee and tea are additional important factors due to wide consumption on a daily basis [4, 67]. According to a prospective study conducted in Denmark between 1989 and 1996 on 18,478 singleton pregnancies, 43% of women did not drink coffee, 34% drank one to three cups a day, with 23% of women categorized as heavy users with four or more cups a day [68]. The results from the Danish National Birth Cohort covering time frame between 1996 and 2002 showed 81.2% of women reported drinking either tea or coffee, with coffee being consumed less (44.7% of women) than tea (63.5% of women), and with the average consumption of two cups per day [69]. The results from the Slone Epidemiology Center Birth Defects Study [70], which covered three periods, that is, 1976–1988, 1998–2005, and 2009–2010, show that tea drinking was more popular in early years with 66% of pregnant women consuming tea, which dropped to 39% in later years. On the other hand, a prospective study by Banjari et al. [67] reports that 68.9% of pregnant women were drinking either coffee, tea, or both during pregnancy, with the highest preference toward coffee (130 out of 153 women). The inhibiting effect of coffee and tea is related to polyphenols (garlic, tannic, and chlorogenic acid). Tea shows higher reduction rate (75–80% for cca 200 ml) than the coffee (by 60% for cca 150 ml). Moreover, the consumption of around 100 g of meat reduces their inhibiting effect by 50% [46, 71, 72]. However, it should be noted that pregnant women tend to cease from their preferred beverage due to nausea or heartburn. Heartburn is experienced by 40–80% of pregnant women sometime during pregnancy, while nausea affects nearly 80–90% of pregnant women followed by vomiting in 50% cases [73]. As reported by Banjari et al. [67], during the first trimester 17.0% of women gave up their preferred beverage due to nausea, while at the third trimester additional 17.7% of coffee drinkers and 26.1% of tea drinkers stopped drinking a particular beverage, referring heartburn as a reason.

Intake of calcium higher than 600 mg/day was found to have the maximum inhibiting effect on iron absorption [46, 74–76]. However, we must emphasize that in terms of a newborn prolonged breastfeeding serves as a protecting agent from IDA [31].

Child's diet especially in that early period solely depends on the mother [31]. Strong evidence supports findings that in both low- and high-income settings omission from breastfeeding contributes to infant mortality, hospitalization for preventable disease, such as gastroenteritis and respiratory disease, increased rates of childhood diabetes and obesity, and adult disease, such as coeliac and cardiovascular disease [77]. Breastfeeding impacts IQ and educational and behavioral outcomes of the child. Importantly, a dose-response relationship was found with the greatest benefit resulting from breastfeeding exclusively, with no added food or fluids, for around 6 months [77], which has been recommended by the WHO [78]. Race and income are major predictors of whether women will exclusively breastfeed for 6 months. The highest rate of breastfeeding is among wealthy whites [77, 78]. However, women with low incomes are often financially compelled to quickly return to the workforce [7], and for them formula is a convenience. But in a time of prolonged economic poverty child's dietary patterns worsen, and mothers even return to earlier practice of giving cow's milk which worsens the symptoms of IDA [3, 6, 31, 74].

On the other hand, intake of vitamin C (ascorbic acid) which has the most promoting effect on iron absorption is especially effective when the most powerful inhibitors are present in a meal [46, 79]. Besides important correlation with the gastric acidity [79], which has immense importance for the overall absorption of iron (**Figure 2**), ascorbic acid prevents the formation of low soluble ferric compounds by a reduction process [46] and this important promoting effect has been observed with or without the presence of phytates [80] or polyphenols [46]. The promoting effect of ascorbic acid depends on the meal composition [81].

Besides already discussed inhibiting and promoting factors, two factors have combined effect on iron absorption. Alcohol increases the absorption of ferric but not of ferrous iron, and this effect has been attributed to enhanced gastric acid secretion [46]. However, the effect was not found in red wine, probably due to high polyphenol content [46, 72]. Vitamin A reduces the inhibiting effect of tea or coffee, that is, it overcomes the inhibiting effect of polyphenols in these beverages, as well as the effect by phytates. They form a complex which is soluble even at pH 6, making iron available for absorption in duodenum. An even stronger effect was found for beta-carotene and other carotenoids (lycopene, lutein, and zeaxanthin) [4].

4. Supplementation and other lifestyle habits

Supplementation in pregnancy is highly recommended [2, 24, 38] because of the already mentioned increased needs (**Table 1**), and low dietary intake [28, 32, 38, 51, 52]. Supplementation with iron or iron-folic acid has been widely recommended and practiced [4, 21]; in Croatia, even 82.6% of pregnant women were taking supplements during pregnancy [4]. Still, general supplementation should be avoided [82] especially having in mind that the recent systematic review and meta-analysis conducted by Fernández-Cao et al. [22] found almost 50% increased risk of gestational diabetes in women having high hemoglobin or ferritin levels, especially in the first and the third trimesters. Additionally, supplements formulated specifically for pregnant women differ significantly in their composition, and if only iron is observed, the intake from producer's prescribed dose (1 or 2 tablets per day) varies from 8 mg up to even 60 mg of iron [4]. Findings from clinical trials on how different supplementation formulations affect iron status during pregnancy and pregnancy outcomes (i.e., time of delivery and birth weight) are equivocal. For example, West et al. [83] conducted a cluster randomized, double-masked trial enrolling more than 44,000 pregnant women from rural Bangladesh who were provided with supplements containing 15 micronutrients or iron-folic acid alone. Multiple micronutrient supplementation group had statistically significant reduction in preterm delivery (RR 0.85, $P = 0.02$) and low birth weight (RR 0.88, $P < 0.001$) as compared to iron-folic acid supplementation group [83]. This contradicts earlier findings from a double-masked randomized controlled community trial conducted on pregnant women from rural Nepal [84]. Study results showed that supplementation with iron-folic acid had increased hemoglobin and had a 54% reduction in IDA; the combination of folic acid, zinc, and iron had a 48% reduction, while the combination of folic acid, zinc, iron, and 11 other micronutrients had a 36% reduction, whereas supplementation with folic acid alone had no influence on IDA [84]. The more recent meta-analysis performed by Petry et al. [85] found that supplementation with iron or zinc during pregnancy had no effect on birth outcomes, but did show the positive effect of low dose daily iron and zinc use during 6–23 months of age on child's iron and zinc status, especially weight-for-age and weight-for-height [85]. Supplementation is encouraged due to expected improvement in iron blood status. A study by Scanlon et al. [29] showed that the prevalence of anemia (based on hemoglobin level) among iron-supplemented pregnant women participating in public health nutrition programs is approximately 8% in the first trimester, but this was not confirmed by Banjari [4] reporting that 3.6% of pregnant women were IDA with additional 10.8% being ID at the first trimester.

One of the most detrimental lifestyle habits during pregnancy is smoking. It has been associated with the increased risk for spontaneous abortion, especially during the first trimester, reduced birth weight, and perinatal mortality [86, 87]. In combination with ID and especially IDA negative effect on pregnancy outcomes is even greater, leading toward low birth weight and preterm delivery [86, 87]. Smoking cessation is very common among pregnant women, and as reported by Banjari [4] even 72.8% of pregnant women decided to stop smoking during pregnancy, while 27.2% of women continue to smoke regardless of all recommendations and the knowledge of its adverse impact on child's health.

5. ID, IDA poverty, and obesity

Iron-rich foods and those that contain nutrients that promote iron absorption fall into a group of foods with the highest price per serving [88]. According to the Food and Drug Administration "healthy foods" are defined as foods based on the protein, fiber, vitamins A and C, calcium, and iron content, and cost analysis showed that grains, dry beans, and eggs are the lowest cost sources of iron [89]. However, those foods contain iron of very low bioavailability [32, 46]. A well-balanced diet with highly bioavailable iron must include foods like meat, fish, and fruits. It is estimated that around one-third of children have low dietary intake of iron [90]. At the time of economic insecurity and fall in socioeconomic status (SES), these foods are the first ones being cut from a diet [91].

At first, the link between iron deficiency and obesity seems farcical. However, in the obesity pandemic era [92], we are experiencing micronutrient deficiencies that are not expected in developed, rich countries [20, 33–35]. The trend affects all population groups; therefore, it is no surprise that overweight/obesity condition is considered the number one priority currently in obstetrics and gynecology [19]. In Croatia, as reported by Banjari [4], 16.7% women start pregnancy as overweight, with additional 10.3% being obese. If we add up excessive weight gain during pregnancy, which was observed among 40.5% of all pregnant women in Croatia [4], the impact of obesity on pregnancy outcomes and future child's health is immense.

The preexistence of overweight/obesity or excessive weight gain during pregnancy represents a significant risk factor for fetal macrosomia and medical complications, including pregnancy-induced hypertension, gestational diabetes, and cesarean delivery [19, 20, 93–99]. Importantly, for women entering pregnancy with a normal body mass index, an inadequate weight gain poses higher risk [20, 94, 95, 100]. Besides, maternal obesity and gestational weight gain are confirmed risk factors for childhood obesity [98, 101], with effects that extend into adulthood [98, 99, 102]. No wonder why childhood obesity rates and predictions seem especially alarming. The predictions say that by 2025 the rate of overweight children is expected to increase to 15.8%, with additional 5.4% of obese children aged 5–18 years by 2025 [103].

A systematic review by Zhao et al. [37] confirmed a significant correlation between ID (including the risk of ID) in obese and overweight individuals. Obese individuals despite their excessive dietary and caloric intake have an unbalanced diet based on carbohydrates and fats [35]. This has also been confirmed for overweight and obese children by Hutchinson [36]. This systematic review concluded that overweight and obese children and adolescents have a higher prevalence or risk of ID, and the evidence is consistent. However, Hutchinson [36] emphasized that the true relationship between body fat mass and iron absorption is still to be clarified. Low-hemoglobin level was found among overweight/obese pregnant women [19].

As already mentioned, pregnancy is observed as a *critical window* for future child's development and considered as an ideal time frame for interventions that would target specific health-related outcomes in child, such as obesity, diabetes, etc. [14, 16, 98, 99, 104]. Evidence supporting this approach accumulates by day. There is no such pretimed intervention, and as nicely emphasized by Gillman and Ludwig [99] *timely intervention during the early, plastic phases of development may lead to improved lifelong health trajectories.*

To sum up on the relation between obesity and ID/IDA, both conditions are more prevalent in population groups with low-quality diet. The relation extends beyond low-SES, consumption of low-cost foods that generally have a low content of essential nutrients [35, 105, 106], and especially iron [88]. Additionally, for pregnant women characteristics, such as younger age, lower level of education, with more children, and with higher pre-pregnancy, body mass index significantly alters diet quality during pregnancy [20, 51, 52]. In other words, this is an infinite loop of ID and IDA [31]. Therefore, targeting pregnant women affected by any of the above-mentioned characteristics/risk factors could significantly improve not only their iron status but also their state of nourishment and the overall health status. By that, we would alter future generations of children, making it a prerequisite for a healthier society.

Author details

Ines Banjari

Address all correspondence to: ines.banjari@ptfos.hr

Faculty of Food Technology Osijek, University of Osijek, Osijek, Croatia

References

[1] WHO/UNICEF/UNU. Iron deficiency anaemia: Assessment, prevention, and control. Geneva (Switzerland): World Health Organization; 2001

[2] Zimmermann MB, Hurrell RF. Nutritional iron deficiency. Lancet. 2007;**370**:511-520

[3] Adamson JW. Iron deficiency and other hypoproliferative anemias. In: Fauci AS, Braunwald E, Kasper DL, Hauser SL, Longo DL, Jameson JL, Loscalzo J, editors. Harrison's Principles of Internal Medicine. 17th ed. New York: Mc-Graw Hill Medical; 2008. pp. 628-634

[4] Banjari I. Dietary intake and iron status and incidence of anaemia in pregnancy [thesis]. Zagreb: University of Zagreb; 2012

[5] Heidemann BH. Changes in maternal physiology during pregnancy. Update in Anaesthesia. 2005;**20**:21-24

[6] Boulpaep EL, Boron W F. Medical Physiology. Philadelphia, PA: Elsevier, Saunders; 2006. p. 1267. ISBN 978-1-4160-3115-4

[7] Drewnowski A, Eichelsdoerfer P. Can low-income Americans afford a healthy diet? Nutrition Today. 2010;**44**(6):246-249

[8] Chepelev NL, Willmore WG. Regulation of iron pathways in response to hypoxia. Free Radical Biology & Medicine. 2011;**50**:645-666

[9] Cairo G, Bernuzzi F, Recalcati S. A precious metal: Iron, an essential nutrient for all cells. Genes & Nutrition. 2006;**1**(1):25-40

[10] Lozoff B, Georgieff MK. Iron deficiency and brain development. Seminars in Pediatric Neurology. 2006;**13**:158-165

[11] Zhou SJ, Gibson RA, Crowther CA, Baghurst P, Makrides M. Effect of iron supplementation during pregnancy on the intelligence quotient and behavior of children at 4 y of age: Long-term follow-up of a randomized controlled trial. The American Journal of Clinical Nutrition. 2006;**83**:1112-1117

[12] Hulthén L. Iron deficiency and cognition. Scandinavian Journal of Nutrition. 2003;**47**(3): 152-156

[13] Grantham-McGregor S, Ani C. A review of studies on the effect of iron deficiency on cognitive development in children. Journal of Nutrition. 2001;**131**:649S-668S

[14] Banjari I. Healthy pregnancy as a foundation for healthy child. Journal of Society of Medical Doctors of Montenegro Medical Essays. 2016;**65**(Suppl 1):88-98

[15] Banjari I, Matoković V, Škoro V. The question is whether intake of folic acid from diet alone during pregnancy is sufficient. Medicinski Pregled. 2014;**67**(9-10):313-321

[16] Langley-Evans SC. Metabolic programming during pregnancy: Implications for personalized nutrition. In: Kok F, Bouwman L, Desire F, editors. Personalized Nutrition. Principles and Applications. Routledge: CRC Press; 2008. p. 101-114

[17] Gambling L, Dunford S, Wallace DI, Zuur G, Solanky N, Srai SKS, McArdle HJ. Iron deficiency during pregnancy affects post-natal blood pressure in the rat. The Journal of Physiology. 2003;**52**(2):603-610

[18] Godfrey KM, Forrester T, Barker DJ, Jackson AA, Landman JP, Hall JS, Cox V, Osmond C. Maternal nutritional status in pregnancy and blood pressure in childhood. British Journal of Obstetrics and Gynaecology. 1994;**101**(5):398-403

[19] Banjari I, Kenjerić D, Šolić K, Mandić ML. Cluster analysis as a prediction tool for pregnancy outcomes. Collegium Antropologicum. 2015;**1**:247-252

[20] Banjari I, Kenjerić D, Mandić ML, Glavaš M, Leko J. Longitudinal observational study on diet quality during pregnancy and its relation to several risk factors for pregnancy complications and outcomes. British Journal of Medicine & Medical Research. 2015;**7**(2):145-154. DOI: 10.9734/BJMMR/2015/15527

[21] Scholl TO. Maternal iron status: Relation to fetal growth, length of gestation, and iron endowment of the neonate. Nutrition Reviews. 2011;**69**(Suppl 1):S23-S29

[22] Fernández-Cao JC, Aranda N, Ribot B, Tous M, Arija V. Elevated iron status and risk of gestational diabetes mellitus: A systematic review and meta-analysis. Maternal & Child Nutrition. 2016; DOI: 10.1111/mcn.12400

[23] Allen LH. Anemia and iron deficiency: Effects on pregnancy outcome. The American Journal of Clinical Nutrition. 2000;**71**(Suppl):1280S-1284S

[24] Milman N, Bergholt T, Eriksen L, Byg K-E, Graudal N, Pedersen P, Hertz J. Iron prophylaxis during pregnancy—How much iron is needed? A randomized dose-response study of 20-80 mg ferrous iron daily in pregnant women. Acta Obstetricia et Gynecologica Scandinavica. 2005;**84**:238-247

[25] Banjari I, Kenjerić D, Mandić M. What is the real public health significance of iron deficiency and iron deficiency anaemia in croatia? A population-based observational study on pregnant women at early pregnancy from eastern Croatia. Central European Journal of Public Health. 2015;**23**(2):122-127

[26] Levy A, Fraser D, Katz M, Mazor M, Sheiner E. Maternal anemia during pregnancy is an independent risk factor for low birth weight and preterm delivery. European Journal of Obstetrics Gynecology and Reproductive Biology. 2005;**122**:182-186

[27] Scholl TO, Hedinger ML, Fischer RL, Shearer JW. Anemia vs iron deficiency: Increased risk of preterm delivery in a prospective study. The American Journal of Clinical Nutrition. 1992;**55**:985-988

[28] Shobeiri F, Begum K, Nazari M. A prospective study of maternal hemoglobin status of Indian women during pregnancy and pregnancy outcome. Nutrition Research. 2006;**26**: 209-213

[29] Scanlon KS, Yip R, Schieve LA, Cogswell ME. High and low hemoglobin levels during pregnancy: Differential risks for preterm birth and small for gestational age. Obstetrics & Gynecology. 2000;**96**(5):741-748

[30] Viteri FE, Berger J. Importance of pre-pregnancy and pregnancy iron status: Can long-term weekly preventive iron and folic acid supplementation achieve desirable and safe status? Nutrition Reviews. 2005;**63**(12):S65-S76

[31] Banjari I. A maternal bond: The story on the infinite loop of iron deficiency anaemia. Medicinski Pregled. 2015;**68**(5-6):211-212

[32] Banjari I, Kenjerić D, Mandić ML. Iron bioavailability in daily meals of pregnant women. Journal of Food and Nutrition Research. 2013;**52**:203-209

[33] Nead KG, Halterman JS, Kaczorowski JM, Auinger P, Weitzman M. Overweight children and adolescents: A risk group for iron deficiency. Pediatrics. 2004;**114**(1):104-108

[34] Turer CB, Lin H, Flores G. Prevalence of vitamin D deficiency among overweight and obese US children. Pediatrics. 2013;**131**(1):e152-e161

[35] Pinhas-Hamiel O, Newfield RS, Koren I, Agmon A, Lilos P, Phillip M. Greater prevalence of iron deficiency in overweight and obese children and adolescents. International Journal of Obesity and Related Metabolic Disorders. 2003;**27**(3):416-418

[36] Hutchinson C. A review of iron studies in overweight and obese children and adolescents: A double burden in the young? European Journal of Nutrition. 2016;**55**(7):2179-2197

[37] Zhao L, Zhang X, Shen Y, Fang X, Wang Y, Wang F. Obesity and iron deficiency: A quantitative meta-analysis. Obesity Reviews. 2015;**16**(12):1081-1093

[38] Lee J-I, Kang SA, Kim S-K, Lim H-S. A cross sectional study of maternal iron status of Korean women during pregnancy. Nutrition Research. 2002;**22**:1377-1388

[39] Berger J, Wieringa FT, Lacroux A, Dijkhuizen MA. Strategies to prevent iron deficiency and improve reproductive health. Nutrition Reviews. 2011;**69**:S78–S86

[40] Wheeler S. Assessment and interpretation of micronutrient status during pregnancy: Symposium on translation of research in nutrition II: The bed. Proceedings of the Nutrition Society;2008;**67**:437-450. https://www.cambridge.org/core/services/aop-cambridge-core/content/view/S0029665108008732

[41] World Health Organization. Assessing the iron status of populations. Geneva (Switzerland): World Health Organization, Department of Nutrition for Health and Development; 2004

[42] Cook J. Diagnosis and management of iron-deficiency anaemia. Best Practice & Research Clinical Haematology. 2005;**18**(2):319-332

[43] Lynch SR. Interaction of iron with other nutrients. Nutrition Reviews. 1997;**55**(4):102-110

[44] Hurrell R, Egli I. Optimizing the bioavailability of iron compounds for food fortification. In: Kraemer K, Zimmermann MB, editors. Nutritional Anemia. Basel: Sight and Life Press; 2007. pp. 77-97

[45] Human vitamin and mineral requirements. Report of a joint FAO/WHO expert consultation Bangkok, Thailand. Rome: Food and Nutrition Division FAO; 2001. p. 286

[46] Hallberg L, Hultén L. Prediction of dietary iron absorption: An algorithm for calculating absorption and bioavailability of dietary iron. The American Journal of Clinical Nutrition. 2000;**71**:1147-1160

[47] Milman N. Iron in pregnancy—A delicate balance. Annals of Hematology. 2006;**85**(9): 559-565

[48] Thompson B. Food-based approaches for combating iron deficiency. In: Kraemer K, Zimmermann MB, editors. Nutritional Anemia. Basel: Sight and Life Press; 2007. pp. 337-358

[49] Tapiero H, Gaté L, Tew KD. Iron: Deficiencies and requirements. Biomedicine & Pharmacotherapy. 2001;**55**(6):324-332

[50] Institute of Medicine. Dietary Reference Intakes for Energy, Carbohydrate, Fiber, Fat, Fatty Acids, Cholesterol, Protein and Amino Acids. Washington, DC: National Academy Press; 2002

[51] Rifas-Shiman SL, Rich-Edwards JW, Kleinman KP, Oken E, Gillman MW. Dietary quality during pregnancy varies by maternal characteristics in project Viva: A US cohort. Journal of the American Dietetic Association. 2009;**109**(6):1004-1011

[52] Petrakos G, Panagopoulos P, Koutras I, Kazis A, Panagiotakos D, Economou A, Kanellopoulos N, Salamalekis E, Zabelas A. A comparison of the dietary and total intake of micronutrients in a group of pregnant Greek women with the dietary reference intakes. European Journal of Obstetrics Gynecology and Reproductive Biology. 2006;**127**:166-171

[53] Viteri FE. Iron endowment at birth: Maternal iron status and other influences. Nutrition Reviews. 2011;**69**:S3-S16

[54] Verbeke W, De Bourdeaudhuij I. Dietary behaviour of pregnant versus non-pregnant women. Appetite. 2007;**48**:78-86

[55] Black MM, Quigg AM, Hurley KM, Reese Pepper M. Iron deficiency and iron-deficiency anemia in the first two years of life: Strategies to prevent loss of developmental potential. Nutrition Reviews. 2011;**69**:S64-S70

[56] Patterson AJ, Brown WJ, Roberts DCK, Seldon MR. Dietary treatment of iron deficiency in women of childbearing age. The American Journal of Clinical Nutrition. 2001;**74**:650-656

[57] Barett JFR, Whittaker PG, Williams JG, Lind T. Absorption of non-haem iron from food during normal pregnancy. British Medical Journal. 1994;**309**:79-82

[58] Hoppe M, Sjöberg A, Hallberg L, Hulthén L. Iron status in Swedish teenage girls: Impact of low dietary iron bioavailability. Nutrition. 2008;**24**:638-645

[59] Johnston J, Prynne CJ, Stephen AM, Wadsworth MEJ. Haem and non-haem iron intake through 17 years of adult life of a British Birth Cohort. British Journal of Nutrition. 2007;**98**(5):1021-1028

[60] Hallberg L, Hultén L. Perspectives on iron absorption. Blood Cells, Molecules and Diseases. 2002;**29**(3):562-573

[61] Reddy MB, Hurrell RF, Cook JD. Meat consumption in a varied diet marginally influences nonheme iron absorption in normal individuals. Journal of Nutrition. 2006;**136**(3):576-581

[62] Kristensen MB, Tetens I, Alstrup Jørgensen AB, Dal Thomsen A, Milman N, Hels O, Sandström B, Hansen M. A decrease in iron status in young healthy women after long-term daily consumption of the recommended intake of fibre-rich wheat bread. European Journal of Nutrition. 2005;**44**(6):334-340

[63] Banjari I, Kenjerić D, Mandić ML. Cereals and their products as source of energy and nutrients in early pregnancy. In: Proceedings of the 6th International Congress FLOUR-BREAD'11. Osijek, Croatia: Faculty of Food Technology Osijek; 2012. pp. 110-117

[64] Cecić I, Colić Barić I, Kuvačić S, Batinić M. Diet quality and grains intake in Croatian pregnant women. In: Proceedings of the 5th International Congress Flour-Bread '09. Osijek, Croatia: Faculty of Food Technology Osijek; 2010. pp. 463-470

[65] Snook Parrott M, Bodnar LM, Simhan HN, Harger G, Markovic N, Roberts JM. Maternal cereal consumption and adequacy of micronutrient intake in the periconceptional period. Public Health Nutrition. 2008;**12**(8):1276-1283

[66] Miler JL. Iron Deficiency Anemia: A Common and Curable Disease. Cold Spring Harbor Perspectives in Medicine. 2013;**3**(7):a011866. DOI: 10.1101/cshperspect.a011866

[67] Banjari I, Kenjerić D, Mandić ML. Intake of tannic acid from tea and coffee as a risk factor for low iron bioavailability in pregnant women. Food in Health and Disease. 2013;**2**(1):10-16

[68] Wisborg K, Kesmodel U, Bech BH, Hedegaard M, Henriksen TB. Maternal consumption of coffee during pregnancy and stillbirth and infant death in first year of life: Prospective study. British Medical Journal. 2003;**326**:420

[69] Hinkle SN, Laughon SK, Catov JM, Olsen J, Bech BH. First trimester coffee and tea intake and risk of gestational diabetes mellitus: A study within a national birth cohort. An International Journal of Obstetrics and Gynaecology. 2014;**122**(3):420-428. DOI: 10.1111/1471-0528.12930

[70] Yazdy MM, Tinker SC, Mitchell AA, Demmer LA, Werler MM. Maternal tea consumption during early pregnancy and the risk of spina bifida. Birth Defects Research Part A Clinical and Molecular Teratology. 2012;**94**(10):756-761. DOI: 10.1002/bdra.23025

[71] Hurrell RF, Reddy M, Cook JD. Inhibition of non-haem iron absorption in man by polyphenolic-containing beverages. British Journal of Nutrition. 1999;**81**(4):289-295

[72] Manach C, Scalbert A, Morand C, Rémésy C, Jiménez L. Polyphenols: Food sources and bioavailability. The American Journal of Clinical Nutrition. 2004;**79**(5):727-747

[73] Keller J, Frederking D, Layer P. The spectrum and treatment of gastrointestinal disorders during pregnancy. Nature Clinical Practice Gastroenterology & Hepatology. 2008;**5**(8):430-443. DOI: 10.1038/ncpgasthep1197

[74] Ziegler EE. Consumption of cow's milk as a cause of iron deficiency in infants and toddlers. Nutrition Reviews. 2011;**69**:S37-S42

[75] Lynch SR. The effect of calcium on iron absorption. Nutrition Research Reviews. 2000;**13**: 141-158

[76] Gleerup A, Rossander-Hulthen L, Gramatkovski E, Hallberg L. Iron absorption from the whole diet: Comparison of the effect of two different distributions of daily calcium intake. The American Journal of Clinical Nutrition. 1995;**61**:97-104

[77] Renfrew MJ, McCormick FM, Wade A, Quinn B, Dowswell T. Support for healthy breastfeeding mothers with healthy term babies. Cochrane Database of Systematic Reviews. May 16, 2012;(5):CD001141. DOI: 10.1002/14651858.CD001141.pub4

[78] World Health Organization. WHO Global Data Bank on Infant and Young Child Feeding (IYCF) [Internet]. 2009. Available from: http://www.who.int/nutrition/databases/infantfeeding/countries/en/ [Accessed: Februray 19, 2015]

[79] Aditi A, Graham DY. Vitamin C, gastritis, and gastric disease: A historical review and update. Digestive Diseases and Sciences. 2012;**57**(10):2504-2515. DOI: 10.1007/s10620-012-2203-7

[80] Olivares M, Pizarro F, Hertrampf E, Fuenmayor G, Estevez E. Iron absorption from wheat flour: Effects of lemonade and chamomile infusion. Nutrition. 2007;**23**:296-300

[81] Cook JD, Reddy MB. Effect of ascorbic acid intake on nonheme-iron absorption from a complete diet. The American Journal of Clinical Nutrition. 2001;**73**:93-98

[82] Banjari I. Ditch and Switch: How much supplements do we actually need? Medicinski Pregled. 2014;**67**(7-8):261-263

[83] West Jr KP, Shamim AA, Mehra S, Labrique AB, Ali H, Shaikh S et al. Effect of maternal multiple micronutrient vs iron-folic acid supplementation on infant mortality and adverse birth outcomes in rural Bangladesh. The JiVitA-3 randomised trial. Journal of the American Medical Association. 2014;**312**(24):2649-2658

[84] Christian P, Shrestha J, LeClerq SC, Khatry SK, Jiang T, Wagner T et al. Supplementation with micronutrients in addition to iron and folic acid does not further improve the hematologic status of pregnant women in rural Nepal. Journal of Nutrition. 2003;**133**:3492-3498

[85] Petry N, Olofin I, Boy E, Donahue Angel M, Rohner F. The effect of low dose iron and zinc intake on child micronutrient status and development during the first 1000 days of life: A systematic review and meta-analysis. Nutrients. 2016;**8**:773

[86] Rasmussen S, Bergsjø P, Jacobsen G, Haram K, Bakketeig LS. Haemoglobin and serum ferritin in pregnancy—Correlation with smoking and body mass index. European Journal of Obstetrics Gynecology and Reproductive Biology. 2005;**123**:27-34

[87] Kallen K. The impact of maternal smoking during pregnancy on delivery outcome. European Journal of Public Health. 2001;**11**(3):329-333

[88] Drewnowski A. The cost of US foods as related to their nutritive value. The American Journal of Clinical Nutrition. 2010;**92**:1181-1188

[89] Drewnowski A. The Nutrient Rich Foods Index helps to identify healthy, affordable foods. The American Journal of Clinical Nutrition. 2010;**91**(Suppl):1095S-1101S

[90] Bucholz EM, Desai MM, Rosenthal MS. Dietary intake in head start vs non-head start preschool-aged children: Results from the 1999-2004 National Health and Nutrition Examination Survey. Journal of the American Dietetic Association. 2011;**111**(7):1021-1030

[91] Drewnowski A. Obesity and the food environment: Dietary energy density and diet costs. American Journal of Preventive Medicine. 2004;**27**(3S):154-162

[92] Ng M, Fleming T, Robinson M, Thomson B, Graetz N, Margono C et al. Global, regional, and national prevalence of overweight and obesity in children and adults during 1980-2013: A systematic analysis for the Global Burden of Disease Study 2013. Lancet. 2014;**384**:766-781

[93] Raatikainen K, Heiskanen N, Heinonen S. Transition from overweight to obesity worsens pregnancy outcome in a BMI-dependent manner. Obesity. 2006;**14**(1):165-171

[94] DeVader SR, Neeley HL, Myles TD, Leet TL. Evaluation of gestational weight gain guidelines for women with normal prepregnancy body mass index. Obstetrics & Gynecology. 2007;**110**:745-751

[95] Morken N-H, Klungsøyr K, Magnus P, Skjærven R. Pre-pregnant body mass index, gestational weight gain and the risk of operative delivery. Acta Obstetricia et Gynecologica Scandinavica. 2013;**92**:809-815

[96] Hutcheon JA, Lisonkova S, Joseph KS. Epidemiology of pre-eclampsia and the other hypertensive disorders of pregnancy. Best Practice & Research Clinical Obstetrics & Gynaecology. 2011;**25**:391-403

[97] Flick AA, Brookfield KF, de la Torre L, Tudela CM, Duthely L, González-Quintero VH. Excessive weight gain among obese women and pregnancy outcomes. American Journal of Perinatology. 2010;**27**(4):333-338

[98] Godfrey KM, Reynolds RM, Prescott SL, Nyirenda M, Jaddoe VW, Eriksson JG, Broekman BF. Influence of maternal obesity on the longterm health of offspring. Lancet Diabetes Endocrinol. 2017;**5**(1):53-64. DOI: 10.1016/S22138587(16)301073

[99] Gillman MW, Ludwig DS. How early should obesity prevention start? The New England Journal of Medicine. 2013;**369**(23):2173-2175

[100] Choi S-K, Park I-Y, Shin J-C. The effects of pre-pregnancy body mass index and gestational weight gain on perinatal outcomes in Korean women: A retrospective cohort study. Reproductive Biology and Endocrinology. 2011;**9**:6. DOI: 10.1186/1477-7827-9-6

[101] Trandafir LM, Temneanu OR. Pre and post-natal risk and determination of factors for child obesity. Journal of Medicine and Life. 2016;**9**(4):386-391

[102] Eriksson JG, Sandboge S, Salonen MK, Kajantie E, Osmond C. Longterm consequences of maternal overweight in pregnancy on offspring later health: Findings from the Helsinki Birth Cohort Study. Annals of Medicine. 2014;**46**(6):434-438. DOI: 10.3109/07853890.2014.919728

[103] Lobstein T, Jackson-Leach R. Planning for the worst: Estimates of obesity and comorbidities in school-age children in 2025. Pediatric Obesity. 2016;**11**:321-325

[104] Hanson M, Barker M, Dodd JM, Kumanyika S, Norris S, Steegers E et al. Interventions to prevent maternal obesity before conception, during pregnancy, and post partum. Lancet Diabetes Endocrinol. 2017;**5**(1):65-76. DOI: 10.1016/S2213-8587(16)30108-5

[105] Grow HMG, Cook AJ, Arterburn DE, Saelens BE, Drewnowski A, Lozano P. Child obesity associated with social disadvantage of children's neighborhoods. Social Science & Medicine. 2010;**71**(3):584-591

[106] Monsivais P, Aggarwal A, Drewnowski A. Are socioeconomic disparities in diet quality explained by diet cost? Journal of Epidemiology and Community Health. 2012;**66**(6):530-535

Chapter 5

Anemia in Women of Reproductive Age

Alina V. Solovyova, Viola Gace,
Kristina S. Ermolenko and Vadim A. Khorolskiy

Additional information is available at the end of the chapter

http://dx.doi.org/10.5772/intechopen.71520

Abstract

Anemia is a common condition in women of childbearing age which is associated with wide spread hyperplastic processes in the uterus (leiomyomas, etc.) and abnormal and/or abundant uterine bleeding (AUB). Our study has considered the main causes of bleeding and the therapy aimed on limiting the amount of blood loss, as well as preoperative treatment of iron deficiency in women with uterine leiomyomas, planning for pregnancy. The combination of anemia with other abnormalities in the woman's health status is associated with complications during pregnancy such as premature births, the birth of small children and failure of the formation of neural tube in iron deficiency and hypoxia. During the treatment of iron deficiency anemia (IDA) with saline iron, we noted severity and pain in the stomach in 11.9% of patients, nausea in 13.1%, constipation in 21.4%, and diarrhea in 7.1% of women. Such complications did not occur while treating with ferric iron. The use of drugs Iron III hydroxide polymaltozate in women after the end of lactation resulted in normalization of the blood hemoglobin within 30 days and the number of erythrocytes and of serum ferritin by the 90th day.

Keywords: anemia, reproductive age, premature birth, uterine leiomyomas, abnormal uterine bleeding

1. Introduction

Anemia in women of reproductive age is the most common condition during pregnancy and post pregnancy days. Iron deficiency is associated with serious health problems such as impaired working capacity, weakness, malaise, headaches, cognitive impairment, decreased concentration or attention, etc. [1]. The lack of iron in the body can be due to inadequate intake, impaired absorption, increased needs and excessive losses. Inadequate intake of iron is often associated with a vegetarian (or vegan) diet, malnutrition or lack of iron in the diet. Same food with a predominant fat and sugar content, fast food, various diets used to maintain low body weight eventually lead to iron deficiency and/or anemia. In India, for example, about 30% of people are vegan; in Russia, this indicator is more modest—about 3–4%, as in most countries of Europe (Switzerland, Spain, Portugal, Poland, etc.). Impaired absorption of iron in the gastrointestinal tract (GIT) plays an important role in the development of iron deficiency and/or anemia. Diseases of the GIT are found in 20–24% of women of reproductive age [2]. Increased iron needs arise in children which is associated with their active growth. In adolescents, this is associated with an increase in the total mass of red blood cells and muscle mass. In young men, however, iron deficiency is less common than in girls, although their growth and growth rate are higher. In girls the high incidence of iron deficiency anemia is associated with the additional factor of blood losing during menstruation. Chronic blood loss and iron deficiency initiate in puberty if there is a disturbance of the development of menstrual function and they occur in a quarter of girls and adolescents [3]. Chronic repeated blood loss is the most common cause of iron deficiency anemia. The highest rates of iron deficiency are characteristic for women of childbirth age which is associated with monthly blood loss, pregnancy, parturition and lactation. A study conducted in 1998, by S. Kagamimori et al. has shown that 78% of Japanese schoolgirls have iron deficiency anemia (IDA) of varying severity 3 years after the onset of menstruation [4]. Women of childbearing age are at risk of developing IDA.

Many of them have chronic latent iron deficiency which remains undiagnosed for a long time as there are no expressed clinical symptoms and the body is well adapted to it. The content of iron and ferritin in the serum during pregnancy decreases as a result of an increase in the volume of plasma and an increase in total iron-binding capacity (TIBC), the percentage of transferrin is also reduced. Increased needs are only partially counter balanced by increased absorption in the intestine and mobilization of iron stores. If iron stores are partially or completely depleted at the beginning of pregnancy; which is observed with frequent and/or profuse menstruation, iron deficiency can be relative or absolute by the time of delivery. Up to 50–60% of women do not have enough iron reserves during pregnancy [5, 6] which is associated with adverse perinatal outcomes.

The data of Rosstat (2014) indicate that the number of women with abundant menstrual bleeding increased by 1.5 to 2 times in 10–15 years [26]. Women often do not consult a specialist for example, 59% of patients with heavy menstruation consider them normal and 41% are sure that they are not amenable to treatment [7]. Regular excessive loss of blood (more than 60–80 ml per cycle) disrupts the whole complex of physiological parameters, hemoglobin levels fall in erythrocytes and iron in plasma [8].

With physiological blood loss these changes are not observed. Adequate nutrition and a healthy lifestyle allow the body to independently restore the volume of blood and iron stores.

The consequence of monthly excessive menstrual blood loss with insufficient intake of iron is iron deficiency anemia which is confirmed by the following inferences [9]:

1. Patients with iron deficiency anemia lose a higher amount of menstrual blood in comparison with healthy women.

2. The users of hormonal contraceptives (even in the presence of a menstrual-like reaction), the iron content in the body is higher than in women who do not take estrogen-progestational agents and who have spontaneous menstruation.

With the purpose of revealing abundant menstrual flow (which causes IDA) the FIGO experts advice the gynecologist to ask their patients the following questions [10]:

1. How much bleeding is profuse?
   - Do you have to change the pads at night?
   - Do the protection pads completely soak in after 2 hours during the days of the most profuse bleeding?
2. Does menstrual blood loss affect the physical condition?
   - Do you observe the release of large clots of blood during menstruation?
   - Have you ever experienced any weakness or lack of air (symptoms of iron deficiency) during menstruation?
3. Does menstruation reduce the quality of life?
   - Does social life require correction in these days?
   - Are you worried about the unpleasant moments associated with bleeding?

2. Results of our studies

The duration of more than 7 days and the volume of blood loss over 80 ml as well as the presence of related physical, emotional and other problems are the characteristics of profuse menstruation. Normal menstruation is inherent in the duration of 2–7 days, the amount of blood lost is 50–80 ml and absence of pain that would disrupt the habitual life or require the intake of medication.

Detection of frequent and/or abundant uterine bleeding for more than 6 months should initiate a patient's examination for hemoglobin and other indicators of red blood cells. The greatest need for iron occurs during pregnancy and lactation. Iron deficiency or IDA leads to many numerical obstetrical complications primarily associated with metabolic disorders in the placental tissue.

In cases of iron deficiency during the first trimester of pregnancy, development of "defective" endometrium is observed which is facilitated by the initiation of intensive peroxidation of lipids in its cells followed by a change in the excitability of cell membranes and a decrease in the functional activity of the tissue. This leads to an inadequate implantation of the fetal egg. There is lack of proper rearrangement of the spiral arteries. This process is high energy-intensive and in IDA the cells lack oxygen sufficient for energy metabolism. Without reorganization of the uterine arteries, adequate fetal blood supply is impossible and primary placental insufficiency develops.

In the 2nd trimester, IDA in pregnant women leads to hypoxic disorders [11]. Circulatory disorders in the placenta and a lack of oxygen cause a failure of the second wave of trophoblast invasion. Hypoxia provokes the release of stress hormone cortisol which negatively affects the growth of the fetus. With further progression of pregnancy in iron deficiency, oxygenation of the blood worsens and total pathological disturbances occur in the tissues which affects the fetoplacental complex, fetal growth, pregnancy and parturition. A systematic review of "Maternal anemia and pregnancy outcomes in low- and middle-income countries" according to the scientific data of world-wide publications in 2016 found that anemia during pregnancy is associated with significantly higher risks [12]:

- low birth weight (RR = 1.3);
- premature birth (RR = 1.6);
- perinatal mortality (RR = 1.5);
- neonatal mortality (RR = 2.7).

The course of pregnancy in women with IDA inevitably affects the physical and psychomotor development of her child. Iron deficiency has a significant limiting effect on the brain's potential due to the negative impact on morphological structures.

The nervous system will reach its morphological maturity only then the brain will be ready for full work [13, 14].

All the basic structures of the nervous system are built up in the first trimester [11]. At the 3rd-4th weeks after fertilization a neural plate is formed. During 4–7 weeks neural tube is developed from which the brain and spinal cord are subsequently formed. By the end of the 8th week from the anterior part of the neural tube are formed five brain vesicles that give rise to all the parts of the brain such as the cerebral hemispheres, pons and cerebellum, middle and intermediate brain and medulla. In 5–10 weeks differentiation of some parts of the brain develops the cortex and subcortical structures.

In the second and third trimesters of pregnancy the structures of fetal nervous system are more complex. The neuronal precursor cells and the neuroglia begin to differentiate. From the 20th week nerve centers are formed which ensure the functioning of the main vital organs and begin the myelination processes. Disturbances of neurogenesis due to iron deficiency significantly limit the potential of the brain in the future.

In the third trimester cells differentiate into neurons and glial cells (astrocytes, oligodendrocytes, ependymocytes) grow axons and dendrites of neurons, synaptic contacts are formed and neural processes intensively myelinate. Obviously there should not be any iron deficiency for the prevention of defective morphological and functional development of the brain [11]. The slowdown of energy metabolism in the brain in iron deficiency occurs for two reasons; the activity of iron-requiring enzymes decreases and the amount of oxygen supplied to the cells decreases the expenditure during the intensive development processes increases by a factor of 2.

The results of numerous studies indicate the following facts:

1. Mental and psychological development is particularly affected by iron deficiency during intrauterine growth and/or in the early years of postnatal life.
2. The consequences of iron deficiency are expressed in adulthood, preventing the full realization of the inherent genetic potential [14–18].

Children who lacked iron in utero or infancy compared with peers who did not lack iron in the subsequent years of life especially during the age 19–28:

- lag behind in mental development;
- suffer from mental disorders;
- have delayed neuromotor development, difficult temperament (mettle);
- are depressed and apathetic, more anxious;
- suffer from attention deficit disorder combined with hyperactivity.

Analyzing the long-term studies (2012–2017) regarding the course of pregnancy in 321 women aged 19–45 years (continuous random sample) conducted at the Department of obstetrics and gynecology with the perinatology course of the Peoples Friendship University of Russia (Head of the Department, RAS Corresponding Member V.E. Radzinskiy) (**Table 1**) we found that there was no difference in the incidence of iron deficiency anemia among different age groups of women.

We also studied the frequency of iron deficiency anemia in women with preterm labor (PL). The subject of the study were 132 pregnant women who entered the maternity hospitals in Moscow to acquire medical assistance. Patients were divided into three groups: Group I - women with preterm labor at term of gestation from 22 to 27 weeks ± 6 days (n = 34); Group II - patients who gave birth prematurely at the gestation period of 28–37 weeks ± 6 days (n = 56) and Group III - women with term labor which constituted the control group (n = 42).

The greatest number of complications in all trimesters of pregnancy was observed in patients with PL including iron deficiency anemia (**Figure 1**). In the first trimester IDA was detected in 6 (17.6%) women with early PL and in 6 (10.7%) with PL at a period of 28–36/7 weeks in women who gave birth in time this complication was not observed. In the second trimester mild-to-moderate IDA was diagnosed in 9 (26.5%) of women who gave birth at the gestation age of 22–27/6 weeks, 15 (26.8%) gave birth within 28–36/7 weeks and 3 (7.1%) of women in the control group ($p < 0.05$). In the third trimester mild anemia was observed in group II in 15

Age of women (years)	19–24	25–29	30–34	35–39	40–45
Number of women (n)	65	67	64	63	62
Frequency of IDA n (%)	14 (21.5%)	15 (22.4%)	14 (21.9%)	14 (22.2%)	14 (22.6%)

$p > 0.05$ - the reliability of the differences is not revealed.

Table 1. Frequency of iron deficiency (IDA) anemia in pregnant women.

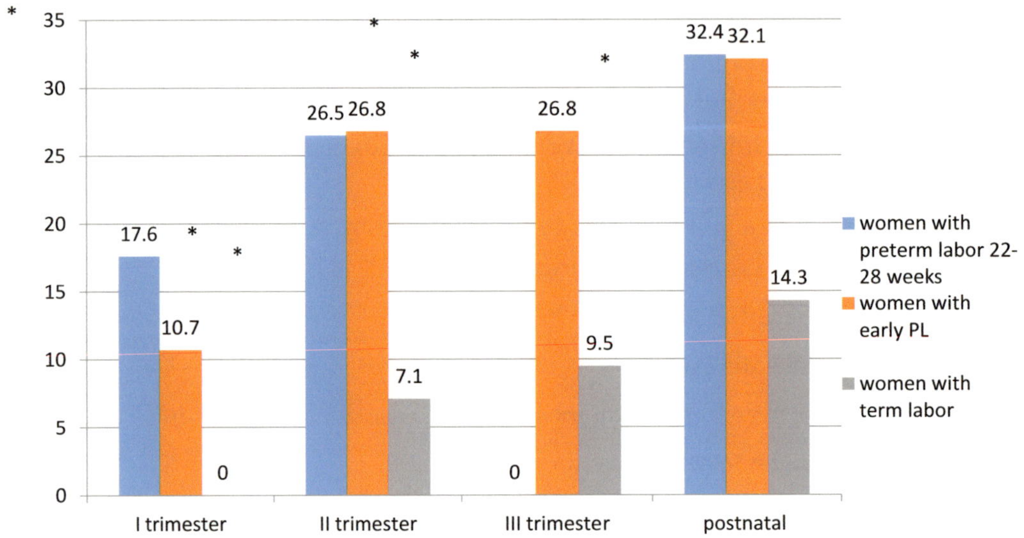

Figure 1. Frequency of iron deficiency anemia in the observed groups. *Reliability of differences was revealed when comparing women with premature and term labor ($p < 0.05$).

(26.8%) women and in 4 (9.5%) between those who gave birth in time. Anemia or iron deficiency is one of the factors of unfavorable perinatal outcomes.

After giving birth the frequency of IDA increased most significantly in women with PL and in women with early PR it was found in 11 (32.4%) of them in patients with preterm labor at a term of 28–36/7 with a frequency of 18 (32.1%). Anemia was found less often in women with term delivery - 5 (14.3%). One third of the women who had premature delivery suffered from IDA and this is not only because anemia developed during pregnancy but also because in women with PL significantly more often the delivery was an operative route (cesarean section). In the group with early PL in 5 (14.7%) in the group with PL in the period of 28–36/7 in 17 (30.3%) and the smallest number 3 (7.1%) of CS was performed in women with term delivery.

The results of the study confirmed the opinion of Professor Serov V.N. (2009) that premature birth is the delivery of a sick child from a sick woman. Anemia was more often diagnosed in women with premature labor.

All women with anemia with both preterm and term ($n = 34$) delivery were examined by the end of lactation (the average duration was 1.8 ± 0.4 years). In the postpartum period they received both bivalent and ferric iron. The number of erythrocytes, hemoglobin level and serum ferritin were measured. In 14 women there were no clinical and laboratory signs of anemia and iron suppression was based on the results of normalization of serum ferritin. Twenty patients were stopped taking iron supplements in the postpartum period on the basis of normalization of hemoglobin and revealed iron deficiency anemia of mild degree after lactation (**Table 2**). When determining the level of hemoglobin in the blood (Hb) it was found that the average level varied from 92 to 109 g/l (101.2 ± 1.3 g/l). Women were examined by a gastroenterologist and physician and treatment was prescribed by a physician. In the observed group there were no patients with blood diseases, inflammatory diseases and autoimmune diseases. Ten (50%) women were diagnosed with diseases of the gastrointestinal tract which was a risk factor for iron absorption and 3 (15%) patients were diagnosed with excessive menstrual bleeding (hormone therapy was prescribed). After 30 days the number of erythrocytes and hemoglobin reached to normal level. Serum ferritin reached normal values by day 90 (**Table 2**).

In the reproductive age anemia is the most common extragenital condition leading to health problems, adverse perinatal outcomes and often associated with organic diseases of the uterus. The International Federation of Gynecology and Obstetrics (FIGO) classification [19] identified the structural and non-structural causes of abnormal uterine bleeding. The results of the work of world-class experts [20] stated that in Russia about 50% of uterine bleeding is due to organic diseases of the uterus. In comparison, in the USA, Canada, Brazil, Korea and China this reason was found in 34–44% of women. Identification and recovery of women with uterine leiomyoma in the pre pregnancy period as in 20–50% of women leiomyoma is the cause of severe, irregular and prolonged uterine bleeding, iron deficiency anemia is a reserve for reducing complications of pregnancy and adverse perinatal outcomes.

A prospective study conducted from 2010 to 2015 included 292 women with uterine leiomyoma in female residents of the Krasnodar Territory. Inclusion criteria to the study were: reproductive age, uterine fibroids, pregnancy planning. Exclusion criteria: extragenital diseases leading to anemia; lack of reproductive plans; pregnancy.

The average age of women was 31.2 ± 1.5 years. Clinical characteristics and anamnesis (the medical history of a patient) of women are presented in **Table 3**. The inhabitants of the city were more than 160 (54.8%) compared to the residents of the village 132 (45.2%). More often women with fibroids had secondary specialized education - 161 (55.1%). Equally women were registered - 144 (49.3%) and unregistered - 135 (46.2%) marriages. 13 (4.5%) patients were unmarried but they planned a pregnancy.

The study of the reproductive anamnesis (**Table 2**) revealed that 179 (61.3%) of women had a history of delivery, i.e. they planned a second or third child. Practically all women 275 (94.2%) had an anamnesis for an official abortion. At the time of the examination none of the participants used any reliable means of contraception (COCs, IUDs). 183 (62.7%) of women reported using interrupted sexual intercourse and condoms the remaining 109 (37.3%) planned a pregnancy so they did not use contraception.

Indicators	Initial indicators	In 30 days	In 60 days	In 90 days
Number of erythrocyte $\times 10^{12}$/l	3.2 ± 0.3	3.9 ± 0.1*	4.1 ± 0.2*	4.2 ± 0.3*
Hemoglobin content (g/l)	101.2 ± 1.3	109.7 ± 1.1*	113.5 ± 1.2*	114 ± 0.9*
Serum ferritin (fl)	23.2 ± 1.1	27.3 ± 1.3*	39.7 ± 1.2*	52.1 ± 0.2*

*$p < 0.05$ in comparison with initial indicators.

Table 2. Indicators of "red" blood smear in women with mild anemia (n = 20) treated with Iron III hydroxide polymaltozate.

Parameter	Amount of women (n = 292)	
	Absolute number	Relative number, %
Social status		
Inhabitants of the city	160	54.8
Inhabitants of the village	132	45.2
Education	125	42.8
Secondary specialized education	161	55.1
Registered marriage	144	49.3
Unregistered marriage	135	46.2
Unmarried	13	4.5

Table 3. Clinical characteristics and anamnesis of women.

The duration of uterine leiomyomas was 4.3 ± 0.2 (2–10 years). The main complaints of women planning pregnancy were bleeding in 201 (68.8%), pain syndrome in 161 (55.1%), disturbance of the function of neighboring organs in 135 (46.2%) and asthenic syndrome in 192 (45.5%).

The number of uterine fibroids per woman varied from 2 to 12 on average 5.4 ± 0.3 and the number differed depending on the localization of the node. Multiple uterine fibroids were found in 266 (91%) women. Subserous localization of leiomyomas was detected in 181 (62%) women, subserous-interstitial and interstitial - in 260 (89%) women. Submucous site localization was determined in 32 (11%) patients. The diameter of the largest fibroid node did not exceed 110 mm an average of 49.8 ± 18.4 mm (15–110 mm).

The average level of hemoglobin in the blood (Hb) varied from 82 to 145 g/l (116.2 ± 2.3 g/l). The lowest level of Hb was observed in women with a predominance of submucous localization of the nodes - 90.8 ± 1.6 g/l (82–99 g/l). Anemia was diagnosed in 158 (54.1%) women. Anemia of mild degree was detected in 79 (27.1%) women. Hemoglobin level in these women was in the range of 109–94 g/l (100.1 ± 0.7 g/l). Anemia of moderate severity was detected in 79 (27.1%) women, the hemoglobin level varied from 91 to 72 g/l (84.4 ± 1.1 g/l). All women experienced profuse menstrual and intermenstrual bleeding.

In 134 (45.9%) women anemia was not detected and the hemoglobin level was determined in the range of 120–145 g/l and averaged 127.5 ± 1.2 g/l. Outpatients with anemia were administrated with divalent (84 - 28.8% women) and ferric iron (50 - 17.1% women). The comparative characteristics of the drugs revealed the following: in the treatment of IDA saline iron causes severity and pain in the stomach in 10 (11.9%), nausea in 11 (13.1%), constipation in 18 (21.4%) and diarrhea in 6 (7.1%) of women.

The average period of preparation for surgery after the administration of iron supplementation was 82.3 ± 0.1 days. In all women with mild anemia (79 - 27.1%) regardless of whether they received two or three-valent iron, normal level of red blood cell values were found. Normalization of the indices was achieved in 8 (2.7%) women with concomitant anemia of medium degree. In 71 (24.3%) compensation indices were impossible due to excessive amount of bleeding. They had to undergo surgery with uncompensated indicators of red blood cells.

3. Discussion of the results

Uterine fibroids and polyps are an indication for surgical treatment and hysteroscopy. However, most abnormal and/or excessive amount of bleeding from the uterus requires medical therapy. The classification of FIGO [19] allows not only to determine the cause of abnormal and/or excessive amount of bleeding from the uterus but also to prescribe a therapy that helps to reduce blood loss:

1. Chronic abnormal uterine bleeding (AUB) is abnormal in terms of volume, regularity, and/or frequency of uterine bleeding during most cycles in the last 6 months. As a rule, this condition does not require immediate medical intervention.
2. Acute AUB is an episode of profuse bleeding in which the specialist has sufficient reason for urgent intervention in order to prevent further blood loss. It can occur against a background of chronic AUB or for the first time in life.
3. Intermenstrual AUB occurs between predictable periods of cyclic menstruation. FIGO experts recommend replacing the term intermenstrual abnormal uterine bleeding on the concept of metrorrhagia.

Classification of causes of AUB called PALM-COEIN relates the causes of uterine bleeding in women of reproductive age to one of the nine categories (**Table 4**). The first four, grouped in the PALM group can be identified visually (structural). The rest are not related to structural anomalies and objectification is not amenable (non-structural).

Diagnostic measures for abnormal uterine bleeding include not only establishing the cause of bleeding and examination but also for the presence of anemia (hemoglobin level, hematocrit, general blood test).

Treatment of IDA in abnormal uterine bleeding cannot include only iron drugs as repeated blood loss will not lead to normalization of blood parameters. In cases of structural changes (polyps, fibroids) surgery is required. Non-steroid anti-inflammatory drugs (NSAIDs) have a high efficiency (blood loss on the background of NSAID intake decreases by an average of 58%),

PALM (structural)	COEIN (non-structural)
Polyp	Coagulopathy
Adenomyosis	Ovulatory dysfunction
Leiomyoma	Endometrial
Malignancy and hyperplasia	Iatrogenic
	Not yet classified

Table 4. Classification of causes of abnormal uterine bleeding (FIGO, 2011).

but it is not safe for the patient especially with prolonged use [8, 21]. The ability of NSAIDs to compensate uterine bleeding is due to inhibition of cyclooxygenase enzyme activity that leads to a decrease in the synthesis of prostacyclin that inhibits platelet aggregation. Tranexamic acid (synthetic lysine derivative) is an effective and a fairly safe drug which reduces blood loss by an average of 58%. The positive effect of tranexamic acid on the quality of life and sexual relations is reported [22, 23]. Contraindication to the administration of tranexamic acid is the presence of an episode of thrombosis. The mechanism of action of tranexamic acid is associated with reversible blocking of plasminogen and prevention of degradation of fibrin. Levonorgestrel-releasing intrauterine system (IUD-LNG) reduces menstrual blood loss by 74–97% [24]. During the first month with the use of IUD-LNG the duration of bleeding may increase. In adolescence IUD-LNG are not used since their mechanism of action is associated with endometrial atrophy.

Combined oral contraceptives (COCs) have a wide spread in reducing blood loss from the uterus. The effectiveness of COC is 43 - 88% [12]. Bleeding when using COC usually stops within 24 hours (the so-called hormonal hemostasis). The effect of COC is associated with the suppression of endometrial proliferation and the indirect reduction in the amount of blood loss.

The use of cyclic gestagens in the luteal phase are ineffective for the treatment of profuse menstruation, however they regulate the menstrual cycle [8]. Admission of medroxyprogesterone acetate (10 mg/day) or norethisterone acetate (2.5–5 mg/day) in a cyclic mode from the 16th to the 25th day provides a predictable bleeding profile.

Gonadotropin-releasing hormone agonists (GnRH agonists) are ineffective in the treatment of profuse menstruation. They are used only for certain indications as second line therapy [8]. These drugs completely block the function of the hypothalamic-pituitary-ovarian axis and cause amenorrhea in 89% of patients which is accompanied by severe side effects such as vaginal dryness, hot flashes, sweating, and with prolonged use (6 months or more) - osteopenia. The mechanism of action of GnRH agonists is associated with a decrease in the number of gonadotropin receptors in the pituitary gland with suppression of gonadotropin release and subsequent decrease in the level of estradiol to the state of hypogonadism.

For having a pregnancy with adequate iron reserves in the body it is extremely important that menstruating women of childbirth age do not experience a deficit in it. For the prevention of iron deficiency in this population in 2016 WHO (World Health Organization) updated the recommendations according to which iron drugs at a dosage of 60 mg/day should be taken to all menstruating women and adolescent girls for 3 months in the year and 3 months before conception. WHO experts recommend to use such preventive measures at the national level in countries where the incidence of anemia reaches 40%.

The optimal choice for women with iron deficiency (latent or already formed anemia), are oral drugs.

1. Bivalent iron drugs are ferrous sulfate, as well as fumarate, gluconate and glyceryl sulfate of iron.
2. Trivalent iron drugs are polymaltose complex of iron hydroxide, iron succinylate protein.

Preparations of two- and trivalent iron are comparatively effective but they have differences in tolerability and compliance.

http://dx.doi.org/10.5772/intechopen.71520

In order to overcome the negative effects of salt iron and improve the tolerance an iron drug based on hydroxide of the polymaltose complex (HPC) was created which has advantages over iron salt drugs with high efficiency, safety, no risk of overdose, intoxication and poisonings and less dyspeptic complications. This allows us to recommend iron preparations based on the hydroxide of the polymaltose complex to women with IDA in their reproductive age [25]. Discontinuation of the treatment with iron drugs is indicated after the normalization of serum ferritin and replenishment of the iron storage.

4. Conclusion

Anemia in women of reproductive age is the most frequent extragenital disease. It impairs the quality of women life and in pregnancy, leads to complications of gestation (miscarriage, placental insufficiency, etc.) and adversely affects the growth and development of the fetus. Iron deficiency before conception will disrupt the formation of the nervous tissue (the brain), which is manifested by a decrease in intelligence, disturbances of psychomotor development and other abnormalities in the future. Often the cause of IDA or iron deficiency in women are the organic diseases of the uterus (polyps, fibroids) and functional disorders - abnormal and/or profuse uterine bleeding. Chronic iron deficiency as a rule remains undiagnosed for a long time as there are no expressed clinical symptoms and the body is well adapted to it. Therefore, role of the gynecologist in diagnosing anemia as well as revealing and treatment of gynecological diseases that led to IDA is important. All the iron drugs have the same efficacy but the fewest side effects (in gastrointestinal tract) have been in trivalent drugs which allows them to be recommended for the treatment of anemia in the reproductive age.

Author details

Alina V. Solovyova[1]*, Viola Gace[1], Kristina S. Ermolenko[1] and Vadim A. Khorolskiy[2]

*Address all correspondence to: av_soloveva@mail.ru

1 Department of Obstetrics and Gynecology with the Course of Perinatology of the Peoples Friendship University of Russia (RUDN University), Moscow, Russian Federation

2 Obstetrics and Gynecology of the Perinatal Center of the Regional Clinical Hospital No. 2, Krasnodar, Russian Federation

References

[1] Pavlov AD, Morshchakova EF, Rumyantsev AG. Erythropoiesis, Erythropoietin, Iron. Moscow: GEOTAR-Media; 2011. 304 p

[2] Radzinsky VE, editor. Guide to Outpatient Care in Obstetrics and Gynecology. 2nd ed., Revised, and additional. Moscow: GEOTAR-Media; 2014. 944 p

[3] A teenage girl as a patient. Endocrine gynecology of physiological pubertal: Optimal correction minimum. In: Kuznetsova IV, editor. Information Bulletin. Moscow: Editorial staff of the magazine Status Praesens; 2014. 20 p

[4] Kagamimori S, Fujita T, Naruse Y, Kurosawa Y, Watanabe M. A longitudinal study of serum ferritin concentration during the female adolescent growth spurt. Annals of Human Biology. 1998;**15**:413-419

[5] Ivanyan AN, Nikiforovich II, Litvinov AV. A modern view of anemia in pregnant women. The Russian Bulletin of the Obstetrician-Gynecologist. 2009;**1**:17-20

[6] Konovodova EN, Yakunina NA. Iron deficiency and pregnancy. RMZ. 2010;(19)

[7] Bitzer J, Serrani M, Lahav A. Women's attitudes to heavy menstrual bleeding, and their impact on quality of life. Open Access Journal of Contraception. 2013;**2013**(4):21-28

[8] Heavy Menstrual Bleeding: Assessment and Management. URL: https://www.nice.org.uk/guidance/cg44/chapter/1-guidance

[9] Toxqui L, Pérez-Granados AM, Blanco-Rojo R, et al. A simple and feasible questionnaire to estimate menstrual blood loss: The relationship with hematological and gynecological parameters in young women. BMC Women's Health. 2014;**14**(71). [PMID: 24886470]

[10] Bushnell DM, Martin ML, Moore KA, et al. Menorrhagia Impact Questionnaire: Assessing the influence of heavy menstrual bleeding on quality of life. Current Medical Research and Opinion. 2010;**26**(12):2745-2755. [PMID: 21043553]

[11] Mutovin GR, Zhilina SS, Umakhanova ZR. Neuroontogenesis and its disorders. Children's Hospital. 2009;(2):36-50

[12] Rahman MM, Abe SK, Rahman MS, et al. Maternal anemia and risk of adverse events in the low- and middle-income countries: Systematic review and meta-analysis. Clinical Nutrition. 2016;**103**(2):495-504. [PMID: 26739036]

[13] Radlowski EC, Johnson RW. Perinatal iron deficiency and neurocognitive development. Frontiers in Human Neuroscience. 2013;**7**:585. [PMID: 24065908]

[14] Hare D, Ayton S, Bush A, Lei P. A delicate balance: Iron metabolism and diseases of the brain. Frontiers in Aging Neuroscience. 2013;**5**:34. [PMID: 23874300]

[15] Beard J. Iron deficiency alters brain development and functioning. The Journal of Nutrition. 2003;**133**(1):1468s-1472s. [PMID: 12730445]

[16] Milward E, Acikyol B, Bassett B, et al. Brain changes in iron loading disorders. In: Linert W, Kozlowski H, editors. Metal Ions in Neurological Systems. Wien: Springer-Verlag; 2012. pp. 17-25

[17] Sadrzadeh SMH, Saffari Y. Iron and brain disorders. American Journal of Clinical Pathology. 2004;**121**(1):s64-s70. [PMID: 15298151]

[18] Burke RM, Leon JS, Suchdev PS. Identification, prevention and treatment of iron deficiency during the first 1000 days. Nutrients. 2014;**6**(10):4093-4114. [PMID: 25310252]

[19] Munro MG, Critchley HO, Fraser IS. The FIGO classification of causes of abnormal uterine bleeding in the reproductive years. Fertility and Sterility. 2011;**95**(7):2204-2208. [PMID: 21496802]

[20] Andreeva EN, Hamoshina MB. Report: Abundant uterine bleeding. In: Educational Seminar "Innovations in Obstetrics and Gynecology from the Perspective of Evidence-based Medicine"; Ufa; 2016

[21] Lethaby A, Duckitt K, Farquhar C. Non-steroidal anti-inflammatory drugs for heavy menstrual bleeding. Cochrane Database of Systematic Reviews. 2013;**1**. Art. CD000400. [PMID: 23440779]

[22] Lethaby A, Farquhar C, Cooke I. Antifibrinolytics for heavy menstrual bleeding. Cochrane Database of Systematic Reviews. 2000;**4**. Art. CD000249. [PMID: 11034679]

[23] Wellington K, Wagstaff AJ. Tranexamic acid: A review of its use in the management of menorrhagia. Drugs. 2003;**63**(13):1417-1433. [PMID: 12825966]

[24] Jensen J, Mansour D, Lukkari-Lax E, et al. Bleeding patterns with the levonorgestrel-releasing intrauterine system when used for heavy menstrual bleeding in women without structural pelvic pathology: A pooled analysis of randomized controlled studies. Contraception. 2013;**87**(1):107-112. [PMID: 23040140]

[25] Chernov VM, Tarasova IS. Efficiency and safety of trivalent iron drugs in the treatment of iron deficiency anemia. The Attending Physician. 2013;(8). www.lvrach.ru

[26] Moscow: Rosstat. 2014

Chapter 6

Nutritional Anemia in Elderly Patients of Developed Countries

Emmanuel Andrès

Additional information is available at the end of the chapter

http://dx.doi.org/10.5772/intechopen.70566

Abstract

In this chapter, we report and discuss the current literature of nutrient-deficiency anemia, also called nutritional anemia, in elderly patients in developed countries. For this purpose, a review of medical literatures was conducted searching PubMed, textbooks of hematology, internal medicine and geriatrics, and information collected from international meetings were also included. The term nutrient deficiency or nutritional anemia covers any anemia, defined by a hemoglobin level <13 g/dL (<130 g/L) in men and <12 g/dL (<120 g/L) in women, resulting from a deficiency of materials essential for erythropoiesis. Patients with nutritional anemia often have mild to moderate anemia, with hemoglobin levels between 8 and 10 g/dL (80 and 100 g/L). In practice, nutritional anemia represents one-third of all anemia in elderly patients. About two-third of nutritional anemia is associated with iron deficiency and most of those cases are the result of chronic blood loss from gastrointestinal lesions. The remaining cases of nutritional anemia are usually associated with vitamin B12 (cobalamin), most frequently related to food-cobalamin malabsorption (especially in case of atrophic gastritis), and Biermer's disease (pernicious anemia); and/or vitamin B9 (folate) deficiency, most frequently related to inadequate dietary intake or malnutrition, several drugs (as methotrexate, cotrimoxazole) and chronic alcohol intake. In clinical practice, recognition of these disorders and deficiencies is essential for optimal treatment (nutrient-deficiency replacement).

Keywords: nutritional anemia, nutrient-deficiency anemia, iron deficiency, vitamin B12 deficiency, cobalamin deficiency, vitamin B9 deficiency, folate deficiency, food

1. Introduction

Anemia is a common condition, especially in elderly patients (≥75 years) and its prevalence increases with age [1]. Anemia affects quality of life in all elderly patients. It also affects cognitive and physical function, especially in frailty patients, and be a factor of aggravation or poor prognosis of chronic diseases, e.g., chronic heart failure (CHF), chronic obstructive pulmonary disease (COPD), chronic renal failure, cerebrovascular disorders [2, 3]. Anemia is even associated with a risk of death. Thus, it should not be accepted as an unavoidable condition or a consequence of aging.

In the elderly, many underlying conditions can lead to anemia such as chronic diseases, renal failure, myelodysplastic syndromes, cancer, and unexplained anemia. However, the most common nutrient deficiencies are iron, vitamin B9 (folic acid), and vitamin B12 (cobalamin) deficiency [4]. In clinical practice, recognition of these disorders and deficiencies is essential for optimal treatment.

In this chapter, we report and discuss the current literatures of nutrient-deficiency anemia, also called nutritional anemia, in elderly patients in developed countries.

2. Bibliographic search strategy

A review of the medical literatures was conducted to identify original studies and review articles concerning nutrient-deficiency anemia in elderly patients. In March 2017, PubMed was searched for English- and French-language articles. The terms used for online bibliographic search included "nutrient-deficiency anemia," "nutritional anemia," "iron deficiency," "vitamin B9 deficiency," "folate deficiency," "vitamin B12 deficiency" or "cobalamin deficiency," and "elderly patients." A total of more than 500 abstracts related to clinical trial and reviews were identified between the years 2007 and 2017. All of the abstracts were reviewed by at least two senior researchers. Only 245 publications were eventually retained and 39 publications were used for this review. These publications have been selected because of the quality or the originality of the text, the excellence of the adopted methodology, and the reputation of the authors.

Textbooks of hematology, internal medicine and geriatrics, and information collected from international meetings were also included.

3. Definition of nutritional anemia

The *World Health Organization* (*WHO*) defines anemia in the adult as hemoglobin (Hb) concentration < 12 g/dL (<120 g/L) for nonpregnant women and <13 g/dL (<130 g/L) for men [2]. In elderly, an Hb concentration < 12 g/dL (<120 g/L) is commonly considered as an "*established*" anemia (under strict sense of the academic definition), regardless of the sex of the patient [5].

Although low hemoglobin levels (approximately 1 g/dL lower than the *WHO* standard) are often seen with advancing age, anemia (called "*unexplained*" anemia) should not be assumed to be a normal consequence of aging. Several age-related physiological changes such as renal insufficiency, stem cell aging, androgen insufficiency, and chronic inflammation may contribute either to a decline in red blood cell production or shortened red blood cell survival.

Age may be associated with compromised hematopoietic reserve and consequently with an increased susceptibility to anemia in the presence of hematopoietic stress induced by an underlying disorder [6].

In clinical practice, an Hb level <10 g/dL is often considered to be a cut off level where investigation in the elderly (*"anemia to explore"*), and treatment should be performed [7]. Indeed, at this Hb level, several recent studies have shown a benefit from investigating the anemia and for treating, in regard to the frequency of discovery of a curable etiology [7].

Nutrient-deficiency or nutritional anemia refers to types of anemia that can be directly attributed to *"nutritional disorders"* [4, 8]. Thus, the term nutrient deficiency or nutritional anemia covers any anemia resulting from a deficiency of nutrients essential for red blood cell formation, for example: iron; vitamins, especially vitamin B9 (folate), but also vitamin B12 (cobalamin) and vitamin C (in scurvy), and more rarely, vitamin A, vitamin E, and vitamin B2 (riboflavin), vitamin B3 (in pellagra), vitamin B6 (pyridoxine); selenium, zinc, and cooper; and protein [8].

4. Prevalence of nutritional anemia

The prevalence of anemia increases with advancing age, especially after age 60–65 years, and rises sharply after the age of 80 years [2, 6]. Currently, anemia in this population represents a public health problem in developed countries.

In the United States (US), results from the third *National Health and Nutrition Examination Survey* (*NHANES III*) indicate that the prevalence of anemia among elderly individuals, living in towns, aged 75 or more and 85 or more, were 15.7% in men and 10.3% in women and 26.1% for men and 20.1% in women, respectively [1]. Survey findings indicate further that most anemia among the middle age and elderly is mild; only 2.8% of women and 1.6% of men had an Hb <11 g/dL [9]. Results from the *NHANES III* also indicate that nutrient-deficiency anemia represents at least one-third of all causes of anemia [1].

In the US, results from the Framingham cohort indicate a lower prevalence of anemia among 1016 subjects within 67–96 years of age. In this group, the prevalence of anemia in men and women was 6.1 and 10.5%, respectively [10]. In this study, in addition to anemia of inflammation and of renal failure, nutritional anemia was also a major cause of anemia.

In a French nationwide study of 1351 patients hospitalized in several departments of Internal Medicine, anemia was present in 874 (65%) patients according to the *WHO* definition, and 573 (42%) patients had an Hb level of <11 g/dL (<11 g/L) [11].

5. Etiology of anemia with a focus on nutritional anemia

Because elderly patients often have several associated co-morbid conditions and are commonly taking a variety of medications, some of which may contribute to anemia, the precise etiology of anemia is frequently difficult to determine, even after extensive investigations, including bone marrow biopsy [3, 13]. Thus, according to the literatures and in our own experience, the etiology of anemia can be identified in only approximately 80% of the cases, in spite of the use of new tools such as video capsule [7, 14]. Moreover, a significant proportion of elderly anemic patients, around 30–50%, are presumed to have multiple causes for their anemia [14, 15]. In cases where the causes of anemia have not been established, an inadequate diagnostic work-up for the patient could be suspected.

In the elderly, causes of anemia are divided into three main broad groups: (1) "nutrient-deficiency or nutritional anemia," mainly in relation with iron deficiency anemia; (2) "anemia of chronic disease," including anemia related to renal failure, chronic inflammation, chronic heart failure; and (3) "unexplained anemia" [2, 3, 9]. In the aforementioned *NHANES III* study, 34% of all anemia in adults and elderly patients were caused by iron, vitamin B9 (folate), and vitamin B12 (cobalamin) deficiency, alone or in combination (nutrient-deficiency anemia) [1]. In this study, 12% of all anemia were related, perhaps at least associated, with renal insufficiency, 20% with chronic diseases, and in 34% of the cases, the cause of anemia remained unexplained.

About 60% of nutritional anemia is associated with iron deficiency and most of those cases are the result of chronic blood loss from gastrointestinal lesions in developed countries [1]. The remaining cases of nutrient-deficiency anemia are usually associated with vitamin B12 and/or vitamin B9 deficiency and are easily treated. In **Table 1**, we report our personal experience (retrospective study) of the etiology of anemia in 300 hospitalized patients of ≥65 years old [4, 7].

Rare unknown causes of nutrient-deficiency anemia include several other vitamin deficiencies (e.g., vitamins A, B2, B3, C, and E), selenium, zinc, or cooper [8]. These later etiologies are nevertheless not well-studied in the literature, and to date, few not well-documented data are available, except for the theoretical and pathological aspects of anemia.

Etiology	**Prevalence (%)**
Chronic inflammation (chronic disease)	23.0
Iron deficiency	18
Renal failure	9
Liver disease and endocrine disease (chronic disease)	7
Posthemorrhagic	7
Folate deficiency	6
Myelodysplasia	5
Vitamin B12 deficiency	4
Unexplained causes	21

Table 1. Etiology of anemia in patients older than 65 years (n = 300), hospitalized in an internal medicine department (tertiary reference center) [7].

6. Iron deficiency anemia in the elderly

Iron deficiency anemia, the most common cause of anemia in the elderly [1], results usually from chronic gastrointestinal (GI) blood loss mainly caused by esophagitis, gastritis, ulcer, related or not related to nonsteroidal anti-inflammatory drug intake, and/or chronic *Helicobacter pylori* infections, varices (portal hypertension), premalignant polyps, colorectal cancer, or angiodysplasia [15, 16].

It is important to keep in mind that GI blood loss is often occult and is not ruled out by negative fecal blood tests. In elderly, GI tract abnormalities can be identified with appropriate investigations (mainly invasive and require general anesthesia) in the majority of patients with iron deficiency anemia [14]. In 40–60% of patients, the source is in the upper GI tract and the identified cause of GI blood loss is benign [18, 19]. In 15–30% of patients, the source of GI blood loss is in the colon, here also with mainly benign lesions. **Table 2** presents our experience of the evaluation of the GI tract in 90 patients with chronic blood loss during their follow-up in an internal medicine department (in a referral center) [7].

The source of bleeding is not found in the remaining 10–40% of patients with GI blood loss. Fortunately, these patients do well with iron replacement and repeated investigation may be only proposed in *"to good health"* elderly patients [15]. In these patients, repeated GI investigation with upper and/or lower endoscopy and video capsule may be of interest, with the detection of the etiology of bleeding in an additional 20% of cases [19, 20]. It is important because one-third of the iron deficiency anemia is related to GI malignancies. In our experience, repeated investigation is not recommended in frailty elderly patients [21].

Etiology	Prevalence (%)
Esophagitis and Mallory Weiss syndrome	4.4
Gastritis, atrophic gastritis and ulcer related or not related to NSAID use and/or *Helicobacter pylori* infection	30
Varices related to portal hypertension	9
Angiodysplasia	2.25
Colon diverticula	4.5
Colorectal benign and pre-malignant polyps	5.5
Colorectal cancer	5.5
Inflammatory bowel disease	2.25
Unexplained causes	36.6

NSAID: nonsteroidal anti-inflammatory drug.

Table 2. Results of the evaluation of the gastrointestinal tract in elderly patients (≥65 years) with chronic blood loss (n = 90), hospitalized in an internal medicine department [14].

H. pylori infection, chronic gastritis (especially atrophic gastritis), and coeliac disease are associated with "*unexplained GI iron deficiency anemia*" [22]. More rarely, large amount of tea (at least 2 L/day), vegetarian and theoretically long-term anti-acid medication intake are also associated with this condition [15]. In practice, any elderly subject whose dietary intake is poor and has recent unexplained weight loss is a candidate for increased medical surveillance [23].

Chronic blood loss from the genitourinary tract and exceptionally from chronic hemoptysis may result in iron deficiency [15]. In this situation, bleeding disorders and particularly anticoagulant and antiplatelet medications may promote the development of iron deficiency in the elderly (around 20% in our experience) [7, 14].

7. Vitamin B9 and vitamin B12 deficiency anemia in the elderly

Both vitamin B9 and B12 deficiencies are common among elderly, each occurring in at least 5% of the patients [15]. The Framingham study demonstrated an incidence of 12% among elderly people living in the community [24].

Vitamin B9 deficiency usually develops as a result of inadequate dietary intake and malnutrition, quiet frequent in elderly patients of malabsorption, as in coeliac disease [1, 15]. In fact, a regular diet contains 500–700 μg of vitamin B9 and the body contains very little vitamin B9 with stocks expected to last 4–6 months. The affected patients usually have a history of weight loss, poor weight gain, and weakness. This is particularly the case in Alzheimer's patient or in patients with advanced dementia. In addition, several drugs (methotrexate, cotrimoxazole, sulfasalazine, anticonvulsants) and alcohol—even in elderly—may cause deficiency of folic acid [7].

In elderly patients, the etiologies of vitamin B12 deficiency are represented primarily by food-cobalamin malabsorption (FCM) and Biermer's disease, also called pernicious anemia. The FCM is not a real malabsorption in view of physiopathology, but a maldigestion of vitamin B12 (linked to food). More rarely, the etiologies of vitamin B12 deficiency include intake deficiency and true malabsorption, related for example, to digestive tract surgery [25]. In a study by our group (n = 200), FCM accounted for about 60–70% of the etiologies of vitamin B12 deficiency and about 15–25% in Biermer's disease [26, 27]. **Figure 1** presents the principal causes of vitamin B12 deficiency in 172 elderly patients (median age: 70 years) hospitalized in the University Hospital of Strasbourg, France [26].

FCM is characterized by the inability to release cobalamin from food and/or intestinal transport proteins, particularly in case of hypochlorhydria, where the absorption of "unbound" cobalamin is normal ("*mal digestion*" of the food-cobalamin) [28]. As we have recently indicated, this syndrome is defined by cobalamin deficiency despite sufficient cobalamin intake from food and a normal Schilling test, where the later rules out malabsorption or pernicious anemia [29]. FCM is caused primarily by atrophic gastritis [28]. Other factors that commonly contribute to FCM in elderly people include chronic carriage and infection of *H. pylori*; intestinal microbial proliferation; long-term ingestion of antacids (e.g., proton-pump inhibitors), and biguanides (metformin); chronic alcoholism; surgery or gastric reconstruction (e.g., bypass surgery for obesity); partial and pancreatic exocrine failure [29]. It should be emphasized that

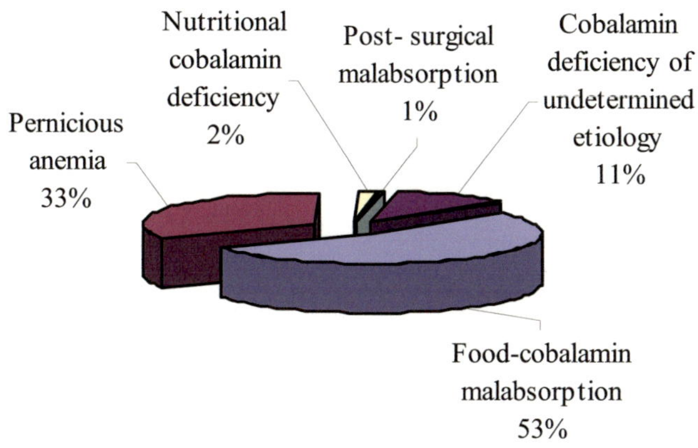

Figure 1 . Etiologies of cobalamin deficiency in 172 elderly patients hospitalized in the University Hospital of Strasbourg, France [25, 29].

Carmel first believed that FCM was associated with moderate cobalamin deficiency, leading to only "subtle" clinical symptoms ("*subtle cobalamin deficiency*") [30]. However in our experience, the clinical manifestations of FCM are not very different from those of cobalamin deficiencies associated with other causes, e.g., Biermer's disease [29].

Biermer's disease is caused by impaired absorption of vitamin B12 due to the neutralization of intrinsic factor action in the setting of immune atrophic gastritis (loss of intrinsic factor in genetic form) [4, 25]. In practice, the diagnosis of Biermer's disease is based on the presence of: (i) intrinsic factor antibodies in serum (specificity: >98%, sensibility: around 50%) and/or (ii) autoimmune atrophic gastritis (the presence of *H. pylori* infection in gastric biopsies is an exclusion factor) [4, 25]. It is to note that Biermer's disease is associated with other immunological diseases, even in the elderly, such as Sjögren's syndrome, Hashimoto's disease, type 1 diabetes mellitus, or coeliac disease.

8. Clinical presentation of nutritional anemia

In elderly patients, the onset of anemic symptoms (fatigue, asthenia) and signs (pallor, palpitations) is usually insidious because majority of these patients adjust their physical activities, stay at home, and take several drugs which mask the anemic symptomatology. Thus, these symptoms may be overlooked and undiagnosed. [15]. In elderly, anemia may be revealed by the exacerbation of chronic-associated conditions or disorders, as dyspnea or edema of the legs related to worsening of cardiac failure. Anemia has also been reported to worsen angina, cognitive dysfunction related to cerebrovascular insufficiency [6].

In elderly patients, anemia has been associated with an increased risk for mortality, a longer hospitalization for elective procedures and a decreased quality of life [6, 31].

Iron, vitamin B9, and vitamin B12 deficiencies may be associated with specific symptoms and clinical manifestations. **Table 3** presents features related to vitamin B12 deficiency

Neuropsychiatric manifestations	Digestive manifestations	Other manifestations
• Frequent: polyneurites (especially sensitive ones), ataxia, Babinski's phenomenon • Classic: combined sclerosis of the spinal cord • Rare: cerebellar syndromes affecting the cranial nerves including optic neuritis, optic atrophy, urinary and/or fecal incontinence Under study: changes in the higher functions, even dementia, stroke and atherosclerosis (hyperhomocysteinemia), parkinsonian syndromes, depression, multiple sclerosis	• Classic: Hunter's glossitis, jaundice, LDH and bilirubin elevation ("intramedullary destruction") • Deba Table: abdominal pain, dyspepsia, nausea, vomiting, diarrhea, disturbances in intestinal functioning • Rare: resistant and recurring mucocutaneous ulcers cobalamin deficiency	• Under study: atrophy of the vaginal mucosa and chronic vaginal and urinary infections (especially mycosis), venous thromboembolic disease, angina (hyperhomocysteinemia)

Table 3. Manifestations related to vitamin B12 deficiency (in addition to hematological manifestations) [25].

in elderly patients [25]. The features of vitamin B9 deficiency are nearly indistinguishable from those of vitamin B12 deficiency, although the symptomatology is generally less severe. Iron deficiency is responsible for changes in hair (hair loss), nails (koilonychias), glossitis, dermatitis herpetiformis, photodermatitis, restless legs syndrome, and/or Plummer's syndrome [32].

9. Biological abnormalities related to nutritional anemia

Patients with nutritional anemia often have mild to moderate anemia, with Hb levels between 8 and 10 g/dL. This anemia is generally hyporegenerative, with a low reticulocyte count ($<50 \times 10^9$/L). This represents the consequence of the reduced activity of the hematopoietic system to replace the peripheral blood loss or deficiency [12, 15].

In elderly, the anemia is frequently "normocytic," with a mean erythrocyte cell volume (MECV) between 80 and 100 fL. This normocytic nature of the anemia is related to the multifactorial etiologies of anemia. In exclusive iron deficiency, the erythrocytes are usually "microcytic," with a MECV <80 fL (main differential diagnoses: chronic inflammation, thalassemia). In exclusive vitamin B9 and/or vitamin B12 deficiency, the erythrocytes are usually "macrocytic," with a MECV >120 fL (main differential diagnosis: alcohol, hypothyroidism, and myelodysplastic syndromes). Other hematological abnormalities and manifestations may also be associated with cobalamin deficiency as listed in **Table 4** [33].

Iron deficiency is documented by a low serum iron level, an increased total iron-binding capacity, and a low serum ferritin level (<15 ng/mL) [17]. In cases associated with chronic inflammation, the transferrin receptor-ferritin index appears to be the most appropriate parameter to discriminate between the two disorders [17].

Parameters	Values
Hemoglobin level (g/dL)	10.3 ± 0.4 (4.9–15.1)
Mean erythrocyte cell volume (fL)	98.9 ± 25.6 (76–142)
Reticulocyte count (%)	15.2 (1–32)
White cell count (/mm^3)	6200 ± 4100 (500–20,000)
Platelet count (10^3/mm^3)	146 ± 42 (27–580)
Anemia with Hb level < 12 g/dL	37%
Anemia with Hb level < 6 g/dL	2.5%
Anemia and macrocytosis (MECV >100 fL)	33.8%
Isolated macrocytosis (MECV >100 fL)	17%
Microcytosis (MECV <80 fL)	5%
White cell count <4000/mm^3	14%
Neutrophil count <1000/mm^3	3%
Thrombopenia (<150 × 10^3/mm^3)	10%
Neutrophil hypersegmentation	32%
Megaloblastosis	60%
Life threatening manifestations	9%

MECV: mean erythrocyte cell volume.

Table 4. Hematological manifestations in patients with documented cobalamin deficiency (n = 201), hospitalized in an internal medicine department (tertiary reference center) [33].

Vitamin B12 deficiency is usually documented by a low serum vitamin B12 level (<200 pg/mL). An increase of the serum methylmalonic acid or homocysteine levels should be established to exclude a false negative result for vitamin B12 [30]. In vitamin B9 deficiency, the red cell vitamin B9 concentration is the recommended investigation [30].

10. Treatment of nutritional anemia

In iron deficiency anemia, iron supplementation should be initiated in association with the treatment of the underlying cause of bleeding. Treatment of nutritional anemia requires particular attention to establish the correct cause in all patients, particularly in elderly patients in a very good general condition of the body or mind [15]. Standard therapy for iron deficiency is an oral administration of 200–300 mg of ferrous sulfate (60 mg of elemental iron) [34, 35]. Oral iron supplementation is usually the first choice for the treatment of iron deficiency anemia because of its effectiveness and low cost. Vitamin C enhances iron absorption. Intravenous iron replacement may be reserved for patients with iron deficiency that fails to respond to oral replacement or in patients with documented malabsorption, inflammatory bowel diseases, malignancies, renal failure, and also perhaps in anemic patients with chronic heart failure. Parenteral iron supplementation may also be used when there is an intolerance or noncompliance with oral preparations. Intravenous iron sucrose is reasonably well tolerated, even when administered in boluses [35].

In elderly patients, vitamin B12 deficiency anemia may be treated by vitamin B12 supplementation, parenterally (commonly intramuscular) or orally [36, 37]. Our team (*CAREnce en vitamine B12* [Care B12]) in the University Hospital of Strasbourg (France) has developed an effective oral treatment for cobalamin deficiency. The main results of our protocol of oral cobalamin therapy studies are summarized in **Table 5** [36] A systematic review conducted under the auspices of the *Cochrane Metabolic and Endocrine Disorders Review Group* also supports the efficacy of oral cobalamin therapy, with: (1) a daily dose of 2000 and 1000 μg for 1 month of crystalline cyanocobalamin

Study characteristics (number of patients)	Therapeutic modalities	Results
Open prospective study of well-documented vitamin B12 deficiency related to food-cobalamin malabsorption (n = 10)	Oral crystalline cyanocobalamin: 650 μg/day, during the condition and continue at least 3 months	• Normalization of serum vitamin B12 levels in 80% of the patients • Significant increase of Hb levels (mean of 1.9 g/dL) and decrease of MECV (mean of 7.8 fL)
Open prospective study of low vitamin B12 levels not related to pernicious anemia (n = 20)	Oral crystalline cyanocobalamin: 1000 μg/day during the condition and continue at least 1 week	• Normalization of serum vitamin B12 levels in 85% of the patients
Open prospective study of well-documented vitamin B12 deficiency related to food-cobalamin malabsorption (n = 30)	Oral crystalline cyanocobalamin: between 1000 and 250 μg/day, during the condition and continue at least 1 month	• Normalization of serum vitamin B12 levels in 87% of the patients • Significant increase of Hb levels (mean of 0.6 g/dL) and decrease of MECV (mean of 3 fL); normalization of Hb levels and MECV in 54 and 100% of the patients, respectively • Dose effect–effectiveness dose of vitamin B12 ≥500 μg/day
Open prospective study of low vitamin B12 levels not related to pernicious anemia (n = 30)	Oral crystalline cyanocobalamin: between 1000 and 125 μg/day during the condition and continue at least 1 week	• Normalization of serum vitamin B12 levels in all patients with at least a dose of vitamin ≥250 μg/day • Dose effect–effectiveness dose of vitamin B12 ≥500 μg/day
Open prospective study of low vitamin B12 levels related to pernicious anemia (n = 10)	Oral crystalline cyanocobalamin: 1000 μg/day, during the condition and continue at least 3 months	• Significant increase of serum vitamin B12 levels in 90% of the patients (mean of 117.4 pg/mL • Significant increase of Hb levels (mean of 2.45 g/dL) and decrease of MECV (mean of 10.4 fL)

Hb: hemoglobin; MECV: mean erythrocyte cell volume.

Table 5. Study by our team on oral cobalamin therapy: Results on hematological manifestations [36].

for FCM and Biermer's disease; and (2) thereafter, a weekly dose between 2000 and 1000 μg of vitamin B12 for FCM and a daily dose of 1000 μg (for all the life) in case of Biermer's disease [37].

In vitamin B9 deficiency, therapeutic doses of vitamin B9 vary between 1 and 5 mg/day [38]. Usually, supplementation is continued for at least 3–6 months, provided that the underlying causes of the deficiencies have been corrected.

Food sources of nutrients are best for prevention of nutritional anemia, but often supplementation is necessary, especially for the elderly [39]. The *USA National Academy of Sciences* recommends that vitamin B9 and vitamin B12 standardized supplementation should be done (fortified cereal) in elderly.

11. Conclusions

In elderly patients, nutritional anemia represents 30–40% of all anemia. About two-third of this nutritional anemia is related to iron deficiency. Iron deficiency anemia is mainly the result of chronic blood loss from gastrointestinal lesions (with benign lesions in two-third of the cases). The remaining cases of nutritional anemia are usually associated with vitamin B12 and/or vitamin B9 deficiency. In elderly patients, vitamin B12 deficiency is most frequently related to food-cobalamin malabsorption; vitamin B9 is related to inadequate dietary intake or malnutrition, several drugs (as methotrexate, cotrimoxazole) and chronic alcohol intake. Treatment of nutritional anemia is simple and involves replacement of the deficient nutrient but requires particular attention to discerning the cause.

Conflict of interest

None related to the content of the present chapter.

Author details

Emmanuel Andrès

Address all correspondence to: emmanuel.andres@chru-strasbourg.fr

Departments of Internal Medicine, Diabetes and Metabolic Disorders, University Hospital of Strasbourg, Strasbourg, France

References

[1] National Health and Nutrition Examination Survey. Anthropometric Reference Data, United States. 1988-1994. Available from: http://www.cdc.gov/nchs/about/major/nhanes/Anthropometric%20Measures. [Accessed: January 7, 2016]

[2] Eisenstaedt R, Penninx BW, Woodman RC. Anemia in the elderly: Current understanding and emerging concepts. Blood Reviews. 2006;**20**:213-226

[3] Woodman R, Ferrucci L, Guralnik J. Anemia in older adults. Current Opinion in Hematology. 2005;**12**:123-128

[4] Andrès E, Federici L, Serraj K, Kaltenbach G. Update of nutrient-deficiency anemia in elderly patients. European Journal of Internal Medicine. 2008;**19**:488-493

[5] Izaks GJ, Westendorp RG, Knook DL. The definition of anemia in older persons. Journal of the American Medical Association. 1999;**281**:1714-1717

[6] Balducci L, Ershler WB, Krantz S. Anemia in the elderly. Clinical findings and impact on health. Critical Reviews in Oncology/Hematology. 2006;**58**:156-165

[7] Andrès E, Serraj K, Federici L, Vogel T, Kaltenbach G. Anemia in elderly patients: New insight into an old disorder. Geriatrics & Gerontology International. 2013;**13**:519-527

[8] Fishman SM, Christian P, Keith PW. The role of vitamins in the prevention and control of anaemia. Public Health Nutrition. 2000;**3**:125-150

[9] Guralnik JM, Eisenstaedt RS, Ferrucci L, Klein HG, Woodman RC. Prevalence of anemia in persons 65 years and older in the United States: Evidence for a high rate of unexplained anemia. Blood. 2004;**104**:2263-2268

[10] Fleming DJ, Jacques PF, Tucker KL, Massaro JM, D'Agostino RB, Wilson PW, et al. Iron status of the free-living, elderly Framingham heart study cohort: An iron-replete population with a high prevalence of elevated iron stores. The American Journal of Clinical Nutrition. 2001;**73**:638-646

[11] Terrier B, Resche-Rigon M, Andrès E, Bonnet F, Hachulla E, Marie I, et al., on behalf of the Groupe de Recherche sur les Anémies en Médecine Interne (GRAMI). Prevalence, characteristics and prognostic significance of anemia in daily practice: Results from a French nationwide cross-sectional and prospective longitudinal study. Quarterly Journal of Medicine: An International Journal of Medicine. 2012;**105**:345-354

[12] Carmel R. Anemia and aging: An overview of clinical, diagnostic and biological issues. Blood Reviews. 2001;**15**:9-18

[13] Joosten E, Pelemans W, Hiele M, Noyen J, Verhaeghe R, Boogaerts MA. Prevalence and causes of anaemia in a geriatric hospitalization population. Gerontology. 1992;**38**:111-117

[14] Petrosyan I, Blaison G, Andrès E, Federici L. Anemia in the elderly: Etiologic profile in a prospective cohort of 95 hospitalized patients. European Journal of Internal Medicine. 2012;**23**:524-528

[15] Smith DL. Anemia in the elderly. American Family Physician. 2000;**62**:1565-1572

[16] Suzuki H, Marshall BJ, Hibi T. Overview: *Helicobacter pylori* and extragastric disease. International Journal of Hematology. 2006;**84**:291-300

[17] Rimon E, Levy S, Sapir A, Gelzer G, Peled R, Ergas D, et al. Diagnosis of iron deficiency anemia in the elderly by transferrin receptor-ferritin index. Archives of Internal Medicine. 2002;**162**:445-449

[18] Rockey DC. Occult and obscure gastrointestinal bleeding: Causes and clinical management. Nature Reviews. Gastroenterology & Hepatology. 2010;**7**:265-279

[19] Liu K, Kaffes AJ. Iron deficiency anaemia: A review of diagnosis, investigation and management. European Journal of Gastroenterology & Hepatology. 2012;**24**:109-116

[20] Muhammad A, Vidyarthi G, Brady P. Role of small bowel capsule endoscopy in the diagnosis and management of iron deficiency anemia in elderly: A comprehensive review of the current literature. World Journal of Gastroenterology. 2014;**20**:8416-8423

[21] Camaschella C. Iron-deficiency anemia. The New England Journal of Medicine. 2015;**372**: 1832-1843

[22] Nahon S, Lahmek P, Massard J, Lesgourgues B, Mariaud de Serre N, Traissac L, et al. *Helicobacter pylori*-associated chronic gastritis and unexplained iron deficiency anemia: A reliable association? Helicobacter. 2003;**8**:573-577

[23] Milman N, Pedersen AN, Ovesen L, Schroll M. Iron status in 358 apparently healthy 80- year-old Danish men and women: Relation to food composition and dietary and supplemental iron intake. Annals of Hematology. 2004;**83**:423-429

[24] Lindenbaum J, Rosenberg IH, Wilson PW, Tabler SP, Allen RH. Prevalence of cobalamin deficiency in the Framingham elderly population. The American Journal of Clinical Nutrition. 1994;**60**:2-11

[25] Andrès E, Loukili NH, Noel E, Kaltenbach G, Ben Abdelgheni M, Perrin AE, et al. Vitamin B12 (cobalamin) deficiency in elderly patients. Canadian Medical Association Journal. 2004;**171**:251-260

[26] Andrès E, Affenberger S, Vinzio S, Kurtz JE, Noel E, Kaltenbach G, et al. Food-cobalamin malabsorption in elderly patients: Clinical manifestations and treatment. The American Journal of Medicine. 2005;**118**:1154-1159

[27] Andrès E, Perrin AE, Demangeat C, Kurtz JE, Vinzio S, Grunenberger F, et al. The syndrome of food-cobalamin malabsorption revisited in a Department of Internal Medicine. A monocentric cohort study of 80 patients. European Journal of Internal Medicine. 2003;**14**:221-226

[28] Carmel R. Malabsorption of food-cobalamin. Bailliere's Clinical Haematology. 1995;**8**: 639-655

[29] Andrès E, Serraj K, Mecili M, Kaltenbach G, Vogel T. The syndrome of food-cobalamin malabsorption: A personal view in a perspective of clinical practice. Journal of Blood Disorders and Transfusion. 2011;**2**:108. DOI: 10.4172/2155-9864.1000108

[30] Carmel R. Diagnosis and management of clinical and subclinical cobalamin deficiencies: Why controversies persist in the age of sensitive metabolic testing. Biochimie. 2013;**95**: 1047-1055

[31] Gabrilove J. Anemia and the elderly: Clinical considerations. Best Practice Research & Clinical Haematology. 2005;**18**:417-422

[32] Sato S. Iron deficiency: Structural and microchemical changes in hair, nails, and skin. Seminars in Dermatology. 1991;**10**:313-319

[33] Federici L, Loukili NH, Zimmer J, Affenberger S, Maloisel F, Andrès E. Manifestations hématologiques de la carence en vitamine B12: données personnelles et revue de la littérature. La Revue de Médecine Interne. 2007;**28**:225-231

[34] Umbreit J. Iron deficiency: A concise review. American Journal of Hematology. 2005;**78**: 225-231

[35] Avni T, Bieber A, Grossman A, Green H, Leibovici L, Gafter-Gvili A. The safety of intravenous iron preparations: Systematic review and meta-analysis. Mayo Clinic Proceedings. 2015;**90**:12-23

[36] Andrès E. Oral cobalamin (vitamin B12) therapy: From empiricism and personal experience to evidence based medicine and perspective of recommendations and guideline. Journal of Blood Disorders and Transfusion. 2012;**3**:e102. DOI: 10.4172/2155-9864.1000e102

[37] Vidal-Alaball J, Butler CC, Cannings-John R, Goringe A, Hood K, McCaddon A, et al. Oral vitamin B12 versus intramuscular vitamin B12 for vitamin B12 deficiency. Cochrane Database of Systematic Reviews. 2005;**20**:CD004655

[38] Wickramasinghe SN. Diagnosis of megaloblastic anaemias. Blood Reviews. 2006;**20**: 299-318

[39] Yen PK. Nutritional anemia. Geriatric Nursing. 2000;**21**:111-112

Section 3

Anemia in Different Diseases

Chapter 7

Anemia and IBD: Current Status and Future Prospectives

Ana Isabel Lopes and Sara Azevedo

Additional information is available at the end of the chapter

http://dx.doi.org/10.5772/intechopen.69203

Abstract

Anemia is a common complication of inflammatory bowel disease (IBD), usually recognized at diagnosis and during flare-ups. However, the exact prevalence of anemia associated to IBD (IBD-A) is unknown. Despite its major clinical relevance and quality of life impact in both adult and pediatric IBD patients, it has been for long time neglected. It is mostly multifactorial, being a unique example of the combination of chronic iron deficiency (ID) and anemia of chronic disease (ACD). The current management of IBD-A represents a paradigm shift in clinical practice, involving several challenges. A pro-active approach is recommended and with the new generation of available iron compounds and recent guidelines, the ultimate goal will be the improvement of the patients' quality of life. Sound data are still lacking, concerning the best treatment/prevention approach for IDA/ID. Based on current evidence, oral iron therapy might be preferred in mild IDA, whereas intravenous iron may be advantageous in more severe IDA/flaring IBD. Long-term prospective clinical trials are needed, to optimize treatment schedule and to better define the clinical and hematological long-term outcomes, both in adults and in children. They should demonstrate the efficacy, safety, and tolerance profile of different available iron formulas, as well as their cost-efficacy ratio.

Keywords: anemia, iron deficiency, anemia of chronic disease, inflammatory bowel disease, Crohn's disease, pediatrics, childhood, adulthood

1. Introduction

Anemia is the most common systemic complication and extraintestinal manifestation of inflammatory bowel disease (IBD), particularly in Crohn's disease (CD) patients [1–3]. Although it may be present anytime along the disease course, it is usually recognized at diagnosis and during flare-ups. However, despite its major clinical relevance and quality of life (QoL) impact in both adult and pediatric IBD patients, it has been for long time neglected in this clinical setting [4].

Following the introduction in the last decade of new intravenous (IV) and oral iron therapies, IBD-associated anemia (IBD-A) has been deserving major attention from the scientific community. Furthermore, the increasing focus on extra-digestive features of IBD, in parallel with the recent emergence of specific management guidelines concerning IBD-A from the European Crohn's and Colitis Organisation (ECCO) [5], has also contributed to a paradigm shift in the clinical approach of this clinical entity.

In fact, anemia in IBD is not just a laboratory marker; it is a complication of IBD that requires increased awareness and needs appropriate and timely diagnostic and therapeutic approaches. The impact of anemia on the quality of life of IBD patients is substantial, as it affects several aspects of quality of life, such as physical, emotional, and cognitive functions, work or school absenteeism, hospitalization rate, and health-care costs [4, 6]. Thus, it seems to be reasonable that both in adult and in pediatric IBD patients, anemia should be recognized, comprehensively evaluated, and treated. Furthermore, not only a disease-specific treatment has to be administered but in particular iron-deficiency anemia should be treated, as there is a sound body of evidence demonstrating its beneficial impact in patients' quality of life [4, 6].

2. Prevalence of anemia in IBD setting

The exact prevalence of IBD-A is unknown [3, 4, 6]. Reported prevalence rates of anemia in IBD adult patients widely range from 6 to 74%, depending on the definition of anemia, the study design, the patient population considered (e.g., hospitalized patients versus outpatients), and the standards of screening and treatment [4, 6]. In a recent systematic review, the mean prevalence of anemia in adult patients treated in tertiary referral centers with CD was 27% (95% confidence interval 19–35) and 21% (95% confidence interval 15–27) for ulcerative colitis (UC) [6]. Not surprisingly, anemia is reported more frequently in hospitalized patients with IBD and occurs more frequently in CD as compared to UC. In fact, according to recent published studies, the calculated mean prevalence was 20% among outpatients and 68% among hospitalized IBD patients. Furthermore, women with CD are at a higher risk for anemia. It also appears that hemoglobin (Hb) concentrations increase in the years after diagnosis which may be explained by the remission of disease following successful medical or surgical treatment.

The currently used World Health Organization (WHO) definition of anemia (**Table 1**) applies also to patients with IBD [7–9]. As mentioned in the subsequent text, anemia in IBD is mainly the expression of a mixed pathogenesis with iron deficiency (ID) and anemia of chronic disease (ACD) as the most prominent factors, often coexisting [10]. However, ID is the most frequent cause, with a reported prevalence between 36 and 90% [4, 7]. Recent Scandinavian data in adults indicated the prevalence of iron deficiency anemia (IDA) at 20% and of isolated iron deficiency at 30% (without anemia). After treatment is stopped, IDA has been reported to recur after a 10-month period and iron deficiency after 19 months after treatment [1–4].

Iron deficiency anemia
1. Mucosal inflammation
2. Chronic GI lost
3. Low absorption
4. Poor appetite/malnutrition
5. Dietary restrictions
Anemia of chronic disease
1. Disturbed iron deposit distribution
2. Immuno-mediated modification of iron transportation: iron retention in macrophages; functional iron deficiency: iron deficiency erythropoiesis
3. Inhibition of erythropoietin activity
Drug-induced anemia
1. Differentiation and proliferation inhibition of erythroid progenitor cells
2. Myelosuppressor effect of drugs—direct effect: thiopurines (azathioprine); indirect effect "anti-folic": salazopyrine
3. Sulfasalazine effect: impaired folic acid absorption; hemolysis; medullary aplasia
Vitamin B12 e folic acid deficiency anemia

Table 1. Major causes of anemia in IBD and underlying pathophysiology.

Recognized limitations concerning most studies on the prevalence of IDA in patients with IBD are their retrospective nature or the fact of being surveys from referral centers. Recently, Ott et al. [10] have prospectively assessed the prevalence of IDA in a population-based cohort at the time of first diagnosis and during the early course of the disease. A high prevalence of IDA at different points during the early course of disease was reported. At first diagnosis, anemia of chronic disease was predominant, whereas during follow-up, iron deficiency became the most relevant reason of anemia. These findings are in line with data of other groups [4, 6], also describing a strong association between the severity of anemia and disease activity.

A possible explanation of these findings might be the population-based character of Ott et al. study [10], as not only outpatients of a tertiary referral center were included in this study but also patients with less severe forms of IBD, which are mainly treated by their family doctors. In this setting, reasons for the insufficient response to the treatment might have been underdosing of iron supplementation, subclinical inflammation of the underlying disease, or lack of adherence of the patient. Surprisingly, only in one-third of patients with proven anemia, further diagnostic approach was undertaken. Even patients with diagnosed iron-deficiency anemia were infrequently and inconsequently treated with iron preparations, despite the high impact on quality of life.

Limited previous data suggest that anemia is more prevalent in children than in adults with IBD [7–10], although, to date, there have been no good comparative studies. Although anemia and iron deficiency might be at least as common in pediatric as in adult patients with IBD, the true prevalence in childhood is not known. In fact, IBD-A has been recently estimated more common (about 70%) in children than in adults (about 30–40%) [10, 11]. In a recent cross-sectional observational study, including pediatric and adult IBD patients, Goodhand et al. [11] found a prevalence of anemia of 70% (41/59) in children, 42% (24/54) in adolescents, and 40% (49/124) in adults ($P < 0.01$). Furthermore, children (88% (36/41)) and adolescents (83% (20/24)) were more frequently iron-deficient than adults (55% (27/49)).

Recent population-based studies have demonstrated that the phenotype of IBD presenting in the young patient differs from that of adult-onset disease [5, 6]. Children and adolescents are more likely to be diagnosed with CD than UC, with a more severe and extensive disease distribution at presentation and more frequent extension of disease during the first 2 years [5, 6]. Since they tend to have more severe IBD, it has been hypothesized that the prevalence of anemia would be predictably greater in children and adolescents than in adults attending IBD outpatient clinics. Although in 2007, Gasche et al. have published the first guidelines on the diagnosis and management of iron deficiency and IBD-IDA [12], only recently the first ECCO guidelines on the management of IDA and ID have emerged. Both guidelines concern IBD-associated anemia, but no specific considerations on the treatment of pediatric IBD patients have yet been included [5, 13].

3. Pathophysiology of anemia

In the majority of cases, IBD-A is mostly multifactorial, being a unique example of the combination of chronic ID and anemia of chronic disease (ACD) (**Table 1**) [4, 5]. Iron deficiency anemia occurs when iron stores are exhausted and the supply of iron to the bone marrow is compromised. IDA is a severe stage of ID in which hemoglobin (or the hematocrit) declines below the lower limit of normal (biochemical evidence of iron deficiency). The precise biochemical definition agreed on by the experts group is given below [5, 7]. In active disease, inflammatory mediators may alter iron metabolism (by retaining iron in the reticular-endothelial system), erythropoiesis, and erythrocyte survival. This condition is termed anemia of chronic disease. Anemia due to iron retention in macrophages driven by pro-inflammatory cytokines and hepcidin is also called functional iron deficiency (FID) [14–16].

Anemia in IBD (an particularly IDA) thus results (a) on the one hand, from low intestinal bioavailability of iron due to chronic intestinal blood loss from inflamed intestinal mucosa; (b) on the other hand, from the combination with impaired iron absorption, either as a consequence of malabsorption and/or short bowel syndrome, or as a consequence of inflammation-driven blockage of intestinal iron acquisition and macrophage iron reutilization; (c) also, impaired dietary iron uptake might be involved, due to therapeutic or voluntary dietary restrictions and anorexia. Among other possible factors, intake of proton pump inhibitors, persisting *H. pylori* infection, may be additionally involved.

Other more rare causes of anemia in IBD include vitamin B12 deficiency (particularly after resection of the ileum), folate deficiency, and potential toxic effects of medications (such as proton pump inhibitors, sulfasalazine, methotrexate, and thiopurines; all these may aggravate anemia by negatively affecting iron absorption or erythropoiesis [5–7]. In fact, methotrexate and sulfasalazine interfere with the absorption of folate and may mediate folate deficiency [5–7]; sulfasalazine may also induce hemolysis or bone marrow aplasia; thiopurines and methotrexate can induce bone marrow toxicity in a minority of patients. Finally, other causes may include renal insufficiency, hemolysis, and innate hemoglobinopathies [5–7].

The average adult harbors at least 3–4 g of stored iron that is balanced between physiologic iron loss and dietary intake. Most iron is incorporated into hemoglobin, whereas the remainder is stored as ferritin, myoglobin, or within iron-containing enzymes. It is estimated that about 20–25 mg of iron is needed daily for heme synthesis; approximately 1–2 mg of this requirement comes from dietary intake and the remainder is acquired from senescent erythrocytes (recycling) [8, 9]. Total iron loss averages about 1–2 mg/day, mostly via fecal losses, skin, and intestine cellular desquamation, as well as through menstruation.

Body iron homeostasis is finely regulated by multiple and sophisticated mechanisms, the interaction of the liver-derived peptide hepcidin with the major cellular iron exporter ferroportin [15–17] being of major relevance. The synthesis and release of hepcidin are induced by iron loading and inflammatory stimuli such as interleukin 1 (IL-1) or IL-6, whereas its synthesis is blocked by ID, hypoxia, and anemia. Hepcidin targets ferroportin on the cell surface (enterocytes and macrophages), resulting in ferroportin internalization and degradation and blockage of cellular iron entry. Low circulating hepcidin levels enable an efficient transfer of iron from enterocytes and macrophages to the circulation, aiming to overcome ID; on the other hand, iron is retained in these cells when hepcidin levels are high and serum iron levels drop [15–17].

Furthermore, inflammatory cytokines can directly inhibit iron absorption and stimulate the uptake and retention of iron in macrophages via hepcidin-independent pathways. Interestingly, there is clinical evidence that circulating hepcidin levels have an impact on the efficacy of oral iron therapy and can predict its nonresponsiveness; this is consistent with experimental data demonstrating reduced intestinal ferroportin expression and iron absorption in individuals with increased hepcidin levels primarily due to inflammation [17]. As a result, anemia develops and is characterized by low circulating iron levels and an iron-restricted erythropoiesis in the presence of high iron stores in the reticuloendothelial system, reflected by normal or high levels of ferritin.

Hepcidin expression mediated through cytokine and the direct effects of cytokines on iron trafficking in macrophages play a decisive role in the development of this type of anemia (i.e., ACD or the anemia of inflammation), by retaining iron in the reticuloendothelial system and blocking iron absorption, which results in an iron-limited erythropoiesis [15,16]. This is reflected clinically by a reduced transferrin saturation (value below 16–20%). In addition, cytokines and chemokines further contribute to anemia by negatively affecting the activity of erythropoietin and an inflammation-driven impairment of erythroid progenitor cell proliferation [15–17].

As previously mentioned, patients with active IBD may have true ID due to chronic blood loss, as reflected by low ferritin levels. Moreover, true ID and anemia reduce hepcidin expression. These effects drive an iron-deficiency-mediated inhibition of SMAD signaling in hepatocytes and erythropoiesis-driven formation of hepcidin inhibitors such as erythroferron and growth differentiation factor 15 (GDF-15) [15, 16]. Thus, in the presence of both inflammation and true ID, circulating hepcidin levels decrease because inflammation-driven hepcidin induction is largely regulated by anemia and ID. Therefore, in truly iron-deficient patients, despite the presence of systemic inflammation, considerable amounts of iron might still be absorbed from the intestine.

4. Diagnostic criteria and differential diagnosis

As stated, in IBD patients, anemia is often multifactorial, being IDA, the most common cause. ACD is also an important etiology, and usually is associated with poor disease control or severe disease. Other causes contributing to anemia in IBD include vitamin B12 and folic acid deficiency as well as adverse effects of certain drugs (salazopyrine sulfasalazine and azathioprine). In both adult and pediatric patients with IBD, other chronic conditions should also be considered (i.e., renal insufficiency, hemolysis, and innate hemoglobinopathies).

In pediatric-IBD setting, other mechanisms of IDA, non-IBD related, must be considered, as this is a high-risk group of ID and IDA, namely characterized by high growth periods, insufficient ingestion due to dietetic choices, parasitic infestations, low socioeconomic level, and migrant families. It should also be noticed that ID in the absence of anemia is more common than IDA, as normal Hb levels do not necessarily mean adequate iron stores [5, 7].

World Health Organization anemia definition (**Table 2**) is considered valid in both adult and pediatric patients with IDA and current ECCO guidelines recommend its application to the establishment of anemia diagnosis.

Hemoglobin levels are influenced by age, gender, pregnancy, ethnicity, altitude, and smoking habits. Interpretation of Hb and hematocrit levels should take these factors into account.

All patients with IBD should be screened regularly for anemia, especially in the presence of active disease, as ACD can coexist with IDA. The initial workup to establish anemia diagnosis (and to differentiate IDA from ACD) should include complete blood count, C-reactive protein (C-RP) or erythrocyte sedimentation rate (ERS), serum ferritin, and transferrin saturation. A mean corpuscular volume (MCV) and reticulocytes are also helpful in the classification and differential diagnosis of anemia in IBD setting (**Table 3**). In some situations, microcytosis and macrocytosis may coexist, neutralizing each other and resulting in a normal MCV. In this case, a wide size range of the red cells (red cell distribution width) (RDW) is an indicator of ID, further contributing to the differential diagnosis. Platelet and white blood cell counts, also available within the complete blood count, are important to distinguish isolated anemia from pancytopenia.

By definition, IDA presents as anemia associated with low serum ferritin (referred as the most important laboratory parameter in the definition of IDA), low serum iron, low transferrin saturation, and elevated total iron-binding capacity. Other hematological parameters, such as RDW, mean corpuscular volume, and mean corpuscular hemoglobin (MCH), might also contribute to IDA diagnosis; high RDW, low MCV, and MCH corroborate IDA. These parameters

Age/gender	Hb (g/dL)	Ht (%)
6 months to 5 years	11.0	33
6–11 years	11.5	34
12–13 years	12.0	36
Female ≥14 years non-pregnant	12.0	36
Female ≥14 years pregnant	11.0	33
Male ≥14 years	13.0	39

Table 2. Minimum Hb and hematocrit (Ht) levels according to age and gender use for anemia definition (WHO) [9].

Microcytic anemia with normal or low reticulocytes
Iron deficiency anemia, anemia of chronic disease, hereditary microcytic anemia, lead poisoning
Microcytic anemia with elevated reticulocytes
Hemoglobinopathies
Normocytic anemia with normal or low reticulocytes
Anemia of chronic disease, acute hemorrhage, renal disease anemia, aplastic anemia, pure red cell aplasia, primary bone marrow diseases, bone marrow infiltration by cancer, combination of iron deficiency, and B12/folate deficiency
Normocytic anemia with elevated reticulocytes
Hemolytic anemia
Macrocytic anemia with normal or low reticulocytes
Myelodysplastic syndrome, vitamin B12 deficiency, folate deficiency, long-term cytostatic medication, hypothyroidism, alcoholism thiamine-responsive megaloblastic anemia syndrome
Macrocytic anemia with elevated reticulocytes
Hemolytic anemia, myelodysplastic syndrome with hemolysis

Table 3. Classification of anemia by MCV and reticulocytes (adapted from Refs. [5, 7]).

may be normal in ACD. In the presence of inflammation (such as acute exacerbation or poorly controlled disease), it should be recognized that ferritin levels are usually high. New promising markers, such as a soluble form of transferrin receptor (elevated in iron deficiency despite the presence of inflammation) are particularly helpful in the presence of active disease, being currently available in some centers [17]. Other markers, such as serum hepcidin and red blood cell size factor, may further contribute to differential diagnosis of IDA and ACD [15, 16].

Currently, it has been proposed that, in the absence of inflammation/active disease, serum ferritin levels of <30 μg/L reflect depleted iron stores; during active disease, serum ferritin levels of <100 μg/L should be considered as depleted iron stores. In both settings, transferrin saturation of <16% has been associated with poor iron stores. IDA should be considered in the presence of elevated inflammation parameters and normochromic and normocytic anemia or microcytic and hypochromic anemia with serum ferritin of >100 μg/L.

If, after initial workup, the cause of anemia remains unclear, other tests should be performed according to the most plausible cause of anemia, such as determination of serum B12 vitamin, folic acid, blood smear, haptoglobin, lactate dehydrogenase, urea, creatinine, and electrophoresis of Hb [5].

5. Evolving treatment strategies

5.1. Treatment goals and options

The treatment strategies of IDA in IBD both in adult and in pediatric patients are evolving from an expectant approach, which is no longer acceptable, to a more interventive approach. A pediatric retrospective study [13] including 80 children with active IBD and IDA evaluated the hematological recovery associated with an expectant management (for a median period of 12 weeks, in parallel with induction therapy). The authors concluded that this approach caused only a modest increase in hemoglobin levels, and that the proportion of children with exclusive IDA had increased within the follow-up period.

In adult IBD setting, the available evidence also supports an interventive attitude as having better outcomes. In one retrospective population-based cohort study [11] (with 279 both adult and pediatric IBD patients: 183 CD, 90 UC, and six indeterminate colitis) that aimed to assess the prevalence of anemia at first diagnosis and during the early course of the disease (during the 5 years of study period), anemia was found at any time during the study time in 90/279 patients (32.2%). At the time of initial IBD diagnosis, 68 patients were anemic (75.5% of all patients with anemia) and 44 patients develop anemia at the first year. IDA was found in 63 (70%) of 90 patients (all anemic patients) and 26 (38.2%) of 68 anemic patients with anemia at diagnosis and in 27/44 patients at 1 year after diagnosis. Considering IDA treatment, only nine patients with IDA at diagnosis (35%) received iron therapy and 18 patients with anemia at 1 year after diagnosis. Overall, considering the study period, only 32 patients with IDA at any time of the study received iron treatment (IV iron was only prescribed in five patients) and 38 remaining patients with IDA did not receive any treatment. The authors concluded that despite the high prevalence of IDA during the early course of disease and the potential highly negative impact on the quality of life, the treatment was infrequent and inconsequent.

IDA and ID without IDA are associated with poor quality of life that is independent of IBD clinical activity [5, 7, 18]. Several studies document that IDA treatment is associated with better outcomes in quality live assessment [5, 7, 18]. Thus, currently, IDA treatment is a formal recommendation in IBD patients, reflected by the recent ECCO guidelines [5]. The goal of iron supplementation is to normalize hemoglobin levels and iron stores. Current treatment options, in IBD-associated IDA, include both oral and IV iron formulas [5, 19–21] (**Table 4**).

The ECCO guidelines recommend IV iron as first-line treatment in patients with clinically active IBD, with previous intolerance to oral iron and Hb below 10 g/dL, as well as in patients who need erythropoiesis-stimulating agents [5]. These guidelines consider that IV iron is a

http://dx.doi.org/10.5772/intechopen.69203

good treatment option in IDA-IBD patients, as it has demonstrated to be more effective, better tolerated, and to improve quality of life to a greater extent than oral iron supplements. Recently published ECCO guidelines, however, do not take into consideration the pediatric age group and no specific considerations are made considering this age group [5].

Oral iron is available as inorganic ferrous salts, the daily dose ranging between 50 and 200 mg, in adults and 3–5 mg/kg/day up to 100 mg/day in pediatric patients (**Table 4**). Although oral iron supplementation has been traditionally used in IBD patients (adult and pediatrics) in the presence of IDA, IV iron, however, is rapidly becoming the first line of treatment in this setting, mainly based on efficacy data, convenience of administration (especially with the most recent formulations—**Table 4**), and good safety profile [23–28]. At present time, there are several available formulations for this purpose, as previously mentioned [5, 19–22]. At pediatric age, IV formulas currently approved by Food and Drug Administration (FDA) and by European Medicines Agency (EMA) are expressed in **Table 4**.

Regarding dosage of IV iron, Ganzoni's formula [29] [(body weight in kg × [target Hb-actual Hb in g/dL] × 0.24 + 500)], has been used to calculate iron dosage, both in adult and in pediatric patients. However, the formula is complex, difficult to use in clinical practice, and appears to underestimate iron requirements. Alternatively, a simple scheme (**Table 5**) has been proposed in the FERGIcor study (*Note: FERGIcor has no additional definition, as it is the specific name/designation of a randomized controlled trial on ferric carboxymaltose for iron deficiency anemia in IBD*) [25], in which the estimation of IV iron need is based according to pretreatment Hb level and body weight. Although initially used only to calculate FCM dosage, it has currently been used in other IV iron formulations, and is recommended in the ECCO guidelines. Limitations of this scheme include lack of validation in pediatric patients with bodyweight of <35 kg and patients with Hb below 7.0 g/dL, who may require an additional 500 mg. Also, the estimation of iron needs in ID without anemia is not taken into account.

5.2. Efficacy, safety, and tolerance data

The efficacy and safety of IV iron for the treatment of IDA in IBD adult patients is well established and demonstrated by several studies [23–28]. However, evidence regarding the superiority of IV iron versus oral formulas is yet to be proven [30–33]. In fact, there are several studies and systematic reviews comparing oral and different IV formulas, with variable results considering efficacy in improving Hb levels, tolerance, and safety (related to common severe adverse effects) [4, 6]. Particularly in adult IBD patients, data from large published trials are available, concerning iron sucrose (IO), ferric carboxymaltose (FCM), and iron isomaltoside (IS) [6, 23, 24, 26–28].

The first IV formulas (high-molecular-weight iron dextran (HMW ID) were associated with more frequent and severe side effects (anaphylactic reactions), as a consequence of IV iron. It has been initially used in specific settings, such as chronic kidney disease, neoplastic, and gynecologic diseases. In gastroenterological disease, IV iron was traditionally reserved for patients with intolerance or inadequate response to oral iron and/or in whom a rapid increase in iron stores was desired. As new IV iron formulas developed, composed by strongly bound

Products						
IV formulations	**Low Mw* iron dextran (CosmoFer®)**	**Iron gluconate (Ferrlecit®) hemodialysis patients**	**Iron sucrose (Venofer)**	**Iron carboxymaltose (Ferinject®)**	**Ferumoxytol (Feraheme®)****	**Iron isomaltoside 1000 (Monofer®)**
Carbohydrate molecule	Dextran (branched polysaccharides)	Gluconate (monosaccharides)	Sucrose (disaccharides)	Carboxymaltose (branched polysaccharides)	Carboxymethyl dextran (branched polysaccharides)	Isomaltoside 1000 (unbranched linear oligosaccharides)
Complex stability	High	Low	Moderate	High	High	High
Maximum single dose	20 mg/kg Single dose; limit 200 mg	125 mg	200 mg	20 mg/kg Single dose; limit: 1000 mg	510 mg	20 mg/kg
Infusion within 1 h	No	NA	NA	Yes	Yes	Yes
Test dose required	Yes	No	Yes/no	No	No	No
Iron concentration (mg/mL)	50	12.5	20	50	30	100
Vial volume (mL)	2	5	5	2 and 10	17	
Pediatric use/data available	No	Yes (in chronic renal disease) Dosage in 0.12 mL/kg. (maximum dosages 125 mg per dose)	Yes (maximum dose per administration 5–7 mg/kg)	Yes (approved > 14 years old)	No	No

Oral formulations

Ferric hydroxide-polymaltose, iron sulfate (oral solutions 100 mg/5 ml and tablets 50 mg; 100 mg; 200 mg) approved in pediatric patients (3–5 mg/kg/day up to 100 mg/day)

Ferric maltol (30 mg hard capsules): dosage 30 mg bid, no data available in pediatric population, 12-weeks treatment required, it should not be used in patients with IBD flare or in IBD-patients with Hb <9.5 g/dL [22]. www.ema.europa.eu/docs/en_GB//WC500203503.pdf

*Mw, molecular weight.

** Only approved in United States of America (USA).

Table 4. Main characteristics of oral and IV iron formulations available (adapted from Refs. [5, 19–22]).

Hb (g/dL)	Bodyweight 35–70 kg	Bodyweight ≥70 kg
10–12 (female)	1000 mg	1500 mg
10–13 (male)	1000 mg	1500 mg
7–10	1500 mg	2000 mg

Table 5. Simplified scheme to estimate IV iron dosage [5, 7].

iron carbohydrate complex (an iron core is wrapped in a carbohydrate shell), in order to minimize the potential risk of free iron reactions and the high immunogenicity leading to severe adverse reactions of the oldest IV iron formulas, IV iron is becoming a more frequent treatment option in IBD setting. These new formulas largely replaced the use of iron dextrans, as they have better safety profiles (allowing the administration without the need of a test dose), and also allowing a more time-efficient fashion in a single high-dose infusion. Nevertheless, iron reactions may occur with all IV iron preparations, but they are generally not thought to be immune mediated [30–33].

Each IV formula has a different profile of side effects, being the most common hypotension, tachycardia, stridor, nausea, dyspepsia, diarrhea, and skin flushing. Other described side effects include itching, dyspnea, wheezing, and myalgias (especially in the infusion of large-molecule iron complexes); however, it should be referred that an acute myalgia at the first administration of IV (without any other symptoms) that alleviates spontaneously within minutes (i.e., the so-called *Fishbane reaction*) usually does not recur, and rechallenge is unnecessary. Serious side effects are rare and include severe allergic reactions, anaphylactic shock, and cardiac arrest, but such problems are more common with the older IV formulas mostly dextran-containing preparations [30–33].

The new IV iron compounds FCM and IS are currently approved for use in IBD setting in Europe and ferumoxytol in the United States. All three compounds have showed high stability, favorable safety profile, and complete replacement of total doses of iron in 15 min [24–27]. FCM was the first of the new agents to be approved for more rapid administration of large doses. FCM can be administered as an infusion of 500–1500 mg in 15 min; however, it allows only doses up to 1000 mg per single dose. This IV iron formula is approved in both adult and pediatric patients (age >14 years old). IS is a particularly promising IV iron formulation, as it can be administered in high doses with a maximum single dosage of 20 mg/kg body weight, allowing single administration of iron doses exceeding 1000 mg. However, it is only approved in adult patients. In younger pediatric patients (<14 years old), IS is the only approved formula.

In 2013, Gasche et al. [7] recommended that oral iron should be considered a possible treatment options in patients with mild to moderate anemia (Hb ≥10 g/dL, ferritin <30 μg/L), as oral iron formulations have low cost and are administered at home. Current published ECCO guidelines reinforce this recommendation, as they suggest that oral iron is effective in patients with IBD and may be used in patients with mild anemia, whose disease is clinically inactive and who have not been previously intolerant to oral iron.

Nevertheless, though several studies (including adult and pediatric patients) have demonstrated the effectiveness of oral iron formulas in reestablishing normal hemoglobin levels, these compounds have a slow response in Hb levels (as it may take until at least 2 months to achieve the desirable Hb level, and up to 6 months to reestablish adequate iron stores), poor gastrointestinal tolerance (especially if high doses are required), poor absorption (in active disease and in the presence of inflammation iron absorption is further limited due to inflammation-driven blockade as referred before), and low compliance (compromising the treatment goal). Intolerance to oral iron therapy leading to discontinuation has been reported to be as high as 20% [7, 23, 24].

Additionally, there is some evidence in animal model [34] that oral iron might contribute to deterioration of mucosal injury. Furthermore, as absorption of iron from the gastrointestinal tract is limited, the unabsorbed iron is exposed to the ulcerated intestinal surface. One animal model study [35] compared the effect of oral versus IV formulas on inflammatory and oxidative stress markers in colitis induced in rats. The animals were divided in four groups (one healthy control, one colitis-induced control), two of the three colitis rats received 5 mg iron/kg of body weight a day (as oral or IV iron) for 7 days. Histologic and laboratory inflammatory markers were assessed. The authors found that the oral iron-treated group had a significant worsening of histologic and inflammatory markers, as compared with the IV iron treatment group and the two control groups. They proposed that IV iron should be considered in IBD patients, as it has shown negligible effects on systemic oxidative stress and local or systemic inflammation.

Other feature that has negatively influenced the option of treatment with oral iron is the putative reported increased prevalence of intestinal adenomas associated to prolonged oral iron treatment, in murine colitis model [30, 32, 33]. However, the true impact of oral iron on mucosal injury in IBD patients is not well established and the potential risk of colorectal carcinoma in humans remains controversial [36]. So far, these potential adverse effects of oral iron could not be confirmed in several published trials [30, 32, 33]. Only one human study specifically assessed this question [37]. In a small study including 10 CD patients with active disease and 10 healthy controls treated with ferrous fumarate for 7 days, the Crohn's Disease Activity Index (CDAI), gastrointestinal complaints and blood samples for antioxidant status, anemia, inflammation, and iron absorption were evaluated (on days 1 and 8). The authors found an increase in CDAI, and patients reported an increase in diarrhea, abdominal pain, and nausea at day 8; moreover, a deteriorated plasma antioxidant status in CD patients as compared with controls was observed, thus suggesting that oral iron treatment deteriorated plasma antioxidant status and increased specific clinical symptoms in patients with active Crohn disease. However, these data should be interpreted with caution, as it was a small sample, referring to a group of patients in which oral iron was not recommended, according to past and current guidelines.

Another potential negative effect of oral iron is the modification of the gut microbiome. In one recent open-labeled clinical trial, the effects of oral (iron sulfate) versus IV iron (Iron sucrose) over a 3-month period, in adult patients with IBD (CD: 31; UC: 22) versus control subjects with IDA without inflammation and its impact in clinical parameters, gut microbioma, and metabolome [38] were compared. The authors concluded that both oral and IV iron were effective in the correction of Hb levels, and moreover they found that oral iron distinctively affected bacterial phylotypes and fecal metabolites, as compared to IV iron. Although these data should take into consideration that IBD patients have already a disturbed gut microbioma, they highlight the potential additional gut damage of oral iron.

A recently published prospective controlled open-label 6-week non-inferiority trial, including 45 adolescents (aged 13–18 years) and 43 adults (>18 years) with IBD, aimed to assess the effects of oral iron (ferrous sulfate) on Hb level, disease activity (clinical scores and inflammatory parameters—fecal calprotectin and CRP) and also the relationship between baseline serum hepcidin and Hb response [39]. Quality of life was also evaluated. Rampton et al. [39] found that the effectiveness (improvement in Hb level) and tolerance of oral iron were similar in both age groups, and an inverse relationship between Hb response and baseline Hb, CRP, and hepcidin was observed. Also, the disease activity was not affected by oral iron and patients reported an improved quality of life—short IBD questionnaire (IBDQ) and perceived stress questionnaire scores in adults. The authors concluded that oral iron was effective in IDA treatment and that CRP and that hepcidin levels at baseline could be used as additional markers to better decide whether iron should be given orally or IV.

Ferric maltol is a novel oral ferric iron compound, associated with a lower rate of gastrointestinal effects, with potential use to treat iron deficiency anemia in mild-to-moderate IBD, even in those who are intolerant to oral ferrous products [40]. This clinical benefit has the potential to change treatment pathways and increase treatment options. Currently, this compound is only approved in adult patients.

In the last decade, numerous studies aimed to compare oral and IV iron treatment options, regarding safety, tolerance and efficacy, as well as impact in the quality of life [23–28, 41]. There are several published systematic reviews in this subject, as well as single and multicenter studies. All the main IV iron formulations have been compared with oral compounds. However, studies comparing different new IV iron formulas among each other and comparing traditional oral iron with the new formulations are lacking. Also, most data refer to adult IBD population; pediatric evidence, although scare, is emerging.

Considering the studies comparing oral iron sulfate to most used IV formulas (IS, FCM, and II) in IBD adult patients, the published data highlight that all IV formulas are safe, well tolerated, and effective in achieving desirable Hb levels. The superiority of IV versus oral iron in treating IDA-IBD remains unclear, as different results have been published. Studies have found, however, that treatment discontinuation due to adverse events was lower in patients treated with IV iron, as compared to patients treated with oral iron. These data are reflected in the current ECCO recommendations (mentioned previously), as oral iron is still a treatment option.

In the IS versus oral iron trial [23], a randomized 20-week, controlled, evaluator-blind, multicenter study with 91 adult patients with IBD and anemia (Hb <115 g/L), the authors reported that IV iron was more effective in correcting hemoglobin and iron stores, when compared to oral iron. In the oral iron group, only 48% tolerated the prescribed dose (which might had influence in the final result in terms of achieving normal Hb levels).

The FCM versus oral iron multicenter study trial [24] (including 200 adult IBD; follow-up of 12 weeks) attested the safety and effectiveness of FCM IDA-IBD. Although in this study, FCM allowed fast Hb increase and adequate iron stores, it could only demonstrate the non-inferiority of this IV iron formulation in terms of Hb change over the study time. Also, the rate of adverse effects was similar in both iron formulas.

Finally, the IV versus oral iron study, published by Reinisch et al. [28], was a randomized, open-label trial with a total of 338 adult IBD patients in clinical remission or with mild disease and an Hb of <12 g/dL. They aimed to prove the non-inferiority of IV iron when compared to oral iron regarding the correction of IDA, as well as to document the number of patients who discontinued the study because of lack of response or intolerance of investigational drugs, change in total quality of life, and safety. This study could not demonstrate the non-inferiority in changing Hb at week 8 post treatment. Indeed, there was a trend for oral iron sulfate being more effective in increasing Hb than IV. The authors suggested that the results might have been influenced by the underestimation of true iron needs by the Ganzoni formula.

Two systematic reviews and meta-analysis of iron replacement therapy in IBD patients with IDA recently published compared the efficacy of oral versus iron therapy in the treatment of IDA in adult IBD patients [21, 30]. One review identified 757 articles. The total sample size included 333 patients, with 203 patients receiving IV iron treatment. The primary outcome was the mean change in the hemoglobin and secondary outcomes included the mean change in ferritin, clinical disease activity index, quality of life score, and the adverse reaction rate. The authors concluded that IV iron is better tolerated and more effective than oral iron treatment in improving ferritin levels. Another systematic review published in 2013 [30], including again only adult IBD patients, also highlighted that IV iron was the best option to the treatment for IDA-IBD, due to improved Hb response, no added toxicity, and no negative effect on disease activity, when compared with oral iron replacement.

The most recently published systematic review, including only evidence from randomized controlled trials [33] (five studies including 694 adults with IBD), and comparing IV versus oral iron, also concluded that IV iron appears to be more effective and better tolerated than oral iron for the treatment of IBD-associated anemia, as IV iron presented higher efficacy in achieving a hemoglobin rise of ≥2.0 g/dL, lower treatment discontinuation rates due to intolerance or adverse effects (including lower gastrointestinal adverse events).

In pediatric patients with IBD-associated IDA, the evidence concerning the different treatment strategies, namely the use of IV iron formulas, is still scare. Also, as previously mentioned, only IS and FCM IV iron formulations are currently approved, wherein FCM is only recommended in pediatric patients of >14 years old (**Table 4**). In the pediatric IDA-IBD setting, so far three published studies support the efficacy of available IV iron formulas [11, 41, 42]. In these studies, both IS and FCM were used and showed to be equally effective in the treatment of IBD-IDA, achieving both the desirable Hb level and adequate iron stores in most patients.

In a small single-center prospective study, including 19 pediatric CD patients (median age: 15.5 years) with remissive/mild disease, with a follow-up of 40 months, Azevedo et al. [41] evaluated the safety and efficacy (short and long term) of IV iron, as well as the need of re-treatment.

The median Hb before and after IV iron was 10.5 and 12.7 g/dL, respectively. No major adverse reactions were documented. This prospective study thus emphasized the efficacy and safety of IV iron in pediatric IBD patients. In a retrospective study, Laass et al. [42] reported the treatment of pediatric patients with IDA associated to several gastrointestinal disorders, including a subset of 52 IBD patients (29 CD patients) with a mean age of 11.8 years. In this pediatric study, all patients were treated with FCM, and the mean Hb level after treatment of 11.9 g/dL was achieved, with good tolerance and minor side effects. In this study, FCM showed efficacy and a good safety profile, although data concerning the disease activity and long-term follow-up of the patients were not reported.

The safety and effectiveness of IV iron (IS) in the pediatric setting were also recently reported in another prospective single-center study (conducted in 24 children with IBD treated with infliximab) [43]. In this study, IS was administered after infliximab and no adverse reactions were documented.

6. Prevention

The recurrence of IDA in IBD is well recognized, occurring in about 50% of the adult patients within 10 months after IV iron treatment [5, 7, 44, 45].

Recurrence of IDA is directly related with iron replenishment at the end of IV iron treatment [5, 44–46]. It is admitted that ferritin levels over 400 μg/L might prevent recurrence of IDA in the subsequent 1–5 years.

ECCO guidelines state that IBD patients should be monitored for recurrent iron deficiency every 3 months for at least 1 year after correction, and between 6 and 12 months thereafter [5]. Furthermore, they highlight that recurrence might be associated to persistent intestinal disease activity even if there is clinical remission and remission in inflammatory parameters. An important message is that recurrence of anemia, especially in the setting of ACD, should lead to the evaluation of disease activity and an optimized treatment strategy would be required, as disease control is usually sufficient to correct anemia.

Data concerning recurrence of IDA in pediatric patients are scarce; however, considering the high prevalence of pediatric IBD-IDA anemia, a recurrence rate similar to that reported in adult patients should be expected. So far, these data were only described in one study [41], in which six of 19 (30%) patients needed re-treatment within the 40 months of follow-up (median period of 15.5 months). Re-treatment was proposed when Hb levels fell under the baseline level according to WHO criteria and after excluding other factors than IDA contributing to anemia. This study reinforces the importance of long-term follow-up of the iron status, also in pediatric CD patients.

The most recent ECCO guidelines suggest that after IV iron treatment, re-treatment should be initiated as soon as serum ferritin drops below 100 μg/L or Hb drops below cutoff level according to WHO criteria [5]. However, the benefit evidence of treating iron deficiency in the absence of anemia in IBD patients and particularly in pediatric IBD patients is yet unavailable. Currently, there are no guidelines concerning the management of ID without anemia in both adult and pediatric IBD patients. However, ID without anemia and IDA should be closely monitored.

The rational of preventing IDA by treating ID relies on the fact that iron is important to cell function and that ID can cause symptoms with a negative impact on the quality of life [5, 18]. Several symptoms have been associated to ID, such as reduced physical performance and cognitive function, fatigue, headache, sleeping disorders, loss of libido, or restless-legs syndrome among others [47].

The evidence concerning the treatment of ID without anemia in the IBD setting, however, is not yet available. ECCO guidelines recommend that the choice of treating ID without anemia should be considered on an individual basis (according to patients' past medical history and comorbidities, age group, symptoms, and individual/parental preferences) [5]. Data on the effectiveness of periodic IV iron administration as a prevention of IDA in IBD patients are available for FCM and II (in adult patients) [44–46]. In the adult studies, after IDA treatment with IV iron, patients received regular doses of IV iron (300–500 mg of FCM or II) during a 12-month period allowing to maintain stable Hb levels without IDA recurrence and with good tolerance regarding side effects.

In refractory cases of ACD with an insufficient response to intravenous iron and despite optimized IBD, therapy ECCO guidelines propose that these patients may be considered for erythropoiesis-stimulating agent treatment. The recommendation is supported by studies demonstrating the improvement of Hb levels; follow-up data, however, are lacking and these agents should be used with caution [5]. There are no pediatric data on the use of erythropoiesis-stimulating agents in IBD patients.

Red blood cell transfusion may be considered when Hb concentration is below 7 g/dL, or above if symptoms or particular risk factors are present. ECCO guidelines also recommend that blood transfusions should be followed by subsequent intravenous iron supplementation [5].

7. Final comments and future prospectives

In conclusion, the current management of IBD-A represents a paradigm shift in clinical practice, involving several specific challenges. A pro-active approach is recommended, and both adult and pediatric IBD patients should be regularly assessed for the presence of anemia, because of its high prevalence, impact on quality of life, and comorbidity.

Although both oral and IV formulations have demonstrated efficacy in IBD-A, oral iron might not be an ideal treatment for active IBD-A, with gastrointestinal intolerance occurring in many patients and a long course needed to resolve anemia and replenish stores. Nonadherence to a prescribed course of oral iron is common, and even in adherent patients, poor intestinal absorption fails to compensate for iron need in the presence of ongoing blood losses. In addition, studies in animal models do not exclude the possibility that oral iron formulations might increase disease activity in IBD and even the risk of development of colorectal cancer.

IV iron treatment has shown to be safe and well tolerated in IBD patients with good clinical response in different formulations (prolonged response). However, although the safety of IV iron has been demonstrated in studies comprising thousands of patients with numerous clinical entities associated with ID, safety concerns still exist. All iron products can cause hypersensitivity or other reactions and the comparative frequencies of reactions remain unknown. All involved clinicians should acquaint with the incidence, clinical nature, and significance of reactions to the existing preparations, systematically reporting to a central agency.

Although any IV iron can cause acute severe reactions, the incidence and severity of reactions seem quite low, with the doses commonly administered in clinical practice and currently available dextran-free formulations of intravenous iron (as iron gluconate, IO, and FCM). Similarly, concerns about IV iron therapy potentially increasing the risks for infections and cardiovascular disease have not been confirmed in prospective studies or clinical trials and remain largely unproven hypothesis. There remain, however, some concerns about the potential for long-term harm from repeated iron administration.

Sound data are still lacking, on when to stop iron supplementation therapy in order to avoid iron overloading, which may cause side effects, because of the potential of the metal to catalyze the formation of toxic radicals. Recent guidelines on the management of anemia in dialysis patients suggest that ferritin levels of up to 500 ng/mL appear to be safe and this limit might be a useful upper threshold in the management of patients with IBD-A. Interestingly, in a recently published prospective single-center study, iron supplementation in chronic kidney disease patients was associated with a significant reduction in overall mortality.

Certainly, the control of inflammation is a key objective in the treatment of IBD. Because IDA has a considerable impact on patient quality of life, a thorough and complete diagnostic and therapeutic strategy should be followed to help patients attain as normal a life as possible. Given the novel intravenous iron-replacement regimens introduced within the last 10 years, physicians may have some doubts concerning the optimal iron-replacement regimen to be prescribed. Based on the current evidence and guidelines, oral iron therapy should be preferred for patients with mild IDA in quiescent disease stages unless they are intolerant or have an inadequate response, whereas IV iron supplementation may be advantageous in patients with more severe IDA or flaring IBD, because inflammation compromises intestinal iron absorption.

Further well-designed clinical trials, including well-selected patients and clearly detailing primary and secondary outcomes, are warranted, to optimize the treatment schedule in these patients. In particular, considering the small number of published randomized controlled studies in this important area, prospective studies will be necessary to establish the optimal dose for correction and maintenance of target Hb levels and iron stores (definition of clinical end point) and to clarify the impact of anemia correction and iron supplementation on the course of IBD-A and patient outcomes. Ideally, these clinical trials should integrate new surrogate biomarkers, reflecting more precisely the true systemic iron pathways.

Also, prospective clinical trials are needed to better define the clinical and hematological long-term outcomes in patients with IBD-A. In fact, good-quality data are required both in adults and in children, demonstrating the efficacy, safety, and tolerance profile of different available iron formulas (oral and IV) in IBD-IDA, as well as to determine their cost-efficacy ratio.

The importance of long-term follow-up of the iron status in IBD patients, including in those in remission and/or with mild disease, should also be emphasized, as well as the inclusion of quality of life impact as a relevant specific intervention outcome. Finally, the future acquisition of larger pediatric experience in the field will drive the emergence of evidence-based-specific pediatric guidelines.

In summary, all clinicians (particularly gastroenterologists) treating patients with IBD will need to be increasingly aware of the importance of the screening, diagnosis, and management specificities of anemia and IBD, for improvement in their general well-being, a matter which frequently does not yet gain the required attention. With the new generation of available iron compounds and existent guidelines, the ultimate goal will be the improvement of the patients' quality of life.

Author details

Ana Isabel Lopes[1,2]* and Sara Azevedo[2]

*Address all correspondence to: anaisalopes7@gmail.com

1 Medical Faculty of Lisbon, Lisbon Medical Centre, Lisbon, Portugal

2 Pediatric Department, University Hospital Santa Maria, Lisbon Medical Centre, Lisbon, Portugal

References

[1] Gasche C, Reinisch W, Lochs H, Parsaei B, Bakos S, Wyatt J, et al. Anemia in Crohn's disease. Importance of inadequate erythropoietin production and iron deficiency. Digestive Diseases and Science. 1994;**39**(9):1930-1934

[2] Gisbert JP, Gomollon F, Gisbert JP, Gomollon F. Common misconceptions in the diagnosis and management of anemia in inflammatory bowel disease. American Journal of Gastroenterology. 2008;**103**(5):1299-1307

[3] Bager P, Befrits R, Wikman O, Lindgren S, Moum B, Hjortswang H, et al. The prevalence of anemia and iron deficiency in IBD outpatients in Scandinavia. Scandinavian Journal of Gastroenterology. 2011;**46**(3):304-309. DOI: 10.3109/00365521.2010.533382. Epub 2010 Nov 15

[4] Kulnigg S, Gasche C. Systematic review: managing anaemia in Crohn's disease. Alimentary Pharmacology & Therapeutics. 2006;**24**:1507-1523

[5] Dignass AU, Gasche C, Bettenworth D, Birgegård G, Danese S, Gisbert JP et al. European Crohn's and Colitis Organisation [ECCO]. European consensus on the diagnosis and management of iron deficiency and anaemia in inflammatory bowel diseases. J Crohns Colitis. 2015;**9**(3):211-22. DOI: 10.1093/ecco-jcc/jju009

[6] Nielsen OH, Ainsworth M, Coskun M, Weiss G. Management of iron deficiency in inflammatory bowel disease. A systematic review. Medicine. 2015;**94**(23):1-14

[7] Reinisch W, Staun M, Bhandari S, Muñoz M. State of the iron: How to diagnose and efficiently treat iron deficiency anemia in inflammatory bowel disease. Journal of Crohn's and Colitis. 2013 Jul;**7**(6):429-440. DOI: 10.1016/j.crohns.2012.07.031. Epub 2012 Aug 20

[8] WHO, UNICEF, UNU. Iron Deficiency Anemia: Assessment, Prevention and Control. Report of a joint WHO/UNICEF/UNU consultation. Geneva: World Health Organization; 1998

[9] WHO. Haemoglobin concentrations for the diagnosis of anaemia and assessment of severity. Vitamin and Mineral Nutrition Information System. Geneva: World Health Organization; 2011 (WHO/NMH/NHD/MNM/11.1)

[10] Ott C, Liebold A, Takses A, Strauch U, Obermeier F. High prevalence but insufficient treatment of iron-deficiency anemia in patients with inflammatory bowel disease: Results of a population-based cohort. Gastroenterology Research and Practice. 2012;**2012**:595970. DOI: 10.1155/2012/595970. Epub 2012 Jul 30

[11] Goodhand JR, Kamperidis N, Rao A, Laskaratos F, McDermott A, Rampton DS, et al. Prevalence and management of anemia in children, adolescents, and adults with inflammatory bowel disease. Inflammatory Bowel Diseases. 2012 Mar;**18**(3):513-519. DOI: 10.1002/ibd.21740. Epub 2011 May 20

[12] Gasche C, Berstad A, Befrits R, Beglinger C, Dignass A, Van Assche G, et al. Guidelines on the diagnosis and management of iron deficiency and anemia in inflammatory bowel diseases. Inflammatory Bowel Diseases. 2007;**13**(12):1545-1553

[13] Wiskin AE, Fleming BJ, Wootton SA, Beattie RM. Anaemia and iron deficiency in children with inflammatory bowel disease. Journal of Crohn's and Colitis. 2012 Jul;**6**(6):687-691. DOI: 10.1016/j.crohns.2011.12.001. Epub 2012 Jan 17

[14] Gasche C, Lomer MC, Cavill I, Weiss G. Iron, anemia and inflammatory bowel diseases. Gut. 2004;**53**:1190-1197

[15] Wrighting DM, Adrews NC. Interleukine-6 induces hepcidine expression through STAT3. Blood 2006;**108**(9):3204-3209

[16] Vermeulen E, Vermeersch P. Hepcidin as a biomarker for the diagnosis of iron metabolism disorders: a review. Acta Clinica Belgica. 2012;**67**(3):190-197

[17] Munoz M, Garcia-Erce JA, Remacha AF. Disorders of iron metabolism. Part 1: Molecular basis of iron homoeostasis. Journal of Clinical Pathology. 2011;**64**(4):281-286

[18] Wells CW, Lewis S, Barton JR, Corbett S. Effects of changes in hemoglobin level on quality of life and cognitive function in inflammatory bowel disease patients. Inflammatory Bowel Diseases. 2006;**12**(2):123-130

[19] Auerbach M, Ballard H. Clinical use of intravenous iron: Administration, efficacy, and safety. Hematology. 2010;**1**:338-347

[20] Munoz M, Gomez-Ramirez S, Garcia-Erce JA. Intravenous iron in inflammatory bowel disease. World Journal of Gastroenterology. 2009;**15**(37):4666-4674

[21] Lee TW, Kolber MR, Fedorak RN, Veldhuyzen van Zantena S. Iron replacement therapy in inflammatory bowel disease patients with iron deficiency anemia: A systematic review and meta-analysis. Journal of Crohn's and Colitis. 2012;**6**:267-275

[22] Available from: www.ema.europa.eu/docs/WC500203503.pdf

[23] Gisbert JP, Bermejo F, Pajares R, Pérez-Calle JL, Rodríguez M, Maté J et al. Oral and intravenous iron treatment in inflammatory bowel disease: Hematological response and quality of live. Inflammatory Bowel Diseases. 2009;**15**(10):1485-1491

[24] Schröder O, Mickisch O, Seidler U, de Weerth A, Dignass AU, Herfarth H, et al. Intravenous iron sucrose versus oral supplementation for the treatment of iron deficiency anemia in patients with inflammatory bowel disease—a randomized controlled, open-label, multicenter study. American Journal of Gastroenterology. 2005;**100**:2503-2509

[25] Lindgren S, Wikman O, Befrits R, Blom H, Eriksson A, Grännö C, Ung KA, Hjortswang H, Lindgren A, Unge P. Intravenous iron sucrose is superior to oral iron sulphate for correcting anaemia and restoring iron stores in IBD patients: A randomized, controlled, evaluator-blind, multicentre study. Scandinavian Journal of Gastroenterology. 2009;**44**(7):838-845. DOI: 10.1080/00365520902839667

[26] Kulnigg S, Stoinov S, Simanenkov V, Dudar LV, Karnafel W, Garcia LC, Sambuelli AM, D'Haens G, Gasche C. A novel intravenous iron formulation for treatment of anemia in inflammatory bowel disease: The ferric carboxymaltose (FERINJECT) randomized controlled trial. American Journal of Gastroenterology. 2008 May;**103**(5):1182-1192. DOI: 10.1111/j.1572-0241.2007.01744.x. Epub 2008 Mar 26.

[27] Evstatiev R, Marteau P, Iqbal T, et al. FERGIcor, a randomized controlled trial on ferric carboxymaltose for iron deficiency anemia in inflammatory bowel disease. Gastroenterology. 2011;**141**:846-853, e841-42

[28] Reinisch W1, Staun M, Tandon RK, Altorjay I, Thillainayagam AV, Gratzer C, Nijhawan S, Thomsen LL. A randomized, open-label, non-inferiority study of intravenous iron isomaltoside 1,000 (Monofer) compared with oral iron for treatment of anemia in IBD (PROCEED). American Journal of Gastroenterology. 2013;**108**(12):1877-1888. DOI: 10.1038/ajg.2013.335. Epub 2013 Oct 22. PMID: 27932449. DOI: 10.1093/ecco-jcc/jjw208

[29] Ganzoni AM. Intravenous iron-dextran: Therapeutic and experimental possibilities. Schweizerische Medizinische Wochenschrift. 1970;**100**:301-303

[30] Thomas WL, Michael RKB, Richard NF, Veldhuyzen van Zanten S. Iron replacement therapy in inflammatory bowel disease patients with iron deficiency anemia: A systematic review and meta-analysis. Journal of Crohn's and Colitis. 2012;**6**:267-275. http://dx.doi.org/10.1016/j.crohns.2011.09.010

[31] Warsch S1, Byrnes J. Emerging causes of iron deficiency anemia refractory to oral iron supplementation. World Journal of Gastrointestinal & Pharmacological Therapy. 2013;**4**(3):49-53. DOI: 10.4292/wjgpt.v4.i3.49

[32] Avni T, Bieber A, Steinmetz T, Leibovici L, Gafter-Gvili A. Treatment of anemia in inflammatory bowel disease– systematic review and meta-analysis. PLoS One. 2013;**8**(12):e75540. DOI:10.1371/journal.pone.0075540

[33] Bonovas S, Fiorino G, Allocca M, Lytras T, Tsantes A, Peyrin-Biroulet L, Danese S. Intravenous versus oral iron for the treatment of anemia in inflammatory bowel disease: A systematic review and meta-analysis of randomized controlled trials. Medicine (Baltimore). 2016 Jan;**95**(2):e2308. DOI: 10.1097/MD.0000000000002308

[34] Toblli JE, Cao G1, Angerosa M1. Ferrous sulfate, but not iron polymaltose complex, aggravates local and systemic inflammation and oxidative stress in dextran sodium sulfate-induced colitis in rats. Drug Design, Development and Therapy. 2015 May 7;**9**:2585-2597. DOI: 10.2147/DDDT.S81863. eCollection 201

[35] Seril DN, Liao J, Ho KL, Warsi A, Yang CS, Yang GY. Dietary iron supplementation enhances DSS-induced colitis and associated colorectal carcinoma development in mice. Digestive Diseases and Science. 2002;**47**(6):1266-1278

[36] Seril DN, Liao J, Yang CS, Yang GY. Systemic iron supplementation replenishes iron stores without enhancing colon carcinogenesis in murine models of ulcerative colitis: Comparison with iron-enriched diet. Digestive Diseases and Science. 2005;**50**(4):696-707

[37] Erichsen K, Hausken T, Ulvik RJ, Svardal A, Berstad A, Berge RK. Ferrous fumarate deteriorated plasma antioxidant status in patients with Crohn disease. Scandinavian Journal of Gastroenterology. 2003;**38**(5):543-548

[38] Lee T, Clavel T, Smirnov K, Schmidt A, Lagkouvardos I, Walker A et al. Oral versus intravenous iron replacement therapy distinctly alters the gut microbiota and metabolome in patients with IBD. Gut. 2017;**66**(5):863-871. DOI: 10.1136/gutjnl-2015-309940

[39] Rampton DS, Goodhand JR, Joshi NM, Karim AB, Koodun Y, Barakat FM et al. Oral Iron Treatment Response and Predictors in Anaemic Adolescents and Adults with IBD: A Prospective Controlled Open-Label Trial. J Crohns Colitis. 2016 Dec 7. pii: jjw208. [Epub ahead of print]

[40] Stallmach A, Büning C. Ferric maltol (ST10): A novel oral iron supplement for the treatment of iron deficiency anemia in inflammatory bowel disease. Expert Opinion on Pharmacotherapy. 2015;**16**(18):2859-2867. DOI:10.1517/14656566.2015.1096929. Epub 2015 Nov 23

[41] Azevedo S, Maltez C, Lopes Ana I. Pediatric Crohn's disease, iron deficiency anemia and intravenous iron treatment: A follow-up study. Scandinavian Journal of Gastroenterology. 2016;**31**:1-5

[42] Laass MW, Straub S, Chainey S, Virgin G, Cushway T. Effectiveness and safety of ferric carboxymaltose treatment in children and adolescents with inflammatory bowel disease and other gastrointestinal diseases. BMC Gastroenterology. 2014;**14**:184

[43] Danko I, Weidkamp M. Correction of iron deficiency anemia with intravenous iron sucrose in children with inflammatory bowel disease. Journal of Pediatric & Gastroenterology Nutrition. 2016;**63**(5):e107–e111

[44] Kulnigg S, Teischinger L, Dejaco C, Waldhor T, Gasche C. Rapid recurrence of IBD-associated anemia and iron deficiency after intravenous iron sucrose and erythropoietin treatment. American Journal of Gastroenterology. 2009;**104**(6):1460-1467

[45] Evstatiev R, Alexeeva O, Bokemeyer B, et al. Ferric carboxymaltose prevents recurrence of anemia in patients with inflammatory bowel disease. Clinical Gastroenterology and Hepatology. 2013;**11**:269-277

[46] Reinisch W, Altorjay I, Zsigmond F, Primas C, Vogelsang H, Novacek G, Reinisch S, Thomsen LL. A 1-year trial of repeated high-dose intravenous iron isomaltoside 1000 to maintain stable hemoglobin levels in inflammatory bowel disease. Scandinavian Journal of Gastroenterology. 2015;**50**(10):1226-1233. DOI: 10.3109/00365521.2015.1031168. Epub 2015 Apr 21

[47] Weinstock LB, Bosworth BP, Scherl EJ, et al. Crohn's disease is associated with restless legs syndrome. Inflammatory Bowel Diseases. 2010;**16**:275-279

Chapter 8

Anemia in Chronic Kidney Disease and After Kidney Allotransplantation (Systematic Review)

Yuriy S. Milovanov, Lidia V. Lysenko (Kozlovskaya), Ludmila Y. Milovanova, Victor Fomin, Nikolay A. Mukhin, Elena I. Kozevnikova, Marina V. Taranova, Marina V. Lebedeva, Svetlana Y. Milovanova, Vasiliy V. Kozlov and Aigul Zh. Usubalieva

Additional information is available at the end of the chapter

http://dx.doi.org/10.5772/intechopen.69746

Abstract

Anemia in chronic kidney disease (CKD) has been recognized as a separate independent risk factor of cardiovascular (CV) events. The aim of the review is to provide a literature summary concerning early diagnosis and treatment of anemia in CKD that may be useful for clinicians and contribute to decrease CV mortality. Literature searches were made in such major databases as: PubMed, Medline, Embase, Cochrane Library, CINAHL, Wiley Online Library, Scopus, Web of Science, e-library, and website of WHO. This search encompassed original articles, systematic reviews, and meta-analyses relevant to CKD and anemia over recent 15 years. A total of 54 references from 562 reviewed articles were selected as they met to the search criteria (anemia and CKD, including diabetes mellitus, systemic diseases and post-transplant anemia). The publications included 27 randomized controlled trials, 20 experimental studies representing new data on the links of CKD anemia and cardiovascular risk markers (cytokines, Klotho, fibroblast growth factor (FGF-23), hyperglycemia, hypoalbuminemia and some others), 4 systematic reviews and 3 clinical practice guidelines. The main attention was devoted to the analysis of the studies provided an early diagnosis of anemia, an ability to minimize the factors contributing to its severity that have allowed to improve CV and total outcomes and to reduce costs of hospital treatment of CKD patients with anemia.

Keywords: chronic kidney disease, anemia, post-transplant anemia, HIF, sKlotho, FGF-23

1. Introduction

Anemia associated with chronic kidney disease (CKD) has been recognized over recent years as a powerful independent predictor of cardiovascular (CV) complications which is the main cause of mortality in CKD patients [1–3].

Numerous studies demonstrated the multifactorial causes of anemia in CKD. Some CKD patients have more severe anemia than it would be expected according to their degree of severity of renal insufficiency [4–7]. In these cases, it is necessary to consider other factors that may contribute to the renal anemia, such as inflammation and infection (excessive production of cytokines), effect of drugs (renin-angiotensin-aldosterone system (RAAS) blockers, cytostatics and some others), nutritional disorders (hypoalbuminemia, deficiency of vitamin B_{12}, folic acid, iron) [2, 8, 9]. Chronic inflammation and pro-inflammatory cytokines (IL-1β, TNF-α, INF-γ) are the factors that may aggravate anemia development in patients with diabetes mellitus (DM), as well as in CKD due to systemic diseases (systemic lupus erythematosus (SLE) and systemic vasculitis) [5, 7].

The role of hypoxia inducible factor (HIF) in renal anemia genesis has been better identified. HIF regulates oxygen-sensitive genes' transcription erythropoietins (EPO gene) and activity of the others important mediators, particularly vascular endothelial growth factor (VEGF), glucose transporters, and nitrogen oxide synthetases [10]. It was studied the relation of HIF with the main iron homeostasis regulator—hepcidin [11]. Active oxygen radicals, which content is always increased in CKD, accelerate HIF degradation and inhibit EPO gene expression, depressing tubular cells adaptation to hypoxia [12]. Hyperglycemia may also lead to HIF degradation and incomplete EPO production, especially in autonomous polyneuropathy in DM [5, 6].

It is discussed the role of lowering sKlotho in CKD anemia that significantly contributes to CV risk increase [13]. Hemoglobin (Hb) levels ≥ 110 g/l was associated with more increased sKlotho levels as a cardiorenoprotective factor in anemia management with epoetin and iron in CKD patients with renal anemia [7, 9].

CKD anemia has normocytic normochromic character. During the course of long-term hemodialysis treatment, anemia may transforms into the hypochromic microcytic iron deficiency anemia due to blood losses and EPO treatment that requires a proper treatment [9, 14].

In recent decades, indications for kidney transplantation have been extended by the taking of high-risk patients (diabetic nephropathy, rapidly progressive glomerulonephritis-RPGN, elderly age) that lead to an increase in the prevalence of post-transplant anemia [15] and increase in CV risk.

If long-term anemia is not completely corrected in CKD patients, eccentric left ventricular hypertrophy (LVH) is formed with developing chronic heart failure (CHF) [1, 16, 17] because of decreased Hb level and an insufficient O_2 supply to the tissues leading to the sympathetic nervous system activation, to the increased heartbeat, the renin-angiotensin system and antidiuretic hormone activation, sodium and water retention and edema occurrence, to the increased venous return to heart and the eccentric LVH. In addition, lowering sKlotho leads to increasing serum fibroblast growth factor (FGF-23), which is considered now as a new uremic toxin, which level elevates earlier than parathyroid hormone (PTH) as the progression of the CKD [18, 19]. Increased FGF-23 and lack oxygen supply to cardiomyocytes enhance their apoptosis with the development of myocardial fibrosis and CHF [18, 19].

Early diagnosis of anemia, minimizing and eliminating as much as possible the factors contributing to its development and timely initiation of treatment are considered today as an important strategy to reduce CV and total mortality of patients, to improve their quality of life, and to reduce costs of a hospital treatment of CKD patients with anemia [1, 9, 20, 21]. However, since the publication of the KDIGO 'Clinical Practice Guideline for Anemia' in 2012, significant advancement has been achieved in our understanding of anemia mechanisms in CKD including kidney transplant patients. At the same time, there is a burning need for randomized clinical trials for better informed decisions and future optimization of CKD patients care. The aim of the review is to provide a literature summary concerning the early diagnosis and treatment of anemia in CKD and after kidney transplantation, which may be useful for clinicians in their clinical practice.

2. Methods

Literature searches were made in 10 major databases: Pubmed, Medline, Embase, Cochrane Library, CINAHL, e-library, Wiley Online Library, Scopus, Web of Science, and website of WHO ICTRP. The search was carried out to find all articles relevant to CKD and anemia, including diabetes mellitus, systemic diseases and transplant patients, as well as original experimental data. This search encompassed original articles, systematic reviews and meta-analyses. There was no language restriction.

2.1. Agreed criteria for article inclusion into the review

- Articles should be full text. Brief publications and abstracts were not included
- Research should include at least 20 patients in each group. The minimum mean duration of study was 6 months
- Analyzed literature over last 15 years
- The article should have the detailed research protocol for assessing of its quality
- Patients examination must meet KDIGO 2012 guidelines
- Randomized controlled trials
- Original experimental data over recent years representing the link of CKD anemia and the markers of cardiovascular risk (cytokines, Klotho, FGF-23, hyperglyceamia, hypoalbuminemia and some others)
- Systematic reviews and meta-analyses in this field

3. Results

A total of 54 references from 562 reviewed articles which met to the search criteria (anemia and CKD, including diabetes mellitus, systemic diseases, and transplanted patients, as well as original experimental data) were selected. The publications included 27 randomized controlled trials, 20 experimental studies representing new data over recent years on the link of the anemia in CKD and the markers of cardiovascular risk (cytokines, Klotho, FGF-23, hyperglycemia, hypoalbuminemia, active oxygen radicals, angiotensin II, interleukin-1,TNF-alpha, NO, and some others), 4 systematic reviews and 3 clinical practice guidelines. There were 10 studies in pre-dialysis patients, 10 in dialysis, and 7 after transplantation among selected studies relevant to the prevention and treatment of anemia in CKD. The main attention was devoted to the analysis of the studies on early diagnosis of anemia, ability to minimize the factors contributing to its severity, timely treatment initiation, that have allowed improving CV and total outcomes, as well as reducing costs of hospital treatment of CKD patients with anemia.

4. Anemia in chronic kidney disease

Renal anemia (defined as serum Hb levels <130 g/l for men and <120 g/l for women) is an obligatory complication of CKD progression [1, 2], which is usually occurring when glomerular filtration rate (GFR) decreases below 60 ml/min/1.73 m^2 (CKD stage 3–5). At GFR below 43 ml/min/1.73 m^2, linear relationship between GFR and Hb level is noted (decreased GFR of 5 ml/min/1.73 m^2 is accompanied by a fall in Hb level of 3 g/l) [1, 2, 20]. Importantly, the degree of Hb decreasing is not just a marker of CKD progression, but now, it is considered as also a direct independent predictor of cardiovascular (CV) complications, which are the main causes of mortality in CKD patients [1–3].

Appearance of anemia in CKD may be due to the lowering of endogenous erythropoietin (EPO) production, shortening of the survival time of red blood cells, decreasing in erythroid progenitors receptors' sensitivity to EPO, and diminution of iron supply to bone marrow because of iron deficiency or its decreased availability, caused mainly by increased levels of hepcidin, due to inflammation accompanying to the chronic uremia [1, 2, 8]. In addition, the pathogenic mechanism of CKD anemia development may involve folate and vitamin B_{12} deficiency due to malnutrition and chronic inflammation resulting in immature erythroblasts apoptosis [22, 23].

Some CKD patients have more severe anemia than it would be expected according to their degree of renal insufficiency severity [4, 5, 23]. In these patients other factors contributing to the anemia should be considered: inflammation and infection (excess cytokines production), effect of drugs (RAAS blockers, cytostatic agents), nutritional disorders (hypoalbuminemia, vitamin B_{12}, folic acid, iron deficiency). In diabetes mellitus (DM) patients, some other factors may also aggravate anemia: chronic inflammation and pro-inflammatory cytokines (IL-1β, TNF-α, INF-γ), their elevated levels are detected even before the renal failure appearance. Anemia has been found in about 10% of DM patients with normal kidney function [24]. In the cohort of >9000 patients without renal disease, DM was an independent determinant of Hb levels [24]. Many factors have been suggested additionally contributing to the pathogenesis of anemia in DM patients, such as erythropoietin deficiency due to efferent sympathetic denervation of the kidney in diabetic neuropathy, chronic inflammatory reaction leading to functional iron deficiency, non-selective urinary protein excretion leading to transferrin and erythropoietin loss and the use of RAAS blockers [5, 25]. A direct comparison of anemia between matched diabetic and non-diabetic CKD patients in the epidemiologic study which included particularly large number of patients at CKD Stage 3A found out the difference between the groups, and diabetic patients had anemia two times more often than patients without diabetes (60.4 vs 26.4%). Serum ferritin levels, but not iron, were higher in diabetic than in non-diabetic patients at all stages; the first ones had also more severe anemia and the increased ferritin as an acute-phase protein may signify higher subclinical inflammation in diabetic patients [6].

In patients with CKD due to systemic diseases (SLE, systemic vasculitis), anemia in 10–20% of cases also develops at the earlier CKD stages (1–2 stage). It is suggested that exacerbation of glomerulonephritis as well as an underlying systemic disease may lead to cytokine-mediated disorders of erythropoiesis with the development of anemia of chronic disease (ACD). Recognition of the ACD based on the analysis of the features of iron metabolism characterized this form of anemia [7, 9, 23]. The disorders of the iron metabolism are mainly associated with increased iron absorption and retention iron by reticuloendothelial system cells (RES), followed to lowering of iron admission to the bone marrow [7, 23, 26].

In recent years, it has determined the role of hypoxia-inducible factor (HIF) in the genesis of renal anemia [10, 12]. It was found that HIF regulates transcription of oxygen-sensitive genes (EPO gene) and activity of other important mediators, particularly VEGF (vascular endothelial growth factor), glucose transporters, and nitrogen oxide synthetases. HIF is a heterodimer constantly expressed in kidney and consists of alpha and beta subunits. Expression of HIF β-subunit occurs constantly and plays an important role in the body's response to xenobiotics when heterodimeric transcription complex with aryl gidrocarbon receptor formed. Expression of α-subunits of HIF-complex (HIF-1α and HIF-2α) is regulated by partial oxygen pressure in tissues. In the case of hypoxia absence, HIF-1α and HIF-2α rapidly degraded. In case of sufficient oxygen supply to tissues, enzyme FIH (factor inhibiting HIF) affects asparagine hydroxylation, thereby preventing increase in transcriptional HIF-1α activity. In case of Hb level fall, α-subunit degradation is inhibited that leads to the formation of HIF-1β—cytochrome P300 complex [10, 22]. As a result, active HIF complex binds to the complementary site of gene EPO locus thereby increasing its production.

Besides hypoxia, transcriptional HIF-1 activation is induced by nitrogen oxide (NO), tumor necrosis factor (TNFα), interleukin-1, and angiotensin II. Thereby, HIF-1 also takes part in the regulation of angiogenesis, glucose, and iron homeostasis [10].

It has been currently established that HIF takes part in EPO production, not only in kidney but also in liver. Liver is also involved in EPO synthesis, but less than kidneys, and extrarenal EPO synthesis cannot compensate its renal production deficiency [27].

The relation of HIF-2α and the main regulator of iron homeostasis—hepcidin has been studied: hypoxia and iron deficiency suppress hepcidin synthesis and thereby increase in the possibility of iron absorption in intestine [11]. It is found that HIF and iron interact by iron-regulated proteins—IRP's: IRP-1 and IRP-2. When iron stores in the body decrease, IRP-IRE complex prevents sequestration of transferrin receptor and thereby enhances intracellular intake of iron. If iron stores in the body are sufficient, IRP-IRE complex is inactivated and undergone to protosomal degradation, and iron is not absorbed. Furthermore, HIF-2α post-translationally prevents the development of more severe iron deficiency [10, 22].

Elevating active oxygen radicals in CKD also promotes HIF-1α degradation and inhibits EPO gene expression, thereby decreasing molecular adaptation of tubular cells to hypoxia [12]. Hyperglycemia accompanying to diabetic neuropathy, and especially in case of autonomous polyneuropathy, also leads to HIF-1α degradation and insufficient EPO production [5, 9, 24].

HIF-1α serum content is decreased in CKD patients with anemia (reference ranges are 1.5–6.0 pg/ml in adults and in children older than 14 years and). The murine antiserum and monoclonal antibodies against HIF-1α molecules are used for HIF detection [1, 12].

4.1. Diagnosis of anemia

According to the World Health Organization, criteria for the diagnosis of anemia are [2, 9]:

- Hb <130 g/l, Hct < 39%, red blood cell count < 4.0 mln/mcl, in men;
- Hb <120 g/l, Hct < 36%, red blood cell count < 3.8 mln/mcl, in women;
- Hb <110 g/l, Hct < 33%, in pregnant women.

In CKD patients for the diagnosis and future dynamic anemia control, it is necessary to check: Hb level, main red blood indexes: mean corpuscular volume (MCV), mean cell Hb (MCH), mean cell Hb concentration (MCHC), number of reticulocytes, ferritin level and transferrin saturation (TSAT), serum vitamin B_{12}, and folates, as well as for the other anemia forms [1, 9, 20].

Anemia in CKD is the normocytic and normochromic one. The number of reticulocytes in renal anemia is usually normal or slightly increased that depends on the degree of bone marrow erythropoiesis activity. It is noted increasing of immature reticulocytes fraction (IRF) that representatives of active bone marrow erythropoiesis, despite the EPO deficiency [1, 20, 22]. Perhaps, constant blood loss, associated with hemodialysis procedures, may activates compensatory medullar erythropoiesis. During the long-term hemodialysis, anemia may transforms into hypochromic microcytic iron deficiency anemia due to blood losses or EPO treatment that requires a proper treatment. In case of hypochromic microcytic anemia development, hemoglobin in reticulocytes (Ret-Hb) decreases [14, 28].

Functional iron deficiency for erythropoiesis may be diagnosed using TSAT coefficient, as well as the hypochromic red blood cells percentage (HRS), determined by flow cytometry [1, 9, 20]. A high serum ferritin level in combination with low-transferrin saturation are the evidence of increased hepcidin activity that may often be caused by inflammation, confirmable by increased C-reactive protein (CRP) concentration (more than 50 mg/dl) [8, 23, 29]. If

CRP level is high, CKD patient should be examined to detect inflammation (acute infection, active systemic inflammatory disease) and subsequent anti-bacterial and/or anti-inflammatory treatment should be provided before starting EPO therapy [1, 9, 20, 23, 29].

Renal anemia is accompanied by various clinical symptoms (dyspnoa, dizziness, poor appetite, depressed mood, decrease in performance, exercise tolerance, breakdown of cognitive, and sexual functions) and led to poor quality of life, increased hospital admissions, progression of kidney, and CV diseases, and increased mortality. Results of observational studies over last years have been strongly confirmed that Hb decreasing is a direct independent predictor of the eccentric LVH and CHF development (**Figure 1**), because of the falling of Hb level in blood and accompanied insufficient oxygen supply to tissues lead to sympathetic nervous system activation, increased heart rate, RAAS and antidiuretic hormone activation, sodium and water retention, appearance of edema, increase in venous return to the heart, and eccentric LVH.

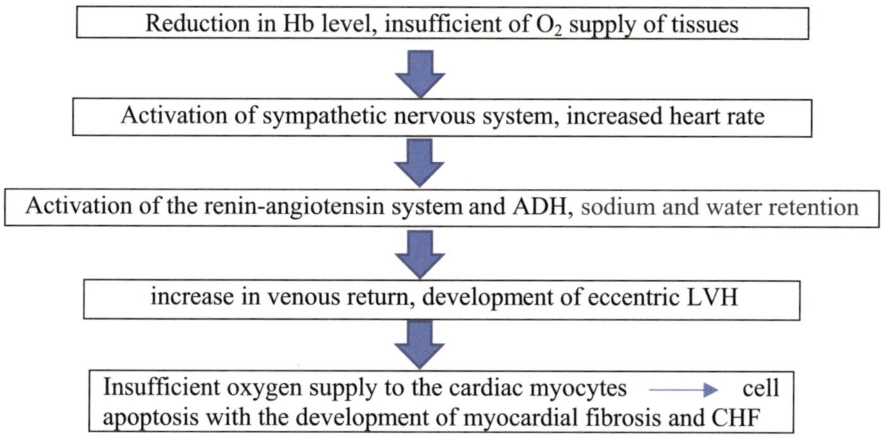

Figure 1. The impact of anemia on the LVH and CHF development in patients with CKD and anemia in the absence of its timely correction.

In addition, changing levels of recently identified new cardiovascular CKD markers such as sKlotho and FGF-23 progressively contribute to the cardiac remodeling in CKD especially in anemia persisting due to CKD progression. Increased FGF-23 and insufficient supply of oxygen to cardiomyocytes lead to cell apoptosis, myocardial fibrosis, and CHF [17–19].

5. Klotho and anemia in chronic kidney disease

It was found that circulating form of Klotho (sKlotho) protein has pleiotropic effects as a humoral factor that protects CV system [13, 30]. Adequate sKlotho expression provides both renal and CV protection. According to our date [31], patients from third stage of CKD have shown a direct linear relation between GFR fall and decreasing in sKlotho level. As it was detected firstly by M. Kuro-o, Klotho is synthesized in kidney tubules. This marker is very sensitive to anemia, oxidative stress, intrarenal increasing of angiotensin II, and inflammation that all take part in reduction of Klotho expression in kidneys [30, 32, 33].

Decrease in serum Klotho may be also a result of inhibition of its extrarenal production. In this regard, it is interesting to know findings of Takeshita et al. [34] that indicate the presence of Klotho gene expression in sinoatrial node and high frequency of sudden cardiac death of mice due to cardiac arrhythmias caused by sinoatrial node's dysfunction with blocked Klotho gene. It has been also recently found the strong correlation of the sKlotho low level with advancing of vascular calcification and CHF in CKD [35, 36]. In addition, it was shown in mice that loss of Klotho results in reduced MCV and MCH in circulating red blood cells (RBC) as well as the expression of HIF-1α and HIF-2α was significantly attenuated in Klotho−/− mice, resulting in suppression of EPO [37]. At the same time, recent studies have shown that administration of recombinant EPO can induce Klotho expression in the rat nephropathy model [37] and in the preliminary clinic studies [32]. Hb levels ≥ 110 g/l were associated with higher serum sKlotho levels in anemia management by epoetin and iron, in patients with anemia at CKD 3B-4 stages ($p < 0.001$) [32]. Moreover, transmembrane Klotho is a co-receptor for FGF-23. FGF-23 is considered now as a new uremic toxin in CKD advancing because of its pathogenic action predominantly on the heart in CKD. In a normal state, FGF-23 produced by osteocytes regulates phosphorus, vitamin D, and PTH metabolism. However, as was later shown, an elevated FGF-23 is associated with a high risk of death from cardiovascular events (CVE) [18]. It is believed, the effects of FGF-23 to the heart may be caused by its nonselective binding to FGF-4-receptors in the myocardium due to the significant increasing of serum FGF-23 along with progressive Klotho deficiency (as co-receptor for FGF-23) during CKD progression, especially if anemia persists [18, 19]. The data, obtained in our clinical center, indicate association between FGF-23 and Troponin-I, which may be a result of FGF-23 cardiotoxic effect on the myocardium, leading to the appearance of the detectable serum Troponin-I levels [19].

So, taking into account that hypoxia is an independent factor in reducing sKlotho synthesis in CKD and an urgent need of Klotho for CV protection, CKD patients with anemia who are managed to achieve the target Hb and to keep it within the reference range by EPO and iron therapy would have been expected to save sKlotho production and accompanied significantly lower CV risk [13, 32, 36].

6. The main practical approaches to the treatment of anemia

6.1. Treatment of anemia at predialysis stages of chronic kidney disease

According to the International Guidelines of Kidney Disease Improving Global Outcomes (KDIGO, 2012), treatment of renal anemia with EPO should be begin if Hb level is decreased under 100 g/l in adults and children 12–14 years old [1].

In patients with comorbid diseases (CV diseases, DM, advanced atherosclerosis, malignant tumors) as well as in case of notes on stroke, malignancies in past medical history, the decision about EPO treatment should be made individually and started if Hb level <100 g/l, firstly by iron medication (intravenous or per os) [1, 20, 38]. Preliminary correction of iron deficiency is obligatory requirement for the EPO therapy [1, 9, 20]. The velocity of Hb level decrement, the need for transfusions, response to the previous iron treatment, the severity of anemia symptoms, as well as the patient's lifestyle (active professional life, intensive school classes in children) should be taken into account at determining time for starting EPO therapy [20].

The upper limit of Hb reference range is determined as 115 g/l for most of the patients. Hb target level should be reached during 4 months [1, 20].

At predialysis CKD stages, short-acting EPO (epoetin-alfa or beta) is administered to patients subcutaneously at a dose of 50–100 IU/kg per week, it is about 6 thousand IU/week subcutaneously [1, 20, 39, 40] (**Figure 2**). Subcutaneous administration way of short-acting EPO is considered as a choice because it allows using lower doses and reducing the treatment cost [21]. The studies of pharmacokinetic of EPO show that subcutaneous administration prolongs half-life period of elimination of short-acting EPO (epoetin alfa and epoetin beta) [40].

At starting therapy, the rate of Hb increasing should be maintained at 10–20 g/l a month. Changes of hemoglobin level less than 10 g/L or more than 20 g/L require to gradual EPO dose correction by 25% weekly up (but not more than 720 IU/kg/week) or downward (**Figure 2**).

The rate of Hb increase >20 g/l per month is undesirable because of increase in risk of thrombosis. In this case, it is necessary to titrate down a total weekly EPO dose by 25–50%. Monitoring Hb level at starting treatment period should be performed every 2 weeks, then once a month. Hb's concentration change less than 10 g/L requires to gradual EPO dose correction by 25% upward [1, 9, 20, 39].

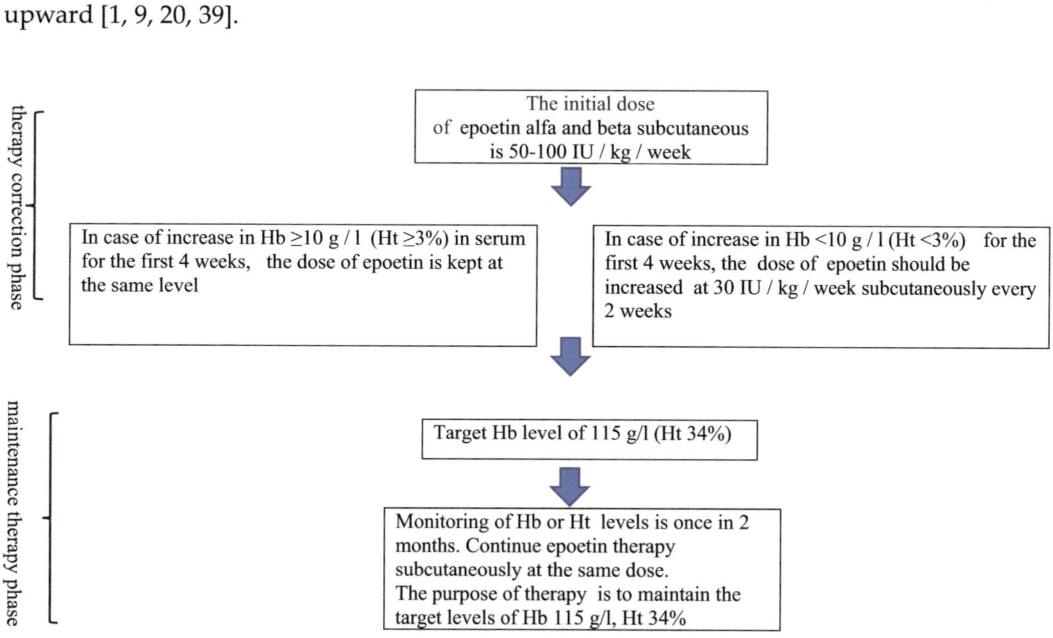

Figure 2. Algorithm for the treatment of anemia with epoetin α or β by subcutaneous administration of the drug at predialysis stages of CKD.

In CKD patients at stages 3–4, iron supplementation is necessary for prevention of iron deficiency, due to increased needs in iron due to EPO treatment, to achieve and maintain Hb level minimum at 115 g/l during EPO treatment. At the CKD stages 3, iron serum balance might be maintained by iron administration per os, for example, ferrum hydroxides (III) polymaltosate, wherein the dose of dietary iron should be at least 200 mg/day [1, 20, 41].

However, in patients with anemia of chronic diseases, it is a good practice to inject iron intravenously only because of insufficient intestinal absorption and iron retention by RES [1, 23, 26].

In addition, it is necessary to control during treatment the residual renal function (GFR and creatinine blood level in the dynamics), blood pressure (ambulatory blood pressure monitoring), hydration (blood volume), and cardiac hemodynamics. Therefore, low-protein diet with sodium restriction that combined with EPO and antihypertensive therapy may also play an important role in Hb maintenance [1, 9, 20]. The lower increasing in Hb level (less than 10 g/l a month or Hct level less than 0.5% a month) is a sign of insufficient effect of EPO treatment.

The most common cause of insufficient response to EPO is an iron deficiency [1, 20, 26, 42]. Adequate correction of iron deficiency is an important part of anemia treatment in patients at predialysis CKD stages and on dialysis [1, 9, 20]. In case of early successful anemia treatment onset in CKD patients, they are required less EPO doses to achieve the target Hb level at hemodialysis reaching as well as a lower incidence of CV complications [9, 39, 43].

6.2. Anemia treatment in CKD patients on maintenance hemodialysis (HD) or continuous ambulatory peritoneal dialysis (CAPD)

Short-acting EPO can be administered to dialysis patients subcutaneously and intravenously as well, but subcutaneous administration way requires lower doses of EPO [1, 20, 44]. Target Hb level is considered as 100–110 g/l (Hct 30–33%) for the majority of hemodialysis (HD) patients [1, 2, 9, 20]. Dose of 100 IU/kg/week of EPO alfa or beta intravenously or of 60 IU/kg/week of EPO alfa or beta subcutaneously is required to achieve and maintain this target Hb level. Subcutaneous EPO administration 1–2 times a week is a way of choice for anemia correction in patients receiving CAPD treatment because it helps to keep conditions for the formation of a fistula in case of further switching to HD treatment[1, 9, 20]. If patients are undergoing CAPD, and neither subcutaneous nor intravenous EPO administration ways can be used, for example, in children, intraperitoneal administration way to the "dry" abdominal cavity is applied, particularly when higher EPO doses are needed than in case of subcutaneous or intravenous injections. Hb level should be monitored every 4–6 weeks in patients on HD and CAPD [1, 9, 20]. Dialysis patients receiving EPO are required iron supplementation intravenously to achieve and maintain target Hb level, for example iron (III) sucrose, low molecular iron dextran or ferric III-hydroxide olygomaltosate intravenously slowly during the last 2 hours of the dialysis session (200 mg once every two weeks) under control of ferritin blood level [1, 45].

Iron deficiency developing during the EPO treatment requires fast correction, which is possible only in case of intravenous administration way of iron. Optimal and tolerance levels of iron metabolism parameters are presented in the **Table 1** (1, 9, 20).

Marker	Optimal level	Tolerance level
Ferritin, mcg/l	200–500	100–800
Transferrin saturation, %	30–40	20–50
Number of hypochromic red blood cells, %	<2.5	<10

Table 1. Optimal and tolerance levels of the iron metabolism parameters.

Iron deficiency is the most definitive for HD patients [1, 22, 23, 26, 45]. The main reason of its development is blood losses during medical manipulations that could be about 3–4 liters, equivalent to 2 g of iron a year: the blood that remains in the extracorporeal circuit (dialyzer, blood tubing line), blood loss from the puncturing locus, blood loss during catheter use, concealed hemorrhage in the gastrointestinal tract, and blood loss during laboratory studies. Young women require more iron supply than men [1, 20, 28].

Efficiency and safety of intravenous iron medications depend on its molecular weight, dose, and ingredients. Complexes of a low molecular weight, such as a ferrum gluconate, are less stable and faster release iron into plasma. Free iron may catalyze reactive oxygen forms generation, causing of lipid peroxidation and tissue damage. The significant portion of a dose of the such drugs is excreted by kidney in the first 4 hours after drug administration and not used for erythropoiesis [1, 45]. Despite of large molecular weight and strength of iron dextran drugs, its disadvantage is the possibility to increase the risk of allergic reactions. Ferric III—hydroxide olygomaltosate [100 mg/ml, 2 ml №5] is not accompanied by free iron release and does not cause antibodies formation and therefore has a good safety profile [1, 9, 20, 45].

The problem of variability of Hb levels during the period of EPO maintenance therapy is important in clinical practice of anemia treatment in CKD patients [4, 28]. According to retrospective analysis of the results of therapy of 281 dialysis patients by short-acting EPO, 90% of those have shown a cyclical variability of Hb levels by more than 15 g/l during 8 weeks. There were three such fluctuations in average during the 1 year observation. These cycles were characterized by increase in average Hb level up to 130 g/l and going down to 103 g/l, and the most common cause (84% of episodes) of it was the changes of EPO dose, 6 times a year in average [46].

One of approaches of solving this problem may be the administration of long-acting EPOs for renal anemia treatment, in particular, darbepoetin alfa and constant erythropoietin receptor activator—methoxypolyethylene glycol epoetin-beta [1, 20, 47, 48]. The starting dose of darbepoetin alfa is 0.45 mcg/kg/weekly in case of subcutaneous or intravenous administration way. It is allowed subcutaneous administration way of a dose of 0.75 mg/kg biweekly [1, 47]. If the increase in Hb levels is less than 10 g/l in 4 weeks, dose of darbepoetin-alfa should be up-titrated by 25%, while the up-titration should not be more often than once every 4 weeks. During maintenance therapy phase, the EPO administration can be continued once a week or biweekly. Darbepoetin alfa could be introduced subcutaneously once a month of a double maintenance dose once biweekly [1, 9, 20].

Starting dose of methoxypolyethylene glycol epoetin-beta is 1.2 mcg/kg once in 4 weeks subcutaneously (baseline Hb level is not taken into account). In case of increase in Hb level less than 10 g/l in 4 weeks, it is necessary titrating dose up by 50%, in case of increase in Hb level more than 20 g/l the dose should be titrated down by 50%. It is important to note that half life of methoxypolyethylene glycol epoetin beta is 139 hours in case of subcutaneous administration way, that is, 7 times longer than half life of epoetin alfa and 3 times longer than half life of darbepoetin alfa [1, 48].

Studies performed in dialysis centers of Germany and the UK have shown that in case of short-acting EPO switching to the long-acting erythropoiesis stimulating agent-methoxypolyethylene glycol epoetin beta (1 injection once a month) or darbepoetin alfa, medical expenses for anemia treatment have been reduced by 58 and 35%, respectively [21].

New classes of erythropoietin-stimulating agents are currently approved. The phase III study of efficacy and safety of Rosksadustat—an inhibitor of prolyl-4-hydroxylase—enzyme, that accelerates HIF deterioration, is carried out. The drug is administered per os. It was shown in preclinical studies that Roksadustat-activated alfa-subunit of HIF and initiated endogenous dose-related EPO secretion, improved iron utilization, and resolved anti-erythropoetin effects of inflammatory cytokines in renal anemia.

7. Anemia after kidney allotransplantation

Despite the impressive successes of transplantation over the last 30 years, 60% of all recipients' deaths occur with a functioning kidney transplant [49, 50]. The cause of death more than a half of these cases is CV complications. In renal transplant recipients, CHF risk factors include DM, age over 65 years, increase in systolic blood pressure, hypoalbuminemia, cytomegalovirus infection, and post-transplant anemia (PTA). There has been an increase in the prevalence of PTA over the recent decades [51]. In addition to the general factors for renal anemia (iron and erythropoietin deficiency), other reasons of PTA are considered [49, 50]:

- widening of indications for renal transplantation for high-risks patients (with diabetic nephropathy, RPGN and etc.)
- elderly age
- renal transplantation from marginal donors
- modification of recipient's immunosuppressive treatment when increased using mycophenolate mofetil, calcineurin inhibitors (tacrolimus, cyclosporine A) and rapamycin that associated with high risk of anemia development.

7.1. The forms of post-transplant anemia

There are relapsing and permanent course of PTA. PTA is also could be of early and late forms, depending on the time after transplantation [50]. Sixty percent of renal transplant recipients show recurrent PTA episodes associated with decreasing of transplant function (GFR < 60 ml/min, serum creatinine more than 190 mmol/l) as well as with recurrent of acute transplant rejection, re-transplantation, that more common in females, in case of donor's age is older than 60 years, in iron deficiency (ferritin <100 mg/l), in patients with DM, secondary hyperparathyroidism, obstinate infections accompanying by increased CRP levels more than 50 mg/ml, in cases of combined administration of rapamycin and mycophenolate mofetil (MMF) or in combined administration of RAAS blockers and azathioprine or allopurinol [1, 9, 50].

Permanent PTA is found in 30–40% of adults and in 60–80% of children as renal transplant recipients [51, 52]. Early PTA develops in the first 6 months after transplantation; it occurs in 2–3 times more often than the late form of PTA that develops after the sixth month from transplantation [51, 53]. The incidence of the early severe PTA form is currently high despite the effective correction of renal anemia with EPO drugs during preparation for transplantation (at regular HD) and rapid increase in EPO synthesis in transplant. This is due to a post-operative blood loss, inflammatory complications, and hyperparathyroid osteodystrophy. Three months later after surgical intervention, PTA severity decreases as erythropoiesis in transplant increases. However, 4–5 years later after transplantation, the risk of anemia development increases (late PTA) because of the progressive dysfunction of transplant (due to chronic rejection, sandimmune nephropathy, nephropathy recurrence in the transplant, nephritis de novo in transplant), as well as appearance of the late transplant complications such as persistent infections, cancerous diseases [54]. There is an inverse relationship between creatinine and Hb levels in the most of recipients with late PTA that is typical for CKD in general [1, 20, 53].

7.2. Causes of post-transplant anemia

Causes of PTA are multifactorial (**Table 2**) [51], but the basic mechanism of either early or late PTA forms is the fall of endogenous EPO synthesis often associated with the absolute or relative iron deficiency. EPO level increases to the normal values after renal transplantation in case of immediate transplant functioning and decreases in case of its delayed start of function. The frequent reason of PTA is a resistance to EPO appears in case of rejection crisis of transplant as well as in severe secondary hyperparathyroidism and particularly often in iron deficiency [50–53]. The absolute or relative iron deficiency is found in 40–50% of recipients, and it is usually associated with PTA. Post-operative blood loss, chronic infections with increased CRP level, absence of iron stores in recipient, and small-scale blood loss may result in iron deficiency [51].

Important causes of PTA are the iatrogenic factors that could impair erythropoiesis, iron metabolism, and aggravate resistance to EPO [51, 52]. Decreased response to EPO may be due to the iron deficiency that could be a result of gastrointestinal erosions, accompanying treatment with non-steroid anti-inflammatory drugs, direct and indirect anticoagulants, and corticosteroids [1, 51]. On the other hand, corticosteroids oppose to myelotoxicity of cytostatics, including iatrogenic hypoplastic PTA, due to both a direct stimulating effect on erythropoiesis and granulocytopoiesis and influence on pharmacodynamic of cytostatics [1, 51]. A number of studies have shown the role of RAAS blockers in the PTA pathogenesis. RAAS blockers diminish EPO synthesis due to blocking renin-angiotensin-aldosterone system and increasing serum level of tetrapeptide AcSDKP as endogenous inhibitor of erythropoiesis. The negative

Anemia pathogenetic mechanism	Causes of the PTA
Iron deficiency	Post-operative blood loss, attenuation of iron stores in case of chronic inflammation, drug-induced erosions of gastrointestinal tract (NSAIDs, glucocorticosteroids)
Erythropoetin deficiency	Acute injury of transplant due to a long period of thermic ischemia, chronic transplant rejection, ciclosporin nehpropathy
Resistance to erythropoetin	Recurrent acute transplant rejection crises, severe hyperparathyroidism, protein-energy malnutrition, pure red-cell aplasia (PRCA)
Disease activity	Systemic disease, bacterial and viral infections
Malignant tumors	B-cell lymphoma, Kaposi sarcoma, hepatocellular carcinoma
Drug-induced disorders of erythrogenesis	Cytostatics (azathioprine, MMF, Sirolimus), RAAS blockers, anti-viral medication (ribavirin, ganciclovir)

Table 2. Causes of anemia prevalence after kidney transplantation.

effect of RAAS blockers on erythropoiesis is a dose-dependent one. Combined administration of RAAS blocker with azathioprine or allopurinol is the most dangerous for erythropoiesis [1, 20, 51, 53].

High doses of sandimmune that are administered in the first few weeks after transplantation enhance EPO synthesis in tardive functioning transplant due to vasoconstriction and activation of renin-angiotensin-aldosterone system, but it does not lead to increase in hemoglobin level. Long term using of calcineurin inhibitors at late stages of transplantation is often accompanied by such complications as progressive tubulointerstitial fibrosis of transplant (sandimmune nephropathy) with EPO deficiency and PTA progression. Myelotoxic effect of sirolimus (rapamycin) has been found in the majority of studies, and it has been more significant that in case of MMF administration. Upon joining the MMF and sirolimus, PTA develops in 30–57% of cases. The degree of decreased in Hb level was correlated with sirolimus dose. Many of new cytostatics used in transplantation require significant increase in EPO dose due to its aggravation of PTA [1, 9, 51, 53].

Rare PTA forms include an autoimmune PTA, a pure red-cell aplasia (PRCA) with autoantibodies to EPO or to its receptor [54]. PRCA appearance as complication of cytostatic therapy (azathioprine, MMF, tacrolimus) with replication of myelotropic parvovirus B19 manifests severe progressive anemia with absolute resistance to EPO and total dependence on blood transfusions.

In recipients, long-term treated by immunodepressants (including polyclonal and monoclonal anti-lymphocyte antibody and anti-cytokine drugs), iatrogenic PTA may be due to manifestation of infectious (tuberculosis, CMV, HBV, HCV replication) or cancer complications of transplantation: malignant lymphoma, hepatocellular carcinoma, Kaposi's sarcoma, melanoma, bladder cancer, parathyroid cancer, and cervical cancer [1, 20, 51]. Iatrogenic PTA (with an increase in the requirement of EPO) often develops in the case of treatment of viral hepatitis by ribavirin, ganciclovir.

7.3. Risk factors of post-transplant anemia

Risk factors of PTA include depression of transplant function (GFR <60 ml/min, blood creatinine > 190 mmol/l), recurrent relapses of acute transplant rejection, retransplantation, female gender, donor age over 60 years, iron deficiency (ferritin < 100 mcg/l), diabetes mellitus, uremic hyperparathyroidism, persistent infection with increase in CRP levels > 50 mg/mL, combined administration of rapamycin and mycophenolate mofetil (MMF), as well as RAAS blockers and azathioprine or allopurinol [1, 51, 53].

On the other hand, PTA is a risk factor of the acute transplant dysfunction and long-term mortality of recipients [49]. Early anemia may aggravate transplant dysfunction immediately after transplantation [50]. So, early PTA aggravates hypoxia of transplant's medullary zone, and ischemia-reperfusion syndrome thereby increases in risk of ischemic acute tubular necrosis, acute transplant abruption reaction, acute pyelonephritis and also slows down regeneration of the epithelium of the convoluted tubules in recipients with delayed transplant function [49]. Extra renal manifestations of early PTA include exacerbation of ischemic heart disease, progressive CHF, arrhythmia, prolonged immobilization with a poor exercise activity, blood transfusion complications, and viral infections [50].

Despite of the fact that the late PTA has a moderate degree in 90% of recipients (Hb level is of 110–115 g/l), it could worsen prognosis by increasing risk of long-term cardiac mortality [53]. A number of studies have shown correlation between PTA severity and survival of recipients [15, 49, 50, 53]. The decrement in hemoglobin level by 10 g/l significantly increases the risk of CHF, cardiovascular, and overall mortality. The data have shown that iron deficiency affect the survival rate of recipients. Recipients with diabetic nephropathy and Hct level of more than 30% have significantly lower risk of CV complications than when Hct < 30% [1, 20, 50].

7.4. Epoetin drugs in post-transplant anemia treatment

The observational studies over the last years did not confirm a detrimental effect of EPO on transplant function and an increase in risk of thrombosis as suggested in 1980–90s. [1, 2, 9, 20]. In the case of early PTA form, despite of presence of factors that may induce resistance to EPO, there is usually an adequate response to EPO treatment with rapid normalization of Hb levels and improving quality of life. In recent years, more preliminary data have been obtained regarding positive effects of early PTA correction with EPO on transplant's function and survival, cardiovascular, immune, and endocrine system of recipient [1, 20, 51].

Response to the EPO treatment of PTA may be enhanced significantly by the modification of drug therapy (**Table 3**): in the case of PRCA, EPO therapy should be cancelled until antibodies to EPO in blood will disappear; in the case of severe hemolysis, the doses of corticosteroids should be increased and plasmapheresis to be carried out [54].

Precedent data have been received are positive about cardioprotective effect of EPO on regression of LVH according to echocardiography and on improving quality of life that was observed in the case of EPO treatment in recipients with blood creatinine less than 190 mmol/l

Drugs	Form of anemia	Therapy approach
NSAIDs, Glucocorticosteroids	Iron-deficiency	The cancel of NSAID, dose decline of glucocorticosteroids, up-titration of iron agents in the presence of the same epoetin dose
Rapamycin, MMF	Hypoplastic	Dose decline of Rapamycin, up-titration of epoetins dose
Azathioprine, MMF, tacrolimus	PRCA	The cancel of cytostatic agents, epoetin and iron agents, high dosage of glucocorticosteroids, plasmapheresis, blood transfusion
RAAS blockers and Azathioprine, Allopurinol	Hypoplastic	The cancel of Azathioprine, Allopurinol, dose decline of ACE inhibitors, its substitution for Angiotensin II Receptor Blockers, calcium antagonists, β-blockers
Ribavirin	Hemolytic	Dose decline of Ribavirin, up-titration of epoetin

Table 3. The principals of the corrections of iatrogenic PTA.

and hematocrit rising (to the level of 33–36%). Cardioprotective effects of EPO are associated as considered with both antianemic and pleiotropic effects: activation of stem endotheliocytes and myocardial neoangiogenesis, as well as with inhibition of myocardiocytes apoptosis and maintenance of sKlotho levels [1, 16, 32, 43].

8. Conclusion

In recent years, renal anemia is considered as not only a risk factor for CKD progression but mainly as a separate independent powerful risk factor for CVD that is the main cause of death in CKD patients. It is recognized not only direct pathogenic effects of anemia on CV system due to its association with increased cardiac output, left ventricular hypertrophy, heart failure but also due to contribution to the reduction of cardiorenoprotective factor's synthesis such as the soluble form of Klotho protein in CKD.

Anemia accompanying CKD in diabetic nephropathy as well as due to systemic diseases occurs earlier than in others patients of CKD populations and requires close attention and control at CKD 2–3a stages.

In dialysis patients along with decreased EPO production and anti-proliferative effects of uremic toxins, chronic immune activation due to the contact of the immune system cells with a dialysis membrane as well as due to frequent episodes of infection, leading to the typical chronic disease anemia, changes of iron metabolism may play a role in the genesis of anemia.

http://dx.doi.org/10.5772/intechopen.69746

In recent decades, an increase in the prevalence of anemia in patients after kidney transplantation has been due to: expanding indications for renal transplantation for high-risk patients, elderly age, renal transplantation from marginal donors («unideal» donors, a donor over 60 years old or over 50 years old and the cause of death whom was cardiovascular disease), modification of recipient's immunosuppressive treatment when mycophenolate mofetil, calcineurin inhibitors (tacrolimus, cyclosporine A) and rapamycin, associated with high risk of anemia development are used more often.

Early diagnosis of anemia, minimizing and eliminating the possible factors contributing to its development, and timely initiation of treatment are considered today as an important strategy to reduce CV and total mortality of patients, to improve their quality of life and to reduce costs of a hospital treatment of CKD patients with anemia.

Acknowledgements

This work was supported by Russian Science Foundation (grant №14-15-00947 2014).

Abbreviations

CKD	Chronic Kidney Disease
CAPD	Continuous Ambulatory Peritoneal Dialysis
CRP	C-reactive protein
CHF	Congestive heart failure
CVC	Cardiovascular complications
CVE	cardiovascular events
DM	diabetes mellitus
EPO	erythropoietin
eGFR	estimated Glomerular Filtration Rate
FGF-23	fibroblast growth factor
HD	Regular Hemodialysis
HIF	hypoxia inducible factor
HRS	hypochromic red blood cells percentage
LVH	left ventricular hypertrophy
MCV	mean corpuscular volume
MCH	mean cell Hb
MCHC	mean cell hemoglobin concentration

MMF	mycophenolate mofetil
PTH	parathyroid hormone
PTA	Post-transplant anemia
PRCA	Pure Red-Cell Aplasia
RCTs	randomized controlled trials
RAAS	renin-angiotensin-aldosterone system
RBCs	red blood cells
SLE	Systemic Lupus Erythematosus
TSAT	transferrin saturation coefficient

Author details

Yuriy S. Milovanov, Lidia V. Lysenko (Kozlovskaya), Ludmila Y. Milovanova*, Victor Fomin, Nikolay A. Mukhin, Elena I. Kozevnikova, Marina V. Taranova, Marina V. Lebedeva, Svetlana Y. Milovanova, Vasiliy V. Kozlov and Aigul Zh. Usubalieva

*Address all correspondence to: ludm.milovanova@gmail.com

I.M. Sechenov First Moscow State Medical University of the Ministry of Health, Moscow, Russian Federation

References

[1] KDIGO. Clinical practice guideline for anemia in chronic kidney disease. Kidney International. 2012;**2**(4):1-335. DOI: 10.1038/kisup.2012.1

[2] Phrommintikul A, Haas SJ, Elsik M, et al. Mortality and target haemoglobin concentrations in anemic patients with chronic kidney disease treated with erythropoietin: A meta-analysis. Lancet. 2007;**369**:381-388. DOI: 10.1016/S0140-6736(07)60194-9

[3] Thorp ML, Johnson ES. Effect of anemia on mortality, cardiovascular hospitalizations and end stage renal disease among patients with chronic renal desease. Nephrology. 2009;**14**:240-246. DOI: 10.1111/j.1440-1797.2008.01065.x

[4] Ebben JP, Gilbertson DT, Foley RN, Collins AJ. Hemoglobin level variability: Association with comorbidity, intrcurrent events, and hospitalizations. Clinical Journal of the American Society of Nephrology. 2006;**1**:1205-1210. DOI: 10.2215/CJN.01110306

[5] Loutradis C, Skodra A, Georgianos P, et al. Diabetes mellitus increases the prevalence of anemia in patients with chronic kidney disease: A nested case-control study. World Journal of Nephrology. 2016;**5**(4):358-366. DOI: 10.5527/wjn.v5.i4.358

[6] Kengne AP, Czernichow S, Hamer M. et al. Anaemia, haemoglobin level and cause-specific mortality in people with and without diabetes. PLoS One. 2012;**7**(8):e41875. DOI: 10.1371/journal.pone.0041875

[7] Milovanov YS, Kozlovskaya (Lysenko) LV, Milovanova LY. et al. Risk factors for anemia development in the early stages of chronic kidney disease. Terapevticheskii Arkhiv. 2017;**6**:(under review)

[8] Keithi-Reddy SR, Addabbo F, Patel TV. et al. Association of anemia and erythropoiesis stimulating agents with inflammatory biomarkers in chronic kidney disease. Kidney International. 2008;**74**(6):782-790. DOI: 10.1038/ki.2008.245

[9] Kozlovskaya (Lysenko) LV, Milovanov Yu S, editors. Anemia. Brief Guide. Moscow: GIOTAR publish group; 2016. p. 120

[10] Volker HH. Regulation of erythropoiesis by hypoxia-inducible factors Blood Reviews. 2013;**27**(1):41-53. DOI: 10.1016/j.blre.2012.12.003

[11] Garrido P, Ribeiro S, Fernandes J et al. Iron-hepcidin dysmetabolism, anemia and renal hypoxia, inflammation and fibrosis in the remnant kidney rat model. PLoS One. 2015;**10**(4):e0124048. DOI: 10.1371/journal.pone.0124048

[12] Volker HH. Hypoxia-inducible factor signaling in the development of kidney fibrosis. Fibrogenesis Tissue Repair. 2012;**5**(Suppl 1):S16. DOI: 10.1186/1755-1536-5-S1-S16

[13] Xie J, Yoon J, An SW. et al. Soluble klotho protects against uremic cardiomyopathy independently of fibroblast growth factor 23 and phosphate. Journal of American Society of Nephrology. 2015;**26**(5):1150-1160. DOI: 10.1681/ASN.2014040325

[14] Kaze FF, Kengne AP, Mambap AT, et al. Anemia in patients on chronic hemodialysis in Cameroon: Prevalence, characteristics and management in low resources setting. African Health Sciences. 2015;**15**(1):253-260. DOI: 10.4314/ahs.v15i1.33

[15] Delville M, Sabbah L, Girard D, et al. Prevalence and predictors of early cardiovascular events after kidney transplantation: Evaluation of pre-transplant cardiovascular work-up. PLoS One. 2015;**10**(6):e0131237. DOI: 10.1371/journal.pone.0131237

[16] Eckardt KU, Scherhag A, Macdougall IC, et al. Left ventricular geometry predicts cardiovascular outcomes associated with anemia correction in CKD. Journal of American Society of Nephrology. 2009;**20**(12):2651-2660. DOI: 10.1681/ASN.2009060631

[17] Li S, Foley RN, Collins AJ. Anemia and cardiovascular disease, hospitalization, and stage renal disease, and death in older patients with chronic kidney disease. International Urology and Nephrology. 2005;**37**(2):395-402. DOI: 10.1007/s11255-004-3068-2

[18] Scialla JJ, Xie H, Rahman M, et al. Fibroblast growth factor-23 and cardiovascular events in CKD, the chronic renal insufficiency cohort (CRIC) study investigators. Journla of American Society of Nephrology. 2014;**25**(2):349-360. DOI: 10.1681/ASN.2013050465

[19] Milovanova LY, Kozlovskaya LV, Milovanova SY, et al. Associations of fibroblast growth factor 23, soluble klotho, troponin i in CKD patients. International Research Journal. 2016;**9**(51):65-69. DOI: 10.18454/IRJ.2016.51.074

[20] Locatelli F, Aljama P, Bárány P, Canaud B, Carrera F, Eckardt KU, Hörl WH, Macdougal IC, Macleod A, Wiecek A, Cameron S; European Best Practice Guidelines Working Group. Revised European best practice guidelines for the management of anemia in patients with cronic renal failure. Nephrology Dialysis Transplantion. 2004;**19**(2):ii2-ii45

[21] Yarnoff BO, Hoerger TJ, Simpson SA, et al. Cost-effectiveness of anemia treatment for persons with chronic kidney disease. PLoS One. 2016;**11**(7):e0157323. DOI: 10.1371/journal.pone.0157323

[22] Babitt JL, Lin HY. Mechanisms of anemia in CKD. Journal of American Society of Nephrology. 2012 Sep 28;**23**(10):1631-1634. DOI: 10.1681/ASN.2011111078

[23] Agarwal N, Prchal JT. Anemia of chronic disease (anemia of inflammation). Acta Haematologica. 2009;**122**(2-3):103-108. DOI: 10.1159/000243794

[24] Grossman C, Dovrish Z, Koren-Morag N et al. Diabetes mellitus with normal renal function is associated with anaemia. Diabetes Metabolism Research and Reviews. 2014;**30**:291-296. DOI: 10.1002/dmrr.2491

[25] Deray G, Heurtier A, Grimaldi A, et al. Anemia and diabetes. American Journal of Nephrology. 2004;**24**:522-526. DOI:10.1159/000081058

[26] Ganz T, Nemeth E. Iron sequestration and the anemia of inflammation. Seminars in Hematology. 2009;**46**:387-393. DOI:10.1053/j.seminhematol.2009.06.001

[27] Kapitsinou PP, Liu Q, Unger TL et al. Hepatic HIF-2 regulates erythropoietic responses to hypoxia in renal anemia. Blood. 2010;21;**116**(16):3039-3048. DOI: 10.1182/blood-2010-02-270322

[28] Feldman HI, Israni RK, Yang W. et al. Hemoglobin variability and mortality among hemodialysis patients. Journal of American Society of Nephrology. 2006;**17**:583A. DOI: 10.2215/CJN.02390508

[29] Yeun JY. C-Reactive protein predicts all-cause and cardiovascular mortality in hemodialysis patients. American Journal of Kidney Diseases. 2000;**35**:469-476. DOI: http://dx.DOI.org/10.1016/S0272-6386(00)70200-9

[30] Hu MC, Kuro-o M, Moe OW. Renal and extra-renal actions of klotho. Seminars in Nephrology. 2013;**33**(2):118-129. DOI: 10.1016/j.semnephrol.2012.12.013

[31] Milovanova LY, Milovanov YS, Kudrjvceva DV. The role of morphogenetic proteins FGF-23, Klotho and glycoprotein sclerostin in the assessment of risk of cardiovascular diseases risk and CKD prognosis. Terapevticheskii Arkhiv. 2015;**6**:10-16. PMID:26281189

[32] Milovanov YS, Mukhin NA, Kozlovskaya LV, Milovanova SY, Markina MM. Impact of anemia correction on the production of the circulating morphogenetic protein α-Klotho in patients with stages 3B-4 chronic kidney disease: A new direction of ardionephroprotection. Terapevticheskii Arkhiv. 2016;**88**(6):21-25. PMID: 27296257

[33] Yoon HE, Ghee JY, Piao SG et al. Angiotensin II blockade upregulates the expression of Klotho, the anti-ageing gene, in an experimental model of chronic cyclosporine nephropathy. Nephrology Dialysis Transplantion. 2011;**26**(3):800-813. DOI: 10.1093/ndt/gfq537

[34] Takeshita K, Fujimori T, Kurotaki Y, et al. Sinoatrial node dysfunction and early unexpected death of mice with a defect of klotho gene expression. Circulation. 2004;**109**(14):1776-1782. DOI: org/10.1161/01.CIR.0000124224.48962

[35] Maltese G, Karalliedde J. The putative role of the antiageing protein Klotho in cardiovascular and renal disease. International Journal of Hypertension. 2012;**2012**:757469. DOI: 10.1155/2012/757469

[36] Hu MC, Shi M, Zhang J, et al. Klotho deficiency causes vascular calcification in chronic kidney disease. Journal of American Society of Nephrology. 2011;**22**(1):124-136. DOI: 10.1681/ASN.2009121311

[37] Madathil SV, Coe LM, Casu C, et al. Klotho deficiency disrupts hematopoietic stem cell development and erythropoiesis. American Journal of Pathology. 2014;**184**(3):827-841. DOI: 10.1016/j.ajpath.2013.11.016

[38] Strippoli GF, Navaneethan SD, Craig JC. Hemoglobin and hematocrit targets for the anemia of chronic kidney disease. Cochrane Database of Systematic Reviews. 2006;**18**(40):CD003967

[39] Cody J, Daly C, Campbell M. et al. Recombinant human erythropoietin for chronic renal failure anemia in pre-dialysis patients. Cochrane Database Systematic Reviews. 2005;**3**:CД 003266. DOI: 10.1002/14651858.CD003266

[40] Halstenson CE, Macres M, Kats SA. et al. Comparative pharmacokinetics and pharmacodynamics of epoetin alfa and epoetin beta. Clinical Pharmacology and Therapeutics. 2004;**39**:602-612

[41] Silverberg DS, Wexler D, Iaina A, et.al. Correction of iron deficiency in the cardiorenal syndrome. International Journal of Nephrology. 2011;**2011**:365301. DOI: 10.4061/2011/365301

[42] Garrido P, Ribeiro S, Fernandes J, et al. Resistance to recombinant human erythropoietin therapy in a rat model of chronic kidney disease associated anemia. International Journal of Molecular Science. 2016;**17**(1):28. DOI: 10.3390/ijms17010028

[43] Green P, Babu BA, Teruya S, et al. Impact of epoetin alfa on LV structure, function, and pressure-volume relations as assessed by cardiac magnetic resonance – The heart failure preserved ejection fraction (HFPEF) anemia trial. Congestive Heart Failure. 2013;**19**(4). 10.1111/chf.12027

[44] Wright DG, Wright EC, Narva AS, et al. Association of erythropoietin dose and route of administration with clinical outcomes for patients on hemodialysis in the United States. Clinical Journal of American Society of Nephrology. 2015;**10**(10):1822-1830. DOI: 10.2215/CJN.01590215

[45] Kalra PA, Bhandari S. Safety of intravenous iron use in chronic kidney disease. Current Opinion in Nephrology and Hypertension. 2016;**25**(6):529-535. DOI: 10.1097/MNH.0000000000000263

[46] Eckardt KU, Kim J, Kronenberg F, et al. Hemoglobin variability does not predict mortality in European hemodialysis patients. Journal of American Society of Nephrology. 2010;**21**(10):1765-1775. DOI: 10.1681/ASN.2009101017

[47] Galle JC, Addison J, Suranyi MG, et al. Outcomes in patients with chronic kidney disease not on dialysis receiving extended dosing regimens of darbepoetin alfa: Long-term results of the EXTEND observational cohort study. Nephrology Dialysis Transplantion. 2016;**31**(12):2073-2085. DOI: 10.1093/ndt/gfw047

[48] Sulowicz W, Locatelli F, Ryckelynck JP, et al. Once-monthly subcutaneous C.E.R.A. maintains stable hemoglobin control in patients with chronic kidney disease on dialysis and converted directly from epoetin one to three times weekly. CJASN. 2007;**2**(4):637-646. DOI: 10.2215/CJN.03631006

[49] Mix TC, Kazmi W, Khan S. et al. Anemia: A continuing problem following kidney transplantation. American Journal of Transplantion. 2003;**3**:1426-1433. DOI: 10.1046/j.1600-6135.2003.00224.x

[50] Vanrenterghem I. Anemia after kidney transplantation. Transplantation. 2009;**87**(9):1265-1267. DOI: 10.1097/TP.0b013e3181a170b7

[51] Winkelmayer WC, Chandraker A. Pottransplantation anemia: Management and rationale. CJASN. 2008;**3**(Suppl 2):49-55. DOI: 10.2215/CJN.03290807

[52] Mitsnefes MM, Subat-Dezulovic M, Khoury PR, et al. Increasing incidence of post-kidney transplant anemia in children. American Journal of Transplantion. 2005;**5**:1713-1718. DOI: 10.1111/j.1600-6143.2005.00919.x

[53] Scandling JD, Belson A. et al. Late post-transplant anemia in adults renal transplant recipients. An under-recognized problem? American Journal of Transplantation. 2002;**2**:429-435. DOI: 10.1034/j.1600-6143.2002.20506.x

[54] Macdougall IC, Casadevall N, Locatelli F, et al. Incidence of erythropoietin antibody-mediated pure red cell aplasia: The prospective immunogenicity surveillance registry (PRIMS). Nephrology Dialysis Transplantation. 2015;**30**(3):451-460. DOI: 10.1093/ndt/gfu297

Chapter 9

The Pattern of Anemia in Lupus

Elena Samohvalov and Sergiu Samohvalov

Additional information is available at the end of the chapter

http://dx.doi.org/10.5772/intechopen.71293

Abstract

Anemia is a frequent incident for patients with systemic lupus erythematosus (SLE), its incidence being reported as 18–80%. Anemia of chronic disease (ACD) is the most common hematological syndrome in the evolutionary context of SLE. In anemia of the chronic disease, cytokines stimulate the production of hepcidin, an acute phase protein, which destroys ferroportin produced by hepatocytes. As a result, Fe (iron) is not able to come out from the erythrocytes and macrophages and is trapped within them. Anemias from chronic disease are usually hypoproliferative processes. This chapter reviews the correlation between systemic lupus erythematosus and anemia of chronic disease in general (but iron-deficiency anemia in particular). This text reviews different important methods of examination used to diagnose the pathological process of lupus as an immune disease and of the hematopoietic system some of these methods include (general blood analysis, Coombs test, serum iron, hematocrit etc.). Furthermore, it will discuss the physiopathological mechanism of anemic syndrome in systemic lupus erythematosus and the changes of the immune system. In conclusion, the relevance of anemia (independent of its cause) is estimated as being both a short-term activity of the disease and long-term prognostic factor for the evolution of SLE.

Keywords: anemia, systemic lupus erythematosus, hematological implications

1. Introduction

In general population, anemia is associated with high morbidity in different clinical conditions. For example, high prenatal risk, developmental anomalies in children, changes in immunological status, high risk of infections and pattern of hormonal and metabolic development are usually associated with anemia. Anemia is an independent risk factor for the development of cardiovascular complications in general population [1–3].

Anemia is present in approximately half of the people with active lupus. Common forms of anemia in these patients are anemia of chronic disease (ACD), followed by iron-deficiency anemia, autoimmune hemolytic anemia, anemia of chronic kidney disease and drug induced. Other types of anemia, such as pure red cell aplasia (PRCA), myelofibrosis, B12-deficiency anemia, sideroblastic anemia, hemophagocytic syndrome and thrombotic microangiopathy, are rare forms described in lupus. Anemias from chronic disease are usually hypoproliferative processes [4, 5]. Recent studies have revealed that resistance to erythropoietin (EPO) in systemic lupus erythematosus (SLE) can be attributed to antibodies against erythropoietin (anti-erythropoietin). Reduced production and resistance to erythropoietin in patients with SLE is hypothetically associated with anemia of chronic disease (ACD) [6, 7]. Normally, red cells live only 120 days (approximately 4 months) and they constantly have to be produced by the bone marrow. The most common explanation of anemia is the production of fewer red blood cells than usual. This can be caused by an inflammation, kidney problems (when kidneys produce insufficient hormone, erythropoietin stimulates the bone marrow to produce more red blood cells), iron deficiency (without iron, hemoglobin cannot be produced—iron deficiency can be caused by excessive menstrual hemorrhage or intestinal hemorrhage caused by non-steroidal anti-inflammatory drugs, such as ibuprofen and aspirin) or diminished bone marrow caused by drugs like azathioprine and cyclophosphamide. Intestinal hemorrhage can be evident if the stool is dark and tarry, but sometimes the hemorrhage is very little and additional analysis are needed for the detection of the hemorrhage [3, 4, 8]. Anemia can be caused by the premature destruction of red blood cells, named hemolytic anemia, or by simple hemolysis. Sometimes patients with hemolysis have paler skin and in these situations the yellowish color of the skin and eyes is not a sign of liver problems. Hemolysis is often caused by specific antibodies of the disease that attach to erythrocytes. When it is accompanied by thrombocytopenia, it causes thrombotic thrombocytopenic purpura. Thrombocytopenia is found in 30–50% patients, and it is caused by antiplatelet antibodies or antiphospholipid antibodies. Both can cause severe thrombocytopenia (<50,000). Platelet transfusion is generally contraindicated in SLE because of the possibility that the patient is exposed to new antigens [5, 9].

Being essential for organ function, a large amount of iron is stored in any organism. Excretion of iron from the body is a very slow process, which occurs through epithelial desquamation and intestinal secretion.

Anemia of chronic disease is the most common hematological syndrome seen in the evolutionary context of SLE. In anemia of chronic disease, cytokines stimulate the production of hepcidin – a protein of the acute phase response, which destroys ferroportin produced by hepatocytes. As a result, iron is unable to be transported out of the erythrocytes and macrophages. Under the influence of hepcidin, iron is trapped [7, 10]. In this condition, in spite of sufficient amount of iron in the body, bone marrow suffers from insufficiency of iron.

Formation of erythrocytes is affected and their duration of life decreases. Erythrocytes are produced in the bone marrow under the influence of erythropoietin, but in anemia of chronic disease the cytokines inhibit the production of erythropoietin.

Anemia in patients with SLE is a common manifestation which can result from many causes such as changes in the immune system, followed by the activation of cytokines, digestive tract bleeding because of chronic consumption of glucocorticoids, various drugs (for example aspirin and ibuprofen), presence of enzyme deficiency that predisposes the fragility of RBCs, poor diet and malabsorption syndrome. Sometimes SLE patients might have multiple etiological factors for their anemia. For that reason, it is important to establish a complete and correct diagnosis, taking into account different therapeutic means [5, 11].

Anemia of chronic disease is determined by a functional deficit of iron, which can be characterized by:

- hyposideremia, despite the adequate/increased amount of iron (increased ferritin in serum);
- direct suppression of erythropoiesis;
- determining the capture of the iron in macrophages;
- limiting the amount of transferrin iron necessary for erythropoiesis makes anemia mild and asymptomatic, making it morphologically normocytic/microcytic and saturation of transferrin low, suggesting the deficit of iron.

Hemoglobin is the protein present in the red blood cells that transports oxygen from lungs to other tissues of the body. Fatigue is a common symptom of lupus and also the first and most common symptom in anemia [12, 13]. Anemia can be measured and followed up in various ways, including calculation of the red blood cells, which emphasizes a reduced number of RBC, a low level of hemoglobin and hematocrit [12, 14].

The diagnosis of a real deficit of iron in a patient with chronic disease can be very difficult to determine because chronic diseases can give false-positive results for hyposideremia despite the presence of stored iron and can also give false-positive results for higher ferritin level in serum, even in the absence of stored iron—the most useful diagnostic test is the soluble transferrin receptor (STfR)/ferritin level. Soluble transferrin level (STfR) and ferritin change in opposite directions during iron deficiency; this value is extremely sensible for the metabolism of iron and can differentiate anemia from chronic disease with the real iron deficit, even if this is accompanied by a chronic disease. This value is not useful in the presence of renal dysfunction or hemodialysis, when the saturation of transferrin is <20% and ferritin <100 μg/l shows the necessity of treatment with iron [2, 14, 15].

2. Physiopathological mechanisms of anemic syndrome in systemic lupus erythematosus

Anemia of chronic disease, the most frequent comorbidity in patients with SLE is normochromic normocytic, mild (Hb < 9.5 g/dl) or moderate form (Hb < 8 g/dl) of hyporegenerative anemia. In its physiopathology, cytokines and SLE cells change the homeostasis of iron; abnormal erythropoietin (EPO) production, inadequate response to the secretion of erythropoietin causes erythroid progenitor abnormalities in the cells and diminished life span of erythrocytes; these are caused by direct toxic effect on progenitors by formation of free radicals like nitric oxide (NO) and superoxide anion (O_2) [16–18].

Changes in the immune system determine the activation of T lymphocytes (CD^{3+}) and monocytes, followed by the production of cytokines such as interleukin-1 (IL-1), interleukin-6

(IL-6), interleukin-10 (IL-10), tumor necrosis factor alpha (TNFα) and interferon-gamma (IFN-gamma), which stimulate the storage of iron in macrophages and synthesis of ferritin (FT), which causes decreased availability of iron for erythropoiesis. IFN-gamma, TNFα and IL-1 have inhibitory effect on the proliferation and differentiation of erythroid progenitors. TNFα and IFN-gamma inhibit the production of erythropoietin in kidney. IL-6 and IL-1 (responsible especially for systemic manifestations in SLE, including anemia) were the first cytokines discovered, implicated in stimulating the secretion of hepatic hepcidin. These cytokines, being the essential elements in the anemia pathogeny of patients with multiple myeloma, acting either independently or through producing hepcidin [10, 17]. Hepcidin represents the link between these two essential mechanisms (immunologic and homeostatic dysfunction) involved in the pathogenicity of ACD.

In conclusion, not all the causes of anemia in the chronic disease SLE are well known. The most characteristic types of anemia are iron-deficiency anemia, autoimmune hemolytic anemia, anemia from chronic kidney failure, vitamin B12-deficiency anemia and other forms. The disease is most frequent in women, does not have a well-known cause and has a special association with some genes of the immune response. Some affected systems are represented by central and peripheral nervous system, lungs, heart, kidneys, serous and other elements of the blood. Other systems of the body may also be affected, infrequently. Some other forms of anemia found in lupus disease are as follows.

2.1. Autoimmune hemolytic anemia (AHA)

- AHA is a rare phenomenon in patients with lupus. Hemolytic anemia may be classified into two major groups: with antibodies at cold and hot temperatures. AHA with hot antibodies is mediated by IgG antibodies that can interact with antigens only at 37°C, and the reaction with cold antibodies can be as low as 4°C. Coomb test is directly positive and involves one of the following elements that interact with the surface of the erythrocytes such as IgG.
- Other hematological disorders such as neutropenia is a common abnormality that amplifies the risk of secondary infections in patients with SLE, but can also be an index of the disease state. In addition to neutropenia, lymphopenia is also reported to be a frequently seen hematological disorder in patients with lupus [4, 9].

2.2. Leucopenia

It is a hematological disturbance that occurs in half of the patients with SLE, circulating granulocytes being decreased because of granulocytopenia by destruction in the peripheral circulation (antigranulocyte antibodies, hypersplenism), bone marrow dysfunction, drug-induced cytopenia (azathioprine), lymphocytopenia through non-immunological mechanisms (drug induced), immunological mechanisms (antilymphocyte-dependent antibodies IgM) and nonspecific antibodies, which interact with lymphocytes. Leucopenia appears in over 50% of patients with SLE and is associated with granulocytopenia or lymphopenia. Most of the times leucopenia can be reversible with adequate immunosuppressive therapy [7, 17, 19].

Often, leucopenia can be a good gravity index regarding the disease activity, and it can also appear as a response to the cytotoxic therapy. Leucopenia and neutropenia are the findings often present in active lupus, but rarely reach such a low level to cause the infections.

The number of cells can be decreased by azathioprine, cyclophosphamide and other drugs. Thus, the number of white cells should always be monitored during the treatment of SLE. If the number of white cells decreases too much, lowering the doses of the drugs or discontinuation of the treatment should be done. Dysfunction of the immune system, which causes widespread infection in SLE, is not reflected in the usual blood tests [11, 12, 19, 20].

2.3. Thrombocytopenia

Mild thrombocytopenia (number of thrombocytes 100,000–150,000/μL) is present in 25–50% of patients with SLE and those with less than 50,000/μL appears to be only 10%. The most common cause of thrombocytopenia in SLE is the autodestruction of thrombocytes.

Impaired production of thrombocytes is drug induced (as a result of bone marrow suppression). The main underlying mechanism of this event is the binding between immunoglobulin and thrombocyte after the destruction in spleen, almost similar to idiopathic thrombocytopenic purpura. Antibodies against thrombocytopenic purpura were detected in the serum of patients with SLE and correlated with thrombocytopenia [10, 13, 21].

Idiopathic thrombocytopenic purpura can be the first sign in SLE, followed by other symptoms that can appear later. In these cases, the presence of high antinuclear factor (ANAs) titer of nuclear antigen increases the possibility of having SLE. A detailed clinical and laboratory examination in many of these cases may reveal the supplementary index of SLE. Patients with lupus suffer frequently from osteoporosis, because they sum up the risk of predominant feminine population and long-term corticosteroid therapy [3, 14].

Specific antibodies for coagulation factors are seen in SLE, which is frequently associated with bleeding. These antibodies are usually present against II, VIII, IX, XI or XII factors. This abnormality is accompanied by hypercoagulation and not by major bleedings. The blood of a SLE patient can be hypercoagulable for various reasons other than procoagulant antibodies; these include inherited deficiency of C, S factors or IIIrd antithrombin. Urinary loss of antithrombin III in patients with nephrotic syndrome also leads to a hypercoagulability state.

3. Methods of investigation

The laboratory examination has particular importance in the diagnosis of the pathological processes of lupus as an immune disease and of the hematopoietic system. Ideally, a peripheral blood analysis is done that includes all the disease manifestation by the quantity and quality index, for example morphological characteristic of erythrocytes, leukocyte, morphological modifications of leukocytes and the presence of the pathological cells. These values provide significant data for establishing the diagnosis for hematological maladies. Investigations of the number of reticulocytes and thrombocytes also have an important role in the diagnosis [1].

General blood analysis. Its purpose is to calculate the number of erythrocytes and leukocyte. Evaluation of the hemoglobin level, erythrocytes and hematocrit index is done for confirmation of anemia. A complete hemogram is performed to evaluate the global hematopoietic system and the presence of inflammation. A particular importance is given to the morphological study of erythrocytes from the blood smear, diameter and the form of erythrocytes (by anisocytosis and poikilocytosis mark) [2, 22].

Hemoglobin is a tetrameric molecule and contains iron with porphyrin structure. Iron is capable of reversible link with oxygen only in ferric phase. Iron oxidation in its ferric phase determines the methemoglobin formation, which alters the absorption and determines the brownish blood coloration. Normal limits of hemoglobin is 120–140 g/l for women.

The majority of authors distinguish three grades of anemia: grade I—the content of hemoglobin varies from 91 to 110 g/l, grade II—hemoglobin values vary from 71 to 90 g/l and grade III—the level of hemoglobin fluctuates from 51 to 70 g/l [1, 17].

Erythrocytes. The number of erythrocytes represents the main test for evaluation of erythropoiesis. Erythrocytes are investigated by measuring the concentration of hemoglobin and hematocrit; based on the values of erythrocyte index: medium erythrocyte volume (MEV), mean corpuscular hemoglobin concentration (MCHC) and mean quantity of hemoglobin in erythrocyte (MCH) are calculated by the analyzer. All these values characterized erythrocytic population qualitatively.

Number of erythrocytes as a single parameter has insignificant diagnostic value, so that the correct evaluation of erythrocyte mass is done through the correlation with hematocrit.

Hematocrit is the volume percentage (vol%) of red blood cells in blood. It is normally 45% for men and 40% for women. It is considered an integral part of a person's complete blood count results, along with hemoglobin concentration, white blood cell count and platelet count. The hematocrit with erythrocytic index is used in the diagnosis of diverse types of anemia [3, 4].

Serum iron is determined using colorimetric method and helps in the diagnosis of iron deficiency. Serum iron is a medical laboratory test that measures the amount of circulating iron that is bound to transferrin. Clinicians carry out this laboratory test when they are concerned about iron deficiency, which can cause anemia and other problems. About 65% of the iron in the body is bound up in hemoglobin molecules in red blood cells. About 4% is bound up in myoglobin molecules. Around 30% of the iron in the body is stored as ferritin or hemosiderin in the spleen, the bone marrow and the liver. Small amounts of iron can be found in other molecules in cells throughout the body. None of this iron is directly measurable from serum level.

However, some iron circulate in the serum. Transferrin is a molecule produced by the liver that binds one or two iron ions, i.e. ferric iron, Fe^{3+}; transferrin is essential if stored iron is to be moved and used. Most of the time, about 30% of the available sites on the transferrin molecule are occupied. The test for serum iron measures the iron molecules that are bound to transferrin and circulating in the blood. The extent at which transferrin molecules are occupied by iron ions can be another helpful clinical indicator, known as percent transferrin saturation. These tests are generally done at the same time. Considering the laboratory results together is an important part of the diagnostic process for conditions such as anemia, iron-deficiency anemia, anemia of chronic disease and hemochromatosis.

It is extremely important to collect the blood correctly for determining the serum iron. It was noted that the tubes washed with distilled water contained traces of iron. Another important matter to be considered is that the patient should not get any iron medication at least 5 days before analysis [8, 23].

Ferritin content in serum facilitates the diagnosis of iron deficiency in pre-latent period. Ferritin is the diagnostic marker in iron deficiency, and the latex-test method is validated for the evaluation of iron storage. Ferritin is measured in the serum using polyclonal antibodies for ferritin absorbed by the latex particles. The established norm is 10.00–160.00 g/l. Values under 10.00 g/l are considered low.

Erythropoietin (EPO), a glycoprotein hormone secreted by the kidney in the adult and by the liver in the fetus, which acts on stem cells of the bone marrow to stimulate red blood cell production (erythropoiesis). The Biometrica EPO ELISA test is a immunofermentative in vivo diagnostic test, which determines the quantity of serum erythropoietin. The glycoprotein hormone erythropoietin (EPO) is an essential growth and survival factor for erythroid progenitor cells, and the rate of red blood cell production is normally determined by the serum EPO concentration. EPO production is inversely related to oxygen availability, so that an effective feedback loop is established, which controls erythropoiesis. Since recombinant EPO became available as an effective therapeutic agent, significant progress has also been made in understanding the basis of this feedback control. The main determinant of EPO synthesis is the transcriptional activity of its gene in liver and kidneys, which is related to local oxygen tensions. This control is achieved by hypoxia-inducible transcription factors (HIF), consisting of a constitutive beta-subunit and one of two alternative oxygen-regulated HIF alpha subunits (HIF-1alpha and HIF-2alpha). In the presence of oxygen (normoxia), the HIF alpha subunits are hydroxylated, which targets them for proteasomal degradation. Under hypoxia, because of the lack of oxygen molecule, HIF cannot be hydroxylated and is thereby stabilized. Although HIF-1alpha was the first transcription factor identified through its ability to bind to an enhancer sequence of the EPO gene, more recent evidence suggests that HIF-2alpha is responsible for the regulation of EPO. Although EPO is a prime example for an oxygen-regulated gene, the role of the HIF system goes far beyond the regulation of EPO, because it operates widely in almost all cells and controls a broad transcriptional response to hypoxia, including genes involved in cell metabolism, angiogenesis and vascular tone. Further evidence suggests that apart from its effect as an erythropoietic hormone, EPO acts as a paracrine, tissue-protective protein in the brain and possibly also in other organs [11].

Coombs test. Circulatory anti-erythrocyte antibodies are detected using indirect Coombs test. Unlike direct Coombs test that uses patient's erythrocytes, indirect test uses serum. At the second phase, this mixture is supplemented with a solution that contains human antiglobulin antibodies. If antibodies exist in the patient's serum, agglutination appears.

Thrombocytes. Normal thrombocytes are represented as small cytoplasmic fragments, light blue colored, with azurophilic diffuse small grains (red-purple), with a diameter of 2–4 μm and oval in shape. The number of thrombocytes can be estimated in the analyzer or in the smear. The normal value of thrombocytes is 180.0–320.0·10/l, and the values under 180 thousand are considered as decreased—thrombocytopenia.

Leukocytes—the white cells from the plasma. Depending on the function and their role, leukocytes are divided in five categories: basophil, eosinophils, lymphocytes, monocytes and neutrophils. Normal values of leukocytes are 4.0–9.0·10/l.

ESR (Westergren)—Erythrocyte sedimentation rate is the rate at which the red blood cells make sediment during 1, 2 hours or 15 minutes.

ESR is regulated by the equilibrium between pro-sedimentary factors, main being fibrinogen, and the negative charge of erythrocytes. The Westergren method is the most frequent method used to determine the erythrocyte sedimentation rate.

The ESR is a simple nonspecific screening test that indirectly measures the presence of inflammation in the body. It reflects the tendency of red blood cells to settle more rapidly in the face of some disease states, usually because of increases in plasma fibrinogen, immunoglobulins and other acute-phase reaction proteins. Changes in red cell shape or numbers may also affect the ESR.

There are two main methods used to measure the ESR: the Westergren method and the Wintrobe Method. Each method produces slightly different results. Most laboratories use the Westergren method.

4. Methods and results

Through analyzing the instruments used for evaluating the SLE activity, we chose the Systemic Lupus Activity Measure (SLAM) index that reflects the clinical and laboratory parameters of SLE. The score of this instrument varies between 0 and 20 points, being considered preferable as compared to Systemic Lupus Erythematosus Disease Activity Index (SLEDAI), for the appreciation of anemia in context with SLE [24]. SLAM is a quantity index that includes 37 parameters, compared to 10 domains that reflect the state of 8 organs and systems (constitutional, reticuloendothelial, pulmonary, cardiovascular, neuromotor, hematological, ocular and articulations) shown by laboratory data. Each domain is marked from 3 to 11 parameters.

We obtained the next distribution: low activity is mentioned till 10 points, medium—10–20 points and high grade—over 20 points [3].

In accordance with the purpose, a group of 110 patients with systemic lupus erythematosus have been selected. About 87 of the investigated patients complied with SLE diagnosis criteria issued by the American College of Rheumatology, which constituted the baseline study group. We had only one male patient, so we excluded him from our research to avoid gender misrepresentation.

In our study, we obtained the data about the onset disease age that ranged from 21 to 62 years (mean age—32.8 ± 1.32), but more often the disease was established at a young age—between 21 and 39 years. The mean age of the patients at the time of examination was 41.37 ± 1.4 (21–65 years), with the onset of the disease at 8.6 years of age. At the moment of examination, patients were mostly between 21 and 39 years and only eight were over 50 years old. We were also interested in analyzing the duration of the disease—from 1 to 365 months (30 years).

In this study, each patient was evaluated individually. We analyzed the obtained results from SLAM compartments—general, clinical and laboratory. In each compartment, we included five possible answer variants: 1—absent or normal; 2—easy; 3—moderate and 4—severe. It is noted that in SLAM the "not examined patient" heading is included.

Fever has been characterized by the levels scored in the SLAM, and the indices like oral and nasal ulcers, alopecia, vasculitis, Raynaud syndrome and anti-DNA antibody-dc had two answers **Yes** or **No**, which signifies **the presence** or **the absence of** them. Other components of SLAM score, which refers to the component status, were represented by a hematological evaluation of some variables such as leukopenia, thrombocytopenia and lymphopenia; stratification of hemoglobin levels and ESR represents the severity of pathological process.

Skin damage was manifested by the nose or mouth sores, rashes, malar erythema and photosensitivity. The detection of at least one of these conditions adds a clinical score SLAM and it is expended to disease activity. Cutaneous manifestations such as maculopapular erythema or deep lupus has denoted with 3 points of damage to more than 50% of the body surface (ASC), with 2 points to extinction of 20–50% and with only 1 point in case of involvement of less than 20% of the area of the manipulation. Similarly, the presence of vasculitis has been noted with the respective score summary area involved. Eye manifestations are presented by corpuscles, bleeding (retinal or colloid) or episcleritis, papillitis or pseudomotor cerebri, and depending on the absence or presence and severity of these events, it produces a score from 0 to 3 points for each clinical index. The central nervous system is affected frequently in lupus patients. The most frequently symptoms were migraine, epilepsy and chorea.

Chronic ulcers, avascular necrosis and hemolytic anemia were observed in our patients with a frequency of 17.4, 8.7 and 8.7%, respectively. Our data on the incidence of avascular necrosis and chronic ulcers are similar to those shown in the literature, and only for hemolytic anemia, the data were lower than the presented percentage of Giannouli [25]. We diagnosed a small number of valvulopathy (8.7%). Referring to confirm secondary APS by laboratory variables, we found that more often anticardiolipin (ACL) IgG antibodies were found than IgM—60.9 vs. 30.4%, which shows that ACL IgG antibodies have sensitivity and high specificity and can be indicated in the research plan of patients with SLE in order to forecast possible thrombosis. Analyzing the results described, we concluded that APS was associated with SLE in 26.7% of cases, which corresponds to the data reported by Duarte [23]—28% of cases, but it differs from some older records invoked by Nossent et al. [7], they detected APS in 54% of patients with SLE. Typical signs of antiphospholipid syndrome—thrombosis—have been developed frequently in 60.9% of patients, including 21.7% of these were recurrent. Antiphospholipid syndrome with concomitant thrombosis in the system of more veins and/or arteries called APS cascading or Asherson's syndrome, which endangers the patient's life or seriously alters the quality of life through complications that may arise. Obstetric pathology was associated frequently in 52.2% of cases examined and negatively affected the prognosis of the disease. This compromises the possibility of a normal pregnancy; therefore, patients with APS associated with SLE can conceive only by an adequate treatment and should be under rigorous surveillance.

We came across a patient with the medical history of systemic lupus erythematosus, iron-deficient anemia and symptoms of antiphospholipid syndrome. From this case, relevance of hematological damage in SLE and APS patients has emerged. So, we continued research analyzing hematologic risk factors that increase individual susceptibility in SLE patients in terms of morbidity and mortality through hematologic damage, including autoimmune hemolytic anemia. Preventive hematology succeeded to prove undoubtedly that by addressing hematologic risk factors significant reduction of the incidence, prevalence, complications and mortality from diseases of the hematopoietic system could be reduced.

Less has been disclosed on the overlapped quantitative influence of hematologic risk factors in patients with autoimmune inflammatory chronic diseases such as idiopathic inflammatory myopathies, Sjogren's syndrome and SLE, as it admits that the risk factors interact between themselves, multiplying the hematological risk, which may impact the patient's condition during the morbid evolution of the disease. For these reasons, we analyzed the morbid hematologic risk factors in two distinct groups by quantifying them, choosing for individuals with SLE and healthy people.

At the next stage, we tried to analyze disease activity and organic damage index depending on the grade of anemia and the presence of anti-DNA antibodies.

According to our results, high SLAM scores (18.78) were associated with severe anemia with Hb level of 51–70 g/l, and they were having organic damage index values of 1.15. In our study, the lowest values of the examined indices were demonstrated in the absence of anemia (SLAM – 7.17, damage index – 0.56) with a background of negative anti-DNA. In the medium and moderate forms of anemia, SLAM score and damage index were moderately elevated.

Analyzing the anticardiolipin antibodies, IgG and IgM, in all these groups, we found that the average IgG antibodies was higher in the group of patients with ACD—12 (35%) cases versus patients in groups with iron-deficient anemia and AHA, where the indices were 5 (25%) and 1 (20%) ($p > 0.05$).

The same frequency was also observed in the level of anticardiolipin IgM antibodies. Patients (20 (33.9%)) with iron-deficient anemia and AHA + ARF (anemia of renal failure) had identical levels of IgM anticardiolipin antibodies in 20% of cases, whereas the ACD patients had a higher rate of 26.5%. We noted that the C3 complement level was reduced to over 80% of cases of anemia in all groups, a situation that indicates high disease activity.

Analyzing the frequency of high titers of anti-DC DNA, we observed that in groups of patients with chronic anemia and iron-deficiency anemia this index was positive in 70% of cases and reported in 44 patients as compared to Group III, where DNA anti-DC was positively observed only in 2 (40%) patients.

In the third group of patients, lupus nephritis was detected more frequently in 60% of cases, whereas in groups of patients with anemia of chronic disease and iron-deficiency anemia, lupus nephritis was detected in 40% of cases. The differences were statistically significant ($p < 0.01$).

For confirming anemia and the quantification of its intensity, we appealed to the index of the disease activity in hematological lupus—Systemic Lupus Activity Measure (SLAM), which is a test that measures the activity of the disease in patients with SLE through the condition of 23 clinical and 7 laboratory parameters commensurate with points. The total possible score of this instrument varies between 0 and 20 points. Unlike SLEDAI, the SLAM index includes not only objective signs and laboratory parameters but also the evaluation of the hemoglobin level and the hematocrit. Analyzing the obtained data, we discovered that of the 59 patients with anemia, 34 (57.6%) were diagnosed with anemia of chronic disease and accumulated an average of 22.6 ± 1.94 according to the SLAM score, a result that is equal to a high activity of the disease; 20 patients (33.9%) with iron-deficiency anemia received 18.9 ± 1.14 score having a moderate-high activity of the disease and 5 (8.5%) of the interviewed patients with other types of anemia obtained 24.9 ± 1.03, a score qualified as a high activity of the disease.

5. Statistical evaluation of the used methods

Data obtained as a result of investigations were processed by computerized analysis (SPSS), correlation and discriminating variation. The degree of correlative relations between the evaluated parameters was assessed using the correlation coefficient R.

Conclusive differences between the mean values of the parameters studied in different batches were estimated using the Student's t test.

Comparing the results of the disease estimated by two questionnaires, it has been inferred that the SLAM, which was drawn up after multiple multidimensional studies, is based on the experience in the field of the assessment of disease activity to patients with lupus, which can be validated as a sensitive instrument in measuring lupus activity and for detection of possible hematological changes in this pathology. The SLAM index is variable, with the instruments and patients included in the study group, and it seems that it has outrun the SLEDAI of being informative in measuring lupus activity, the signs and symptoms activation of pre-existing hematological changes. It should be noted that SLAM evaluates, like the SLEDAI does, light organic manifestations, as well as the serious ones, which define the prognosis of the disease and the amount of organic damage index.

We were interested to estimate general state of health through SLAM, which is not stipulated in the SLEDAI. And that is because a person without neurolupus, but with a poor general condition estimated by the SLEDAI may display a low score, and the same patient assessed after SLAM can display with proper activity according to the index that is constitutionally expended score from hematological changes. We recorded the importance of the accuracy of the applied tool according to the hypothesis, the first-ever SLAM is designed to record only the symptoms reported by the patient due to SLE, but sometimes it becomes difficult to distinguish claims of secondary manifestations of light lupus exacerbations.

In the tests for the evaluation of disease activity in accordance with the questionnaire, in addition to SLAM, clinical examination has taken into account and some laboratory **variables** such as **the number of leucocytes, lymphocytes, platelets, hemoglobin** and **ESR**. Hemoglobin values ranged between 68 and 148 (107.6 ± 2.1) g/l, they being an indication of anemia. Leukocyte index in the batch of examined patients noted in average 1900–8800 (4.38 ± 0.3). The average values of lymphocytes were 9942 ± 0.4 (variations between 565 and 1900 or from 12 to 36%), and the level of platelets has been downsized considerably—246,900 ± 9.2 (numerical variations between 111,200 and 450,000).

We analyzed the ESR as important hematological index, which increased the number of patients to 64% (74.4% advertising and reflecting the high activity of the disease).

We were interested to analyze the titers fractions C3 and C4 of the complement, along with the complement titer, which ranged between 1:4 and 1:128. It is worth noting that complement C3 fraction joined in the range of 6.8 to 130 mg/dl (23.4 ± 3.4), predominantly being low. C4 fraction was found for low and medium (8.22 ± 1.48) with variations between 4.0 and 22.4 mg/dl, the most common being dropped in the majority of patients with systemic lupus erythematosus.

We were interested in comparing the results of two cohorts in the SLAM. Patients included in the study were divided, as we agreed in two batches: with anemia—59 cases (68.6%) and without anemia—27 cases (31.4%).

To analyze anemic syndrome, two groups, which consisted of 59 patients with anemia and 27 patients without anemia, were numerically different to compare, so later we resorted to instrumental indexes included in the scale of assessment of the SLAM disease activity.

Comparing groups through the constitutional component, it was estimated that the patients who had various types of anemia, constitutional abnormalities, included in this section, were detected more frequently than those without anemia ($p < 0.05$). We also found that the skin of the patients in the first group, with anemia were more frequently affected, compared with the group of patients without anemia and fatigability (43.2%) were present in bigger intensity was expressed in the batch of patients with anemia. It could define the basic disease, but precipitated by the presence of anemia.

Collaboration obtained outlined in the following: oral ulcers, periangle erythema and photosensitivity were found in a greater number of patients with anemia—46 (77.9%) in comparison with batch without anemia, where they were detected in 18 (66.7%) patients. In addition to erythema alopecia and discoid lesions being extended to patients with anemia.

After the estimation of lupus activity on cardiovascular impairment, the results revealed higher values in the batch of patients with anemia to 61.0% (versus 29.9% cases), and in the group without anemia, we can summarize that the activity has an impact on disease anemia or maintain this pathology. Speaking about the effect of SLE on central nervous system, it was observed especially in patients with anemia, accounting for 57.6% of cases having an impact on lupus activity. Our data transpose with literature data show that the damage to the nervous system reflects the activity of the disease in patients with anemia [3].

Comparing the values of lymphocytes in both groups of patients, we have revealed that lymphocytopenia was more specific in the group of patients with anemia—49.1% of cases had decreased lymphocyte levels as low as 565 cells. Thrombocytopenia was also more common in patients with the beginning of anemia in lupus. As a matter of fact, the ESR, primarily, is a common index, and it was investigated in terms of different rates of acceleration, depending on the activity of the disease. Defining line was inspired by the study of LIGHT XXIX (Villa, 2005), which divided the ESR values into four categories: <12—normal, 12 to 30—average acceleration, 30 to 50—moderate hike and over 50 mm/hour—marked acceleration, the results being calculated after an hour and the possibility of making a finding after 2 hours (to 6–24 mm).

We were interested in analyzing the disease activity and damage rate index of various categories of ESR. ESR has been determined to be of average elevation—12 to 30, moderate elevation—30 to 50 and marked as acceleration—over 50 mm/hour.

We analyzed whether the activity, SLAM index and IL are reflected in ESR. According to the data, ESR was independently associated with high scores of SLAM. It was found that accelerated ESR associated with both disease activity, as measured by the SLAM, and with high scores of the SF-36, which had been in decline. The relation between index variables and effect on the quality of life as measured by the SF-36 was foreshadowed.

It should be noted that the increase in ESR was not dependent on the organic damage index. We can conclude that the erythrocyte sedimentation speed is a relevant test and can be considered a sensitive index. ESR has been correlated with disease activity, assessed by SLAM and has impact on the quality of life, based on estimates by the SF-36.

6. Risk factors for the development of hematologic manifestations in SLE

We took the risk factors as a research vector in order to highlight and analyze their impact later on the installation of hematological lupus and their interference with the subsequent development of the disease. Data displayed in the recent related literatures highlight both general and specific risk factors for hematological lupus. General risk factors are hypertension, diabetes, obesity, dyslipidemia, smoking (more than 10 cigarettes per day), valvular heart disease and/or atrial fibrillation, cumulative doses of glucocorticosteroids >10 g, oral contraceptives, pathology of thyroid (history of hypo- or hyperthyroidism, antithyroid therapy or HRT) and family history of psychiatric illness [18]. Specific risk factors involve increased levels of antiphospholipid antibodies, the presence of lupus anticoagulant and antiphospholipid syndrome and the presence of Raynaud's phenomenon, livedo reticularis and cutaneous vasculitis [10, 14].

An imperative of assessing anemia is presented by identifying and stratification of the importance of each clinical and serological parameter suggested as a risk factor for hematopoietic system involvement in lupus [13].

From the study, we observed that the most commonly found index in patients with lupus was the antiphospholipid syndrome, which was present both in patients without hematological damage—8 (9.3%) cases and in those with severe hematological damage—15 (17.4%) cases. Our survey data coincide with those stipulated in researches throughout the world, where the association of antiphospholipid syndrome is most often reported anemia pattern in lupus.

According to the following data, the presence of livedo reticularis in patients without anemia was detected in 14 (16.3%) cases and in patients with anemia in 17 (19.7%) cases. Thus, we presume that the presence of livedo reticularis in the study conducted by us is associated with hematologic manifestations and can be considered as a risk factor of a hematopoietic system involvement in patients with lupus. The newest scientific reports present the Raynaud syndrome as a specific risk factor for developing anemia, mainly for ACD (anemia of chronic disease) and iron-deficient anemia [7, 13]. According to our data, Raynaud syndrome was present less—only in 3 (3.5%) patients without anemia and in 6 (6.9%) patients who developed anemia.

Clinical examination of patients noted that cutaneous vasculitis has been associated closely with various events in the development of anemia and was present in 12 (13.9%) patients, since patients without anemia only in 5 (5.8%) cases.

In addition to specific risk factors, we were concerned about examining generic risk factors that were less connected with anemia before. We found a close association between hypertension and hematological manifestations—11 (18.6%) patients. It is important to mention that in 2 (2.3%) cases where diabetes was detected, hematological syndromes were observed simultaneously. Following the examination, we reported that factors such as obesity, dyslipidemia, smoking excessively and cumulative dose of glucocorticosteroids >10 g were identified mainly in patients who developed various hematologic manifestations.

A special role is given to valvulopathy, which was detected in 5 (5.8%) patients without anemia and 6 (6.9%) patients with anemia. The studies in the domain show a high frequency of anemia in patients with valvulopathy of left heart in systemic lupus erythematosus [20]. Other research highlights the frequent association of renal and hematological manifestations in lupus [11, 26]. According to data reported, kidney damage was detected in 4 (4.6%) patients without anemia and in 24 (27.9%) patients with anemia. The risk profile is complemented by another factor, such as compromised neuropsychiatric history detected in 5 (5.8%) patients in the group with hematological antidamage (clarify).

Summarizing the exposed view of the risks of the patients with SLE, we can register that antiphospholipid syndrome, livedo reticularis, skin vasculitis, smoking, cumulative dose of glucocorticosteroids >10 g and kidney damage are more commonly found in the context of a hematological lupus than in those without impaired heme.

7. Synthesis of the obtained results

At the current stage, the study of the hematological manifestations in systemic lupus erythematosus (SLE), which is a severe, multisystem autoimmune disease of unknown etiology with varied clinical and paraclinical expressions associated with a hyper production of auto-antibodies and with a potentially major fatality rate, represents a domain of scientific interest and an important medicosocial issue [19].

In the past 5 years, thanks to immunological and morphopathological achievements and the usage of techniques of fundamental organic research, important progress was obtained in regard to the diagnosis, monitoring and the treatment of autoimmune diseases.

Nevertheless, the diagnosis of this disease [11] and the bearing of the expenses of the social support persist because SLE has a major potential of disablement and thereby affects the quality of life severely. The prevention of relapses transforms into an extension of the remissions leading to a mostly regular social inclusion and reduced social costs through limiting the hospitalization time [24]. Still, the impact of the pathology of the hematopoietic system on the quality of life remains uncertain.

In the presented paper, we intended to analyze the modern research regarding the clinical and paraclinical diagnosis of systemic lupus erythematosus. We have examined a group of patients with lupus by thoroughly researching the hematopoietic system—a clinical criteria discussed in the specialty literature. In the past 10 years, these discussions [12, 13] are related not only to the classically iterated clinical manifestations but also to their quantification through instruments and also using hematological, immunological and paraclinical methods.

In our study, the female/male ratio was 86 (100%), respectively, 0. Analyzing the average age of onset, we have established that the onset of the disease was at various ages—from 21 to 62 years old (average 32.8 ± 1.32) but essentially young people are affected. At the moment of examination, the patients observed were averagely 41.37 ± 1.40 with variation intervals 21–65 years. The analysis of the disease duration detected significant divergences: from 1 month up to 365 months (48 years). In the study, we have examined patients with an average evolution span of the lupus process of 98.28 months (8.6 ± 0.47 years), most frequently between 1 month and 5 years. A study of prospective analysis was accomplished by Harly (1989) [11] but with an average evolution span of the lupus process of 5.4 months and because of the shorter stage, a disparity of results is presumed when it comes to a comparison to our own data regarding the cumulative doses of corticosteroids and the index of organ lesion.

Throughout our study, we were interested in distinguishing the etiological aspect of the moment of onset of SLE, an aim for which we have intended to reflect the specter of triggers through the overlap of anamnestic data that were accurately collected from the patients included in the study and divided into two groups: those with anemia and those without anemia. Our results revealed the presence of stress in 11.1% of those who did not develop anemia and in 10.2% of those who developed hematological syndromes during the disease. This determined us to consider that the psychoemotional stress was significantly involved in both groups included in the study. Exposure to low temperatures was identified both in the evolutionary context of the patients without anemia—18.5% and in that of those with anemia—20.3%. Another trigger, antecedents of exposure to sun, was detected in 33.3% of lupus patients without subsequent hematological manifestations and in 27.1% of those who developed anemia. It seemed that the exposure to sun generated the systemic lupus erythematosus but it somehow was a more protective measure for the following lesion of the hematopoietic system while the vaccination was less actively implicated in the onset of lupus—in 3.7% but those cases presented with a significant potential of hematopoietic system implication in the course of the disease—in 1.7% of cases. Simultaneously, we established that 29.6% of the patients without anemia and 32.2% of those with anemia could not outline any causes that led to SLE, this leaving room for more elaborate studies on this topic in the future.

Thus, the comparative assessment of the conditions which preceded the disease in the study groups revealed that the insolation and the exposure to low temperatures take up the biggest share as triggers for the development of hematological syndromes in systemic lupus erythematosus, while the psycho-emotional stress and the vaccination are not directly responsible for the onset of lupus but their impact on the development of anemia is not excluded.

For the estimation of the activity of lupus, we chose a validated instrument—the SLAM index. The results of the investigation confirmed that the use of this index is also practicable in the dynamic assessment of the activity of the process and the implication of the hematopoietic system rendered through anemia, leukopenia, lymphopenia, thrombocytopenia and accelerated erythrocyte sedimentation rate. Referring to the average score of the SLAM index, it was higher in the patients included in the study than in the prospective study presented by Bertoli (2007) [24], constituting 22.6 ± 1.94 versus 19.4 ± 5.5. It should be noted that on the position of significant discrepancy is the fact that all the patients from our group of study were receiving corticosteroids, whereas in the reference study only 69.2% of the patients were receiving corticosteroids at the moment of the examination.

The clinical picture of lupus presented very diversely by involving different organs and systems. We wanted to compare the frequency of the diagnostic criteria ACR 1997 for SLE met by the patients in our group of study and those from the reference study reported by Giannouli (2006) [23], where the prevalence of anemia between the lupus patients was 50%. Similar data were published by Bertoli (2007) [20]. Considering that we detected a rate of 68.8% of hematopoietic system implication in our study, we continued to compare our results with other studies. In this connection, we discovered that the results obtained by Voulgares (2000) and Alastair [1] proved the hematopoietic system affliction at a rate of 14 and 80%, respectively. It is noteworthy that in the longitudinal study LUMINA LI (2007) [24] carried out on a cohort of 613 patients in the hematological modifications were present in 62.3% of cases. Therefore, our results are similar to the data of some studies, whereas they differ substantially from others. It is difficult to explain the big difference for the hematopoietic system impairment, but we can suppose that the cause has been the recently instituted lupus—only 5 months in the reference group, while the hematopoietic system implication is a rare manifestation.

For obvious reasons, we referred our results to the data from other studies which reported to the presence of lupus diagnostic criteria: oral ulcerations, arthritis and arthralgia, serositis and renal lesions and we deduced that these attest in similar proportions to those appreciated by the prospective study of Harley (1989) [18]. Our data noted that the presence of photosensitivity in 65.1% of the patients and that of the malar erythema in 89.5 versus 36–41.5%, respectively, which were discovered in the study of reference Harley (1989). The data referring to hematological and immunological modifications and the antinuclear antibodies are similar to those appreciated throughout our study—64.3% cases. In all the patients with systemic lupus erythematosus, we remarked the presence of antinuclear autoantibodies (ANA) and anti-double-stranded DNA (anti-dsDNA), at least one of these indexes was found positive in the patients included in the study. According to the criteria defined by the American College of Rheumatology (ACR), the diagnosis of systemic lupus erythematosus was established on the basis of 4 or more criteria from the 11 criteria stated by the ACR, characteristics that were found simultaneously or successively in the patients investigated by our studies.

The study carried out analyzed the lupus patients with a hematological pathology, confirmed by a hematologist and the patients who did not manifest a pathology of the hematopoietic system. Through clinical and paraclinical examination of the hematopoietic system of the patients with SLE from the selected group, we deduced that the disease can affect the hematopoietic system at any level, but has a predilection for these types of ailments: anemia, leukopenia, lymphopenia and thrombocytopenia.

In our study, the number of hematological syndromes has correlated positively with the high score of the SLAM index and the SLICC/ACR score, which suggested that more hematological manifestations could be associated with the high activity of the disease and can predispose to a further organ lesion. Nevertheless, some hematological events in SLE may only be the clinical presentation, persistent even at a low activity of the disease, without specific serological markers.

According to the investigational objectives, we analyzed the possible relations between the clinical manifestation, the activity of the process and the organ lesion. The results of the research under this aspect have estimated that the evolution of the hematological manifestations depends on the activity of the lupus process. The impact of these on the organ lesion index and the quality of life was recorded. The index of organ lesion becomes higher with the display of hematological events: anemia, leukopenia, lymphopenia and thrombocytopenia, which lower the patient's quality of life significantly. Despite the frequent hematological manifestations in SLE, there are no specific clinical or paraclinical tests for the diagnosis of the implication of the hematopoietic system in SLE, and there are also no specific clinical or paraclinical tests for the diagnosis of the implication of the hematopoietic system in the disease evolution, all these imposing the necessity of further research and the imperative demand for finding specific biomarkers for anemia.

With the purpose of establishing the importance of the reduction of erythropoietin level as a hypothetical biomarker that is associated with hematological disorders in lupus, particularly of the anemia of the chronic disease, we stratified the values depending on the obtained results. We examined the level of erythropoietin in 57 patients from the study group, in 3 of whom other types of anemia were found, 20 presenting iron-deficiency anemia of different degrees and 34 patients had the anemia of the chronic disease. Continuing the analysis of the presented data, we discovered that in 43 patients the level of the researched index was subnormal—between 1.12 and 3.22 μIU/ml. In 20 patients, the level of erythropoietin was estimated as normal and the diagnosis emitted—iron-deficiency anemia. We overlapped our records with the results in recent literature and we affiliated towards the principle that the level of erythropoietin may be useful in detecting the anemia in lupus. According to the data of Schett (2010) [3], the low titer of erythropoietin correlates with the anemia of the chronic disease in lupus, and the data only confirmed this statement. All of the findings support the opinion that these patients require a dynamic evaluation and monitoring.

Calculations for the total doses of corticosteroids, also named cumulative dose, preoccupied us into relating it to the involvement of the hematopoietic system in the lupus process. The cumulative dose of corticosteroids was calculated according to the prednisolone dose administered orally throughout the disease, also including the pulse therapy. The cumulative dose, as is known, not only increases during the disease but also includes the pulse therapies which imply the administration of high doses of corticosteroids—1500 to 3000 mg (1.5–3.0 g) in a single cure or the programmed pulse therapy with a dose of 500 mg monthly. We divided the patients according to the quantity of corticosteroids administered and we considered the quantity below 5 g as a low dose, between 5 and 10 g as a medium dose and higher than 10 g as a high dose [11]. After the summary dose of corticosteroids, our patients accumulated mostly medium and high doses of corticosteroids—above 5 g. We did not detect a correlation of the doses of corticosteroids with the disorders of the hematopoietic system in the group of study.

According to the outlined objectives, we were motivated to analyze the damage to the hematopoietic system in accordance with the criteria for SLE elaborated by ACR (1999). The analysis of the results obtained shows a large and diverse specter of hematopoietic system implications in SLE. Of 86 patients examined in the study, the hematopoietic system implication and more precisely anemia were present in 59 (68.6%) patients. At the same time, the same patient may develop one or more hematological syndromes. Our data correspond to the data of the recent scientific methods dedicated to the assessment of the anemia in the context of lupus, including those reported by the cohort study carried out on 345 patients under the supervision of Voulgares and Kokori (2000) [23], which reported the clinical incidence of hematological manifestations in 38.4% of the patients.

From this study of reference, we ascertained that the most frequent hematological syndromes were the anemia of chronic disease—37.1% cases (39.5% in the patients examined by us), iron-deficiency anemia—35.6% (versus 23.2% in our study), followed by autoimmune hemolytic anemia— 14.4% and other types of anemia—12.9% cases. According to these results we observe similarities between the frequency of the hematological syndromes detected in the patients from the study of reference and those enrolled in our study.

Therefore, the diversity of hematopoietic system damage reveals the indubitable value of applying the criteria developed by ACR (1999) for evaluating the patients with SLE.

Continuing the research on this subject, we insisted on the thorough approach of anemia as a form of hematopoietic system affliction in SLE. Anemia and other hematological disorders, such as leukopenia, lymphopenia and thrombocytopenia, are still a challenge for the diagnosticians for reasons which include the fact that they could be either a direct manifestation of SLE or a secondary response to a chronic disease that affects the quality of life.

We tried to assess the indexes important for SLE in the patients without anemia tied to lupus and in those with the anemia of chronic disease. From the data reported before, it can be derived that the average age of onset in the patients without anemia was 34.73 years, whereas in the patients with anemia of chronic disease was 37.2 years. The patients with anemia of the chronic disease also had been sick for a longer period of time—123.4 months compared to those without anemia—80.6 months. It has been determined that the accentuation of anemia happens during the disease. According to the activity of the disease appreciated through the SLAM index, it was established that the patients with anemia of chronic disease had the highest activity of the disease—22.6 points, whereas those without hematological manifestations showed a moderate activity—15.8 points. The index of organ lesion: SLICC was highest in patients with anemia of chronic disease showing values of 1.6 points qualified as an index of moderate organ lesion compared to the first group where the SLICC index was 0.5 points. Our data correspond to those affirmed in a study of reference, Vila (2009) [23] which reveals that anemia and other hematological syndromes occur on the background of active SLE and are associated with a longer age of the disease as well as the organ lesions are more emphasized.

According to the outlined objectives, we evaluated the parameters regarding the patient's quality of life using the SF-36 score. The SF-36 accumulated values were 61 points in the patients without anemia and 41 points in the patients with moderate and severe depression; this being interpreted as a sign of a significantly reduced quality of life. An important study of reference carried out by Stoll (2009) [13] was dedicated to evaluating the quality of life of the patients with SLE and anemia. This study reveals a suggestive detail such as the fact that the routine assessment of the quality of life of the patients with SLE may facilitate the early detection of anemia.

Of course, we were also tempted to analyze the predictors of a reserved prognosis for the patients with SLE who during the disease develop a large variety of hematological syndromes that have an impact on the quality of life. After the analysis of our own data, we cataloged as such the manifestations of renal lesion, thrombocytopenia and a high level of anticardiolipin (aCL) antibodies presented in the patients with SLE and their role in inducing or associating hematological syndromes.

The analysis of diverse clinical manifestations in the hematological lupus was necessary because the persisting clinical indexes may pass on into the class of risk factors. Despite the fact that the paraclinical signs are included in the diagnosis criteria, we analyzed the cases included in the study group by stages. The study carried out by us detected high titers of anti-dsDNA in both groups but only in 6 (23.0%) of the patients without anemia and 56 (94.9%) in those with anemia. Given the fact that aCL (anticardiolipin antibodies) is an index associated with disorders of the hematopoietic system, the analysis of the level of aCL antibodies, Ig and IgM, in the two groups of patients with lupus was a priority. It is to be remarked that in both groups the patients had high levels of anticardiolipin (aCL) IgG antibodies, but in the group without hematological lesions, their frequency was 22.2%, whereas in the patients with hematological lupus it was 28.8% ($p > 0.05$). Continuing the examinations under this aspect, we detected anticardiolipin (aCL) IgM antibodies in 1 (3.7%) patient who did not develop anemia and in 4 (6.8%) patients who manifested anemia; the data obtained in our study being similar to those in a retrospective longitudinal study carried out by Pasero (2009) [14].

The antiphospholipid syndrome was present both in the patients without hematological disorders—8 (29.6%) cases and in those with hematological disorders—in 15 (25.4%) cases. Besides, the data obtained in our study coincide with those stipulated in the research carried out globally, according to which the association of the antiphospholipid syndrome is most frequently reported in relation to the pattern of hematological events. According to the data that analyze the presence of livedo reticularis in the patients without anemia, we discovered 4 (25.9%) of such cases, and in those with anemia this characteristic of the disease was signaled in 21 (35.6%) of the cases. Thereby, we conclude that the presence of livedo reticularis in the study carried out by us was associated to hematological manifestations and may be considered a factor that implies the risk of hematopoietic system affliction in the patients with lupus. Recent investigations report the presence of Raynaud syndrome as a specific risk factor for the development of anemia [18], but according to our data, the Raynaud syndrome was a rarely assessed phenomenon—in 1 (3.7%) patient without anemia and in 4 (6.8%) of those who did not develop anemia.

We intended to use valid instruments for the assessment of the quality of life in the patients with SLE. For this purpose, we applied the SF-36 questionnaire in its short version (short form-36). SF-36 is a brief way of testing but in the special literature there are also other sets of indexes used for reflecting the quality of life such as SF-20. According to the literature data, the SF-36 questionnaire possesses the capacity to evaluate the patients with lupus exhaustively—a quality for which we preferred it in evaluating the impact of the hematopoietic system affliction on the quality of life of the lupus patients. The low quality of life of these people both by the mental health and the physical health, predominantly the physical one conditioned by the hematopoietic system afflictions in 35.6% of the cases. We compared our results with the data presented by Harley and Urowitz (2010) [22, 27], which indicate both the implication of the mental component and the physical one in determining the quality of life of the patients with hematopoietic dysfunctions on the background of lupus.

The data obtained by us after carrying out the study detected similar results with those reported by Harley (1989) [22], especially the ones referring to the vitality domain, physical function, general health and pain, but there were differences regarding affectivity and social function.

We analyzed comparatively the patients with anemia by means of the disease activity index, the organ lesion index and the impact of these on the quality of life. Our results were similar to those obtained in the study done in parallel with ours and recently emitted by other teams of researchers in the world [23], who confirmed that the quality of life index is inversely proportional to the activity of the disease and the organ lesion index for the patients with anemia.

Another study of reference carried out by Nossent and Locatelli (2004) [7] was dedicated to the interrelations of different dimensions and subscales of the generic questionnaire SF-36. Both our data and those from the study of reference denote the prevalence of low scores (<50 points) among the patients with SLE. In contrast to our data, the patients enrolled in the study by Moitinho (2011) [11] accumulated even higher scores—between 81-0 and even 91-100, which were not observed among our patients. Thus, the data provided by the SF-36 questionnaire attest the impact of the hematopoietic system dysfunctions in SLE on the quality of life, most of all through the development of major hematologic syndromes, by affecting all the criteria which characterize it. The low scores among the patients without hematological afflictions invoke that the chronic disease itself implies an important role in the patient's life, the patient being often forced to review some aspects of their daily life, including some in regard to social relations and professional preoccupations.

Even if it is insistently approached in several scientific centers, recognizing the hematological manifestations in the early stages of lupus still remains a challenge for the clinicians. Correctly attributing the hematological syndromes to those caused by the primary disease or to those that present as a reaction to suffering from a chronic and incurable disease or to the adverse reactions to medication or to some metabolic dysfunctions still remains a diagnostic dilemma [5, 13]. Because the physiopathology of these clinical manifestations is not fully elucidated, they cannot be attributed unequivocally to anemia.

An important moment and a problem with a difficult evolution are the subclinical manifestations of the hematopoietic system implication in SLE, which require an early identification and a gradual therapeutic intervention in order to improve upon the further disabilities of the patients. In this connection, the lack of a consensus in regard to the application of different hematological tests with a different potential of sensibility makes its mark. In the absence of a diagnostic standard and potential specific biomarkers for the hematologic affliction, various serological explorations and laboratory investigations are used to support the clinical diagnosis. The results of our study confirm this situation.

Our data correspond to those reported by Bertoli et al. LUMINA LI (2007) [20] and reveal that anemia is strictly associated with the activity of the disease and the organ lesion index both at the disease onset and during its evolution; this association being even closer than that with the anti-dsDNA antibodies. Moreover, anemia is associated with several clinical manifestations including, but not only, those that reflect a more severe disease such as the neuropsychiatric or renal implication. Ideally, the biomarkers have to be standardized and vastly applied especially when the hematocrit assessment is an easy and accessible test and can be considered a cheap indicator of the disease evolution, which allows the clinicians to anticipate the intermediary and long-term consequences of the lupus infection [22].

In our study, the relevance of anemia (independently of its cause) was estimated as being both a short-term prognostic factor (the activity of the disease) and a long-term (lesion index) prognostic factor for the evolution of the disease. The estimated data in the lupus patients with anemia corresponded to those reported in the special literature and invoked the necessity of the improvement of early exploration, including through raising the awareness of the rheumatologists and the cooperation with the general practitioner, the hematologists, etc., who could advisedly get involved in the early detection of hematological dysfunctions, because through their improvement with specific methods, it is possible to maintain a long-term good quality of life.

Author details

Elena Samohvalov[1]* and Sergiu Samohvalov[2]

*Address all correspondence to: elena-samohvalov@rambler.ru

1 Department of Internal Medicine, State Medical and Pharmaceutical University "Nicolae Testemițanu", Chișinău, Moldova

2 Hepato-Surgical Laboratory, State Medical and Pharmaceutical University "Nicolae Testemițanu", Chișinău, Moldova

References

[1] Alastair L et al. The management of peripheral blood cytopenias in systemic lupus erythematosus. Rheumatology. 2010;**49**:2243-2254

[2] Andrade RM et al. Seizures in patients with systemic lupus erythematosus: Data from LUMINA, a multiethnic cohort (LUMINA LIV). Annals of the Rheumatic Diseases. 2008;**67**: 829-834

[3] Hochberg MC. Updating the American College of Rheumatology. Criteria for the classification of systemic lupus erythematosus. Arthritis and Rheumatology. 1997;**40**:1725

[4] Crow MK. Collaboration, genetic associations and lupus Erythematosus. New England Journal of Medicine. 2008;**358**:956-961

[5] Ng WL, Chu CM, Wu AK. Lymphopenia at presentation is associated with increased risk of infections in patients with systemic lupus erythematosus. Quarterly Journal of Medicine. 2009;**99**:37-47

[6] Branch D et al. Antiphospholipid antibodies and the antiphospholipid syndrome: Clinical significance and treatment. În. Seminars in Thrombosis and Hemostasis. 2010;**34**:256-266

[7] Hereng T, Lambert M, Hachulla E. Influence of aspirin on the clinical outcomes of 103 anti-phospholipid antibodies-positive patients. Lupus. 2009;**17**:11-15

[8] Mirzayan MJ, Schmidt RE, Witte T. Prognostic parameters for flare in systemic lupus erythematosus. Rheumatology. 2010;**39**:1316-1319

[9] Castellino G et al. Single photon emission computed tomography and magnetic resonance imaging evaluation in SLE patients with and without neuropsychiatric involvement. Rheumatology (Oxford). 2010;**47**:319-323

[10] Kokori SI, Ioannidis JP, Voulgarelis M. Autoimmune hemolytic anemia in patient with systemic lupus erythematosus. American Journal of Medicine. 2010;**108**(3):198-204

[11] Khamashta M et al. Molecular composition of Ro small ribonucleoprotein complexes in human cells. Intracellular localization of the 60- and 52-kD proteins. Journal of Clinical Investigation. 2010;**93**:1637-1644

[12] Fadz GJ et al. Education, quality of life and immune profile, an integrative perspective of depression in women with lupus. Lupus. 2011;**4**:398

[13] Icen M, Nicola P, Maradit-Kremers H. Systemic lupus erythematosus features in rheumatoid arthritis and their effects on overall mortality. Journal of Rheumatology. 2009;**36**: 50-57

[14] Rosse F, Schreier S, Ebmeier KP. Pattern of impaired working memory during major depression. Journal of Affective Disorders. 2011;**90**:149-161

[15] Cervera R et al. The Euro-Phospholipid project: Epidemiology of the antiphospholipid syndrome in Europe. Lupus. 2009;**18**:889-893

[16] Cuchacovich R, Gedalia A. Pathophysiology and clinical spectrum of infections in systemic lupus erythematosus. Rheumatic Disease Clinics of North America. 2009;**35**:75-93

[17] Moitinho M, Fonseca C, Geraldes R. Systemic lupus erythematosus: A stroke unit diagnosis. Lupus. 2011;**4**:396

[18] Ruchir Agrawal, In: Russell W Steele, chief editor. Complement Deficiency Updated: May 6, 2009

[19] Jacobi AM, Rohde W, Ventz M. Enhanced serum prolactin (PRL) in patients with systemic lupus erythematosus: PRL levels are related to the disease activity. Lupus. 2010;**10**:554

[20] Duarte C et al. Health related quality of life in Portuguese SLE patients: An outcome measure independent of disease activity and cumulative damage. Acta Reumatólogica Portuguesa. 2010;**35**(1):30-35

[21] Alarcon GS et al. Lupus in minority populations, nature versus nurture. Systemic lupus erythematosus in three ethnic groups. IX. Differences in damage accrual. Arthritis and Rheumatism. 2001;**44**:2797-2806

[22] Isenberg D. Updating the tools to assess lupus. Lupus. 2007;**16**:40

[23] Joan TM. Measuring disease activity in systemic lupus: Progress and problems. Journal of Rheumatology. 2009;**25**:42-49

[24] Kokori IG, Ioannidis JPA, Voulgarelis M. Autoimmune hemolytic anemia in patients with systemic lupus erythematosus. American Journal of Medicine. 2011;**115**(7):19-24

[25] Stoll T, Stucki G, Malik J. Association of the Systemic Lupus International Collaborating Clinics/American College of Rheumatology Damage Index with measures of disease activity and health status in patients with systemic lupus erythematosus. Journal of Rheumatology. 2009;**24**:309-313

[26] Stahl Hallengren C, Nived O, Sturfelt G. Outcome of incomplete systemic lupus erythematosus after 10 years. Lupus. 2011;**13**(2):85-88

[27] Valesini G, Tighiouart H, Weiner DE. Anemia as a risk factor for cardiovascular disease and all-cause mortality in diabetes: The impact of chronic kidney disease. Journal of the American Society of Nephrology. 2011;**16**:3403-3410

Chapter 10

Severe Malarial Anemia (SMA) Pathophysiology and the Use of Phytotherapeutics as Treatment Options

Greanious Alfred Mavondo and
Mayibongwe Louis Mzingwane

Additional information is available at the end of the chapter

http://dx.doi.org/10.5772/intechopen.70411

Abstract

Hemolytic anemia results when red blood cells (RBCs) are destroyed prematurely by a number of agents. Obligate intracellular parasites like the Plasmodium species proliferate by infecting RBCs, growing through different stages of their life cycles, expanding their population to unsustainable numbers and eventually rupturing the cell membranes in order to transmit and infect new RBCs. In this manner, more RBCs are infected by the parasites and destroyed together with some nonparasitized cells. Membranes of RBCs are altered and deformed by parasite antigens expressed on the surfaces of both parasitized and nonparasitized cells, which lead to their premature phagocytosis and destruction by the reticuloendothelial system. Parasites and the hemoglobin waste products produced by them are released when the RBCs burst. Activated leukocytes take up the hemoglobin waste (hemozoin which is a polymerized heme), which stimulates the innate immune system leading to the synthesis and secretion of pro- and anti-inflammatory cytokines, chemokines, growth factors and mediators. Together with the destruction of RBCs in malaria, imbalance between pro- and anti-inflammatory events results in the modification of erythroid cell proliferation leading to severe malarial anemia (SMA) and other pathophysiologies of malaria. While current malarial management is targeted at the destruction of the parasite, it is the malaria-related pathophysiology (disease aspect of malaria) like severe malarial anemia that results in the high malaria morbidity and mortality. Antidisease approaches promise to be more effective at malarial management. Triterpenes with antioxidant, pro-oxidant, anti-inflammatory and antiparasitic effect show effects at retarding and abrogating severe malarial anemia. Asiatic acid, amongst other triterpenes like oleanolic acid, masilinic acid administered through oral or transdermal route improves severe malaria anaemia providing promise in the management of malaria pathophysiology.

Keywords: malaria, severe malarial anemia, *Plasmodium falciparum*, pro-inflammation, anti-inflammatory, antidisease, cytokines, chemokines, growth factors, rhoptry protein ring surface protein 2, tumor necrosis factor

1. Introduction

Anemia remains one of the most obdurate diseases affecting the general public in Africa where it contributes close to a quarter of the continent's nutrition-related Disability Adjusted Years (DAILY's) lost for the past decade and half [1]. There are several causes of anemia with micro-nutrient deficiencies, iron deficiency and parasitic infections contributing a major share in Sub-Saharan Africa [2]. Among the parasitic infections that contribute to global anemia, malaria, schistosomiasis and soil transmitted helminth (STH) compose a considerable disease burden in school children in developing countries [3]. There is a similar geographic distribution and polyparasitism of *Plasmodium falciparum*, schistosomiasis and STH infections in different epidemiologic settings in Africa that has been observed to date, with considerable contributions to anemia [4, 5]. With many factors contributing to anemia in general, establishing the relative contribution of malaria to anemia is complex, as malarial anemia is more frequently present in combination with other conditions.

The multifactorial causes of anemia make the disease a continuous and nagging problem to the human populations in different parts of the world, more so in the underdeveloped and developing world. The disease burden contributed by anemia had been projected to decrease worldwide in this century; however, signs on the ground seem to portray a different picture altogether. Hemoglobin (Hb) concentrations are used for the diagnosis of anemia and assessment of its severity.

Anemia can be defined, generally, as a decrease in Hb and related hematologic indices according to the individual's age, gender, physiologic state and geographic location [6].

In pregnant women, premature labor with low birth weight babies may be caused by anemia [7, 8]. Small for age live birth infants, still births and high perinatal maternal and infant mortality are all common features of anaemia [9]. Anemia caused by nutritional inadequacies may result in stunted growth and underweight infants that predisposes to several infectious and noninfectious diseases of childhood [10] and has a phenotypic presentation with chronic severe malarial anemia (SMA).

2. Definitions of severe malarial anemia

Severe malarial anemia (SMA) is defined by an Hb concentration of <5 g/dl or a hematocrit of <15% in children <12 years of age (<7 g/dl and <20%, respectively, in adults) together with a parasite count >10,000/μl, which distinguishes it from other diseases with similar presentations. Besides malnutrition, human immunodeficiency virus (HIV), schistosomiasis, soil transmitted helminth (STH) as causes of anemia, Plasmodium infections (malaria) contribute a major portion of the debilitating illness to the global disease burden [11]. SMA is a complication of severe malaria, which results from infection caused by the apicomplexan protozoan parasite of the genus *Plasmodium*. The Apicomplexa (also called Apicomplexia) are a large phylum of parasitic alveolates. Most of them possess a unique form of organelle that comprises a type of plastid called an apicoplast and an apical complex structure. The organelle is an adaptation that the apicomplexan applies in penetration of a host cell.

Any of the complications such as severe malarial anemia, significant bleeding, shock (compensated or decompensated), nonrespiratory acidosis and hypoglycemia can develop rapidly and progress to death within hours or days [12, 13].

Severe malaria is differentiated from other conditions by the demonstration of asexual forms of the malarial parasites in the blood in a patient with a potentially fatal manifestation or complication of malaria such as SMA in whom other diagnoses have been excluded. Even though the complications have been considered to be almost unique to *P. falciparum* infection, in recent years, many cases of severe malaria, including deaths, have been reported in *Plasmodium vivax* and *Plasmodium knowlesi* malaria. The case fatality of *P. falciparum* malaria is around 1%, and this accounts for more than half a million deaths per year all over the world, in which 80% of these deaths are caused by cerebral malaria. The incidence of complications and deaths due to the other two types is much lower.

Pregnancy anemia or maternal anemia is defined by an Hb of <110 g/L (11 gdL) and a hematocrit less than 31% [14]. In malaria, these values tend to be extremely low making SMA a critical clinical emergency in pregnancy and infancy where it displays distinct physiologic and morphologic characteristics between the two groups.

SMA threatens to kill the next generation. In the pregnant women and children <5 years, malarial infection develops into a fatal SMA more often than in any other population group due to reduced immune protection. This trend is also seen in malaria of endemic areas where natural immunity is supposed to develop over time due to higher exposure to the reinfection.

There is an increased demand for RBC synthesis in pregnancy, and the intrusion by the parasite creates a dilemma from decreased efficiency of nutrient utilization. Under reduced immunity, parasitemia increases persistently, resulting in increased level of parasite toxins that inhibit bone marrow functionality. The anti-immune response of pregnancy is meant to protect the fetus from autoimmune destruction. The same scenario is observed in SMA during infancy; however, the cause of reduced immunity in this case is from immature immune system activation and reduced maternal immunoglobulins.

Compounding the disease prevalence are factors such as parasite virulence, parasite-host interactions, host characteristics, and socio-economic conditions that play out an intricate web resulting in SMA. The production of pro-and anti-inflammatory cytokines, certain genetic traits, α or β-thalassemia, Duffy (Fy) blood groups and sickle cell traits remain the most common predisposing host factors to SMA. Malarial parasite species, disease endemics, Plasmodium multiplication rates, drug resistance and antigenic polymorphism all contribute to parasite factors that lead to SMA.

3. Malarial anemia etiology

Approximately 30–40% of deaths caused by *P. falciparum* are associated with SMA development. The multifactorial causes of SMA range from increased removal of circulating parasitized and nonparasitized red blood cells (pRBC's and npRBC's) to reduced synthesis of erythrocytes in the erythroid germinal centers. While the molecular mechanisms underlying the SMA remain obscure, malarial parasites' ability to remodel RBC's morphology and physiology through ligands found on both the parasite and RBC's membrane has been investigated in the past few years. Immunologic mechanisms associated with malarial pathophysiology seem to be more effective in increasing SMA. Elicitation of immunologic and inflammatory processes by malarial parasite antigens and immunokines plays a major role in the complex milieu that results in SMA. Coinfections with other parasites may increase SMA susceptibility as they aggravate malaria-associated inflammation. A normocytic and normochromic RBCs' morphologic appearance is a common presentation of anemia in malaria, which is characterized by the absence of spherocytes and schistocytes although there may be abundance of fragmentocytes and eliptocytes typifying increased hemolysis. High frequencies of hemoglobinopathies and iron deficiencies in areas of high malarial prevalence may change the picture to microcytytosis and hypochromasia [15].

Severe malarial anemia displays inadequate reticulocytosis in the presence of the anemia signifying that there is reduced synthesis of RBC's and not just increased hemolysis. In malaria, hematocrit gradually decreases, after an apparent initial steady state even with the onset of fever, showing either an increase in reticulocytosis or an absence of hemolysis within the first 24 h after infection. The decrease in hematocrit is independent of treatment initiation and may even occur in the absence of overt parasitemia on peripheral blood films, blood transfusion and adequate antimalarial treatment. In *P. falciparum*, parasite sequestration in the microvasculature may account for the parasite-negative peripheral blood smears accompanying decreasing hematologic indices. These parasites continue to shed soluble antigens, hemoglobin metabolites and derivatives that drive various syndromes of malaria like SMA. This may explain the continued decline in hematologic indices despite the evidently low parasitemia and the malarial anemia pathogenesis, which implicates bone marrow dysfunction as displayed by low reticulocytosis [16, 17]. When Hb decreases, the normal body physiology upregulates the bone marrow erythroid progenitors and reticulocytes are increased as an indicator of this process. Failure to increase immature red blood cells in circulation during overt anemia states indicates dyserythropoiesis and/or ineffective erythropoiesis associated with the myeloid progenitors' proliferation, which is common in malaria. Bone marrow suppression of the erythroid blast cells has been evidenced in children exposed to multiple reinfections, receiving inadequate treatment or experiencing treatment failure that tend to become asymptomatic during acute *P. falciparum* infections showing partial immunocompromised state [18] against an expected hyperimmune reactivity of an inflammatory condition like malaria. Inadequate erythropoietin production or effectiveness, the effect of the inflammasome on erythropoiesis, concomitant parasitic and bacterial infections contribute to the complex milieu culminating in SMA as well. Red blood cell membrane modifications by attached parasite ligands remodel the cells to a phenotype tagged for destruction through phagocytosis.

4. Effects of parasites on cell membranes leading to severe malarial anemia

Anemia is described as a decrease in Hb concentration, which is directly related to RBC's mass within the circulation. Infection with *P. falciparum*, which is associated with a rapid development of SMA, is also known to influence pRBC's sequestration in the microvasculature of different tissues and organs that include skin, lung, gut, muscle, heart, and brain. Parasitized RBCs are commonly sequestered from circulation together with npRBCs that carry parasite antigens. Rosetting (aggregation of pRBCs into rings of four or more cells) and agglutination (combining of pRBCs and npRBCs to form clumps) are common phenomena that occur due to ligands that are found on the surfaces of pRBCs and npRBCs, which result in reduction of freely circulating RBCs and eventually on RBC's mass and Hb concentration. Cytoadherence of pRBC's to the microvasculature, rosetting and cell-cell agglutination are processes facilitated by several ligands of *P. falciparum* trophozoites and schizonts. These pRBC's surface protruding molecules cause pathological cell-cell communication. These ligands such as *P. falciparum* erythrocyte membrane protein 1 (*Pf*EMP-1) [19, 20] enable pRBCs to bind to endothelial cell (EC) receptors, e.g., leukocyte differentiation antigen CD36, intercellular adhesion molecule 1 (ICAM-1), integrin, chondroitin sulfate and hyaluronic acid [21].

Some of these ligands are necessary for the formation of the host cell-parasite connection, which allows invagination of the erythrocyte bilayer leading the parasite engulfed into the RBC. As a result, an intracellular parasite vacuole is formed and provides an environment for parasitic multiple stage growth. During the process of parasite-protein-mediated internalization as well as during the intracellular proliferation, several other parasite proteins bearing a host-targeting (HT) or plasmodial expert element (PEXEL) are also exported into RBCs [22, 23], providing a myriad of host cell-parasite communication paradigms.

Intracellular proliferation and parasite antigens release cause considerable reduction in RBC membrane stability and alters cell surface characteristics leading to eventual pRBC's membrane rupture. The ability of RBCs to change shape allows them to pass through the spleen filtration mechanisms. Infection in the cell membranes causes them to be more rigid and unable to change shape when passing through capillaries and become prone to phagocytosis and hemolysis.

Some of the exported parasite ligands adhere to the membranes of npRBCs. Parasite ligand deposition on npRBC's tags these cells and pRBCs for rapid reticuloendothelial system pooling and sequestration by the spleen, which removes them from circulation resulting in SMA. Cytoadherence and auto-agglutination, emanating from the various ligand-epitope interactions, also removes a considerable amount of cells from circulation exacerbating SMA. Reduced RBC's flexibility occurs with a very few ligands being found on the surface of the cells reducing the half-life of such marked cells. However, such tagging only occurs on a subset of erythrocytes to account for the rapid setting of SMA encountered in malaria meaning that host cell-parasite ligand interactions along with other mechanisms play profound role in the creation of overt SMA.

5. Host cell-parasite ligand interactions and severe malarial anemia

The interaction between host cell and parasite ligands is a complex process of an inefficient invasion mechanism that may be completed in a small fraction of infection-targeted RBCs. As a result, many ligands need to be secreted and shed off into plasma resulting in many of these pRBC-adhesive proteins being present in high concentrations in plasma. These free molecules adhere to npRBCs triggering IgG and complement binding. Subsequently, cells binding immunoglobulin (Ig) and complements are cleared from circulation through phagocytosis by macrophages and hemolysis. This results in a critical hemoglobin reduction. Furthermore, HT/PEXEL-containing-proteins are released into plasma from pRBCs and adhere to npRBCs. These processes are repeated over and over again as the parasite intracellular cycle ends, concomitantly increasing the disease. Aberrant signaling circuits are also increased in the affected cells heralding their apparent need for removal from circulation by macrophages and exacerbating SMA.

Parasite proteins in rhoptries and merozoites surface membranes are candidates associated with SMA development. Merozoites are blood asexual forms of the parasites that are released in the circulation when pRBC's ruptures. As these parasites are intracellular, they invade new cells for the continued propagations of more asexual and sexual forms. To execute invasion, the parasite aligns its apical surface to the surface on RBCs. Rhoptries are structures protruding from the parasites. The merozoite uses the rhoptry proteins for anchoring on the surface of the RBC targeted for invasion. During the invasion processes, merozoites use rhoptries, which are also secretory structures on the merozoites apical end, to release their contents at the junction between the parasite and the erythrocyte. The *P. falciparum* proteins such as rhoptries secretory protein-2 (RSP-2) or rhoptries-associated protein-2 (RAP-2) have been found to be located at the surface of pRBCs as well as on npRBCs [24]. The presence of these proteins on the surface of npRBCs is possibly a result of failed invasion or when they adhere to the surface of these cells, they shed off from the merozoites into the plasma. Specific antibodies then opsonize the adhered RSP-2/RAP-2 complex accelerating complement-mediated RBC's lysis as well as macrophage uptake of targeted npRBCs [25]. In this way, the parasite is able to facilitate hemolysis of both npRBCs and pRBCs without necessarily entering the cell (**Figure 1**).

5.1. Parasite rhoptry protein ring surface protein 2 (RSP-2/RAP-2) and severe malarial anemia

It has been shown that the parasite RSP-2 not only tag npRBC's surfaces, but it extends to erythroid precursor cells in the bone marrow (BM) eliciting SMA [26] (**Figure 1**). The RSP-2 is transferred to the surface of the host cell around the site of contact with the merozoite. Gradually, the protein spreads over the entire surface of the cell by slow, lateral movements in both the npRBCs and pRBCs, leading to their premature identification and destruction by the reticuloendothelial system. *P. falciparum*-infected individuals respond to the infection by increasing the proliferation of phagocytic macrophages and their activity on tagged RSP-2 npRBCs and pRBCs.

There are other nongross RBC's membrane abnormalities that result in RBC's clearance in addition to adhesive-interacting ligands, RSP-2-antibody phagocytosis and complement activation. These changes are not observable by the light microscope as there are no obvious cell membrane morphologic abnormalities that have been noted. The subtle changes are due to oxidative damage of cell membranes, phosphatidylserine (PS) externalization or exposure and reduced deformability, which contribute to increased RBC's clearance leading to SMA. The involvement of ligands in RBC's clearance is mediated through stimulation of the inflammasome and its role in erythropoiesis in malaria [27].

http://dx.doi.org/10.5772/intechopen.70411

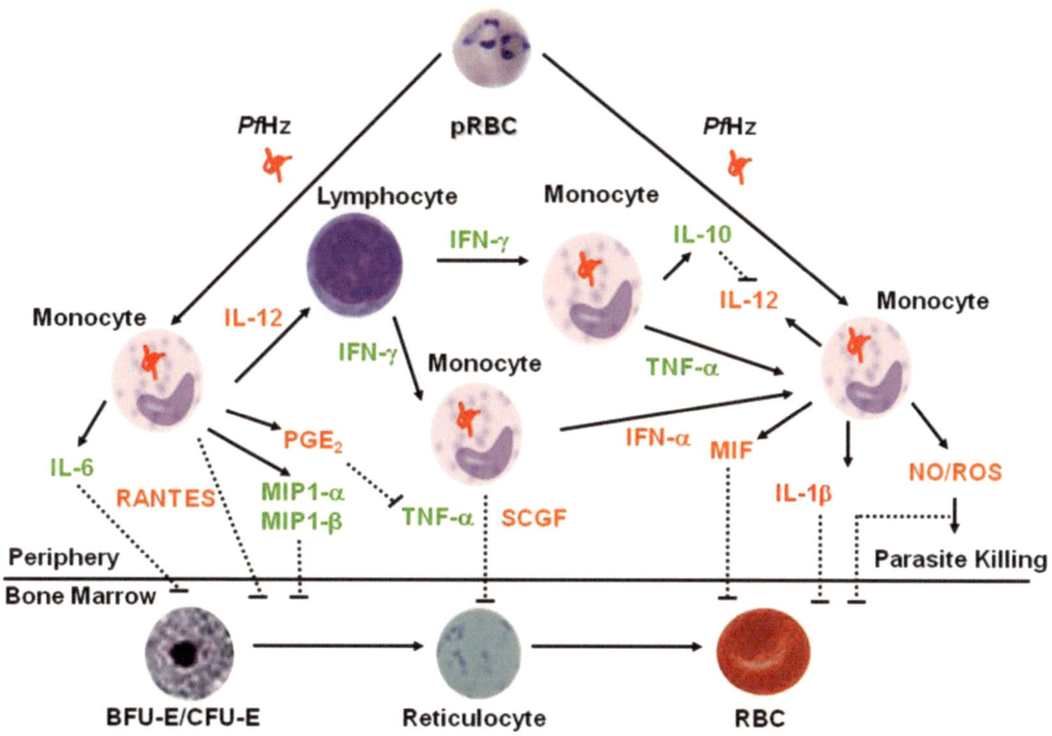

Figure 1. Proposed model of dysregulation in innate immune responses in severe malarial anemia. Based on concomitant measurement of innate inflammatory mediators (using multiplex technologies) in children with varying severities of malarial anemia, a model to describe how dysregulation in innate inflammatory mediators promotes suppression of erythropoiesis in children with SMA was developed. Phagocytosis of hemozoin (*Pf*Hz) by monocytes causes of altered production of innate inflammatory mediators. Elevated inflammatory mediators are shown with an arrow facing up against text, those that are decreased in children with SMA are shown with arrow facing down. Solid lines indicate positive (+) signalling (upregulation), whereas dashed lines indicate suppression (-) (downregulation). Children with SMA have decreased levels of IL-12 in response to ingestion of parasitized red blood cells (pRBC) and/or hemozoin by monocytes. Suppression of IL-12 in children with SMA is due to *Pf*Hz-induced IL-10 over-production. TNF-α can induce PGE2 and nitric oxide (NO); however, these effector molecules are suppressed in children with SMA. Suppression of PGE2 allows over-production of TNF-α, which is associated with enhanced SMA severity. MIF is suppressed in children with falciparum malaria, which is associated with phagocytosis of *Pf*Hz by monocytes and enhanced SMA severity. Levels of IFN-α, IL-1β, RANTES and SCGF are decreased in children with SMA. Reduced production of innate inflammatory mediators, along with increased TNF-α, IL-6, MIP-1α and MIP-β, likely contributes to the development of SMA by suppressing the erythropoietic response. Reduced NO and reactive oxygen species (ROS) generation in children with falciparum malaria may promote ineffective parasite killing and, thereby, prolong parasitemia, and children with malarial anemia have elevated levels of NO and ROS that can directly inhibit erythropoiesis (adapted from open access source: Perkins et al. [27]).

Despite massive RBC's destruction in malarial infection, there is also a delayed compensation of RBCs in overt anemic individuals due to defective erythropoiesis. Acute infection in children shows a picture of normal to small erythroid precursors in bone marrow (BM). There is considerable change noted on the erythroid cells morphology in malaria induced anaemia. These include multinucleated erythroid cells, karyorrhexis, incomplete or unequal mitotic divisions, intercytoplasmic bridges and cytoplasmic budding. A higher proportion of the erythroid progenitors are held in G_2 phase in SMA as compared with healthy individuals.

RSP-2 has been observed to be transferred to erythroid precursors only when there has been a direct contact with merozoites, in vitro. In vivo, these proteins are also known to be tagged to these cells [28]. Subsequently, erythroid precursors tagged with RSP-2 are destroyed through complement activation and cytokine oxidative stress linked apoptosis processes.

Noteworthy is that colony-forming units (CFU's) and other stages of the erythroid lineage suffer the same fate in the presence of cytophilic antibodies accounting for their reduced numbers in SMA. The antibody-RSP-2 complex on the surface of erythroblasts triggers the decline of these cell lines through phagocytosis or morphologic alterations observed in erythroid cells in the BM and the mediators of this process are closely linked to the inflammasome in SMA.

In addition to the described BM involvement in SMA, studies in Gambian children have demonstrated that SMA was defined by erythroid hyperplasia with dyserthropoiesis and a hypercellularity with an inefficient reticulocyte production index (RPI) [29] shown as <2.0. RPI is a measure of the extent to which the reticulocyte count has risen (or not) in response to the level of anemia, which indicates that SMA is the result of erythroid suppression [30], arbitrated by inflammatory molecules. Concomitant erythroid hyperplasia and reduced RPI signifies a cellular maturation check point or bottleneck that is introduced in SMA.

6. Severe malarial anemia and the inflammasome

Inflammation is a process that tends to control the proliferation of hostile entities and foreign bodies when the physiologic aspect of the body is invaded by pathogens or when there is a physical injury at both macroscopic and microscopic levels. The inflammasome is composed, among other mediators, of both pro-inflammatory cytokines typically denoted as T-helper cells type 1 (Th1) and anti-inflammatory cytokines denoted as T-helper cells type 2 (Th2), which tend to counteract each other into a balance state under normal physiologic states. SMA in children shows a close relationship of the disease with an imbalance between the Th1 and Th2 cytokines and chemokines (**Figure 1**). In an attempt to control parasitemia, the host releases an array of pro-and anti-inflammatory cytokines, chemokines, growth factors, and effectors as part of a wholesome innate immune response. Depending on the timing and magnitude of the inflammatory response to the infection and release of the cytokines, parasitemia may be controlled successfully or uncontrolled parasitemia may cause imbalance of the inflammatory milieu with damage to the host and suppress the erythropoietic response [30].

Understanding the context in which inflammatory response to malarial infection culminates in SMA involves a close scrutiny of the microenvironment in which the cellular components and mediator interact. The process by which erythroid progenitors proliferate and differentiate into non-nucleated reticulocytes in the BM is called erythropoiesis. Erythroblastic islands, where erythropoiesis takes place, are specialized cellular niches composed of a central macrophage surrounded by erythroblasts in which cells proliferate, differentiate and enucleate [31]. The pro-erythroblast, which goes through four mitotic cycles, is the earliest recognizable erythroblast that gives rise to reticulocytes. Basophilic polychromatic erythroblasts give rise to orthochromatic erythroblasts, which expel their nuclei to generate reticulocytes. The well-coordinated mechanism is characterized by a decreased cell size, more condensed chromatin material, progressive hemoglobinization and marked membrane organizational alterations. The role of various cytokines and chemokines in the regulation of erythropoiesis is revealed by the intimate interaction of the myeloid progenitors, macrophages and erythroblasts during RBC's production.

The erythroid hyperplasia seen in SMA excludes erythropoietin deficiency as a cause of inadequate erythropoiesis of malaria intimating that the aberrant inflammatory response mounted by the cytokine milieu as the culprit. Associated with the hypercytokinemia is the ingestion by neutrophils, monocytes and macrophages of the inflammatory mediator hemozoin (Hz, a parasite-derived polymerized heme), which is known to influence the dysregulation of inflammatory responses through synthesis of a number of cytokines with subsequent induction of SMA [32]. *P. falciparum* Hz (*Pf*Hz) is a brown/black pigment that accumulates in phagocytic cells in the BM, which is formed during the intraerythrocytic asexual replication cycle when *P. falciparum* metabolizes host Hb as a source of amino acids [33]. During the formation of the insoluble *Pf*Hz, toxic iron-rich heme known as ferriprotoporphyrin IX (FP-IX) is aggregated by heme polymerase. The engulfing of *Pf*Hz is a good indirect measure of sequestered parasite burden, recent schizogony, disease severity, decreased hematocrit and degree of erythropoiesis suppression in children with *P. falciparum*-induced SMA [34, 35].

The phagocytozed *Pf*Hz triggers the innate immune response through the toll-like receptors (TLR's) [36] with downstream cytokine elicitation promoting RANTES suppression by a pathway involving IL-10 [37].

When and how much of interleukin 12 (IL-12), interferon gamma (INF-γ) and tumor necrosis factor alpha (TNF-α) are released is critical to minimize and preserve erythropoiesis. Activation of this pro-inflammatory cytokines elicitation should be timely abrogated by type 2 cytokine IL-10, transforming growth factor beta (TGF-β) and IL-4 to avoid host damage by the inflammatory process [38]. TNF-α is critical for parasite killing and prevention of parasite replication directly as well as through macrophage migration inhibitory factor (MIF) and through nitric oxide synthase type 2 (NOS2-inducible nitric acid synthase) and generation of nitric oxide (NO), which kills parasites directly [39]. Inflammatory responses are commonly exacerbated by the TNF-α induction of cyclooxygenase-2 (COX-2), which drives prostaglandin E synthesis (PGE) with subsequent generation of malarial symptoms such as fever, headache, nausea, vomiting, diarrhea, anorexia, myalgia and thrombocytopenia [40, 41].

During the early phases of malarial infection, natural killer cells, $\alpha\beta$-T cells and regulatory $\gamma\delta$-T are activated to produce IFN-γ [42], a prototypical type 1 cytokine for childhood malaria [43]. Individuals who produce IFN-γ from monocytes when immunized with asexual malarial parasites are able to resist infection by *P. falciparum* as has been seen in West Africa, Mali, Burkina Faso and Sudan as well higher Hb concentration and reduced prevalence of SMA are observed in Kenyan children challenged with pre-erythrocytic antigens [44]. Over-production of the innate inflammatory mediators is associated with anemia, and it has been observed that persistent macrophage activation is significantly greater in children with malarial complications through BM suppression, dyserthropoiesis and erythrophagocytosis [45].

There is a strong alliance between the interleukins Iβ and 1α, potent endogenous pyrogens, which promotes inflammatory response against invading pathogens [46], with TNF-α in the enhancement of NO and IFN-γ production. Sustained release of IL-1β, as experienced in malaria, has the potential of inducing several hematologic and immunologic anomalies with anemia as a candidate [47, 48]. However, cytokine IL-1β has a protective role in certain haplotypes, which are predisposed to produce higher levels of this cytokine and prevents anemia development [49].

One of the cytokines, IL-6, has been demonstrated to be increased in malaria with peripheral blood mononuclear cells (PBMC) being the source of the increased cytokine production during acute malaria [50]. IL-6 mediates the protective immunity against the pre-erythrocytic phases of malaria by inducing Ilβ and TNF-α. During the erythrocytic stage, IL-6 controls parasitemia through boosting up specific immunoglobulin (Ig) G antibodies. However, lack of control over parasitemia and the resulting progression toward severe disease may explain the association between elevated levels of IL-6 and enhanced pathophysiology [27]. Macrophage migration inhibitory factor (MIF) is a ubiquitous molecule produced by T cells, monocytes-macrophages and the anterior pituitary in response to pro-inflammatory stimuli [27]. Notably, there is a rapid mobilization and expression of large concentrations of MIF during acute inflammation as the cytokine is stored in preformed vesicles only to be released without de novo gene expression.

The pro-inflammatory properties of MIF are important for both innate and adaptive immune response in both parasitic and bacterial infections [27, 51]. In animal models, elevated MIF concentrations have strong connexion with SMA while mice with MIF knockout gene have less anemia and higher survival chances when infected with *Plasmodium chabaudi* compared with the wild type [52]. In humans, however, there is an opposite picture of elevated MIF protein (in circulation) and MIF transcripts (in PBMC) being connected to less severe falciparum malaria [53]. Fascinating is the fact that worsening SMA is linked to decreasing circulating MIF concentrations as well as blood leukocytes MIF transcripts in Kenyan children. Remarkably, MIF concentration in peripheral blood was not significantly inter-related to reticulocyte responses in these children. Correction for age, gender and parasitemia, however, did show that elevated levels of monocyte chemotactic protein [MCP] were significantly associated with both SMA and decreased MIF production.

Phagocytosis of *Pf*Hz by PBMC causes dysregulation in MIF production in an apoptosis-independent manner. Consequently, *Pf*Hz presence in malaria suppresses peripheral blood MIF production, thus enhancing severity of anemia. The intricacy by which *Pf*Hz is involved in the malarial parasite life cycle makes it the central molecule to SMA development and other malarial pathophysiologies. Therefore, *Pf*Hz as a heme metabolism waste product deliberately synthesized by the parasite may be regarded as a long-term strategy for its survival.

Interleukin 23 is another pro-inflammatory mediator involved in conditioning the SMA pathogenesis, which is also important in mediating anemia development in autoimmune diseases [54] and chronic inflammation [55]. The subunits making up IL-23 are designated p19 and p40, and this cytokine shares a number of common properties with IL-12. Among these characteristics is the p40 subunit, ability to bind the IL-12Rβ1 receptor, release from activated myeloid antigen presenting cells, type 1 immune response promotion, suppression by both IL-10 and IL-12 p40 homodimers. A striking feature observed with IL-23 is its sustained elevation when both IL-12 and IL-10 are suppressed [56]. In cultured PBMC, hemozoin induces sustained IL-23p19 transcript concentrations for more than 72 h, whereas IL-12p40 and IL-10 transcripts rapidly decline after reaching peak at 24 h [57]. In other words, IL-23 is important in the pathogenesis of SMA (through *Pf*Hz influence), whereas IL-12 and IL-10 play pivotal role in the regulation of IL-23 synthesis in *P. falciparum* infection.

Interleukin 12 is a heterodimer protein made up of 35 and 40 kDa subunits, which is a prototypical cytokine of type 1 immune response interfacing inflammation and immunity. The main IL-12 secreting cells include dendritic cells, monocytes and B-cells, which can be activated by bacterial cell wall components, intracellular pathogens and the ligation of CD40. By stimulating the synthesis of IFN-γ and TNF-α from T-cells and natural killer (NK) cells, IL-12 augments Th1 response to infection. Secretion of IL-12 can be promoted by several cytokines and chemokines to include granulocyte macrophage-colony stimulating factor (GM-CSF) and IFN-γ, while others negatively regulate its production such as IL-4, IL-10, IL-11, IL-13, monocyte chemotactic protein (MCP)-1/CCL2, and TGF-β. Reinfection with *P. falciparum* and development of SMA are averted through the administration of recombinant IL-12 together with the less efficacious chloroquine showing that IL-12 is crucial in the prevention of malarial anemia and dyserythropoiesis. The protective role of IL-12 in malaria lies in its ability to stimulate antibody production and its ability to act as a hematopoietic growth factor. Low concentrations of IL-12 are associated with SMA through, in part, the influence of *Pf*Hz phagocytosis that influences upregulation of monocyte-derived IL-10 which in turn suppresses the IL-12p40 subunits [58].

Cytokine involvement in SMA induction includes influencing iron trafficking. Moreover, cytokines play a critical role in the maturation of erythroid cells. Interleukin 6 (IL-6) induces hepcidin production and expression in the liver, (a master regulator of iron trafficking), resulting in decreased iron availability. Also well-known is the involvement of transforming growth factor beta (TGF-β) in the inhibition of erythroblast proliferation and the maintenance of the hematopoietic stem cells (HSC) in a state of quiescence to preserve the stem cell pool and avoid the exhaustion of the same. Neutralization of TGF-β results in the release of early HSC progenitors from quiescence [59].

Tumor necrosis factor alpha (TNF-α) is involved in the cleavage of GATA-1, which is a major erythroid transcription factor. Interferon gamma (IFN-γ) induces production of TNF-related apoptosis-inducing ligand (TRAIL) by macrophages, which inhibits erythroblast differentiation. This is suggestive of a critical role of these cytokines in SMA. Furthermore, suppression of IL-12, which is strongly associated with pediatric SMA, decreases the production of IFN-γ and IFN-α. Infection induces IL-10 synthesis which in turn suppresses IL-12 associated with hemozoin (Hz) acquisition by monocytes [58, 60].

SMA in children is, therefore, invariably associated with increased circulating concentrations of TNF, IL-6, IL-1b, interleukin-1-receptor agonist (IL-1RA), macrophage inflammatory protein 1alpha (MIP-1α) and macrophage inflammatory protein 1beta (MIP-1β) [61, 62]. What is astonishing is the finding that prostaglandin E (PGE) and nitric oxide (NO) are suppressed in

SMA even though the increased TNF level is expected to induce higher concentration of these inflammatory mediators. However, reduction in PGE may permit over synthesis of TNF-α enhancing anemia severity. Suppression of NO in children with SMA promotes ineffective parasite eradication while suppressing erythropoiesis in the BM. In pediatric SMA, IL-12p70 and INF are associated with positive prediction of Hb (elevated Hb) whereas IL-2R, IL-13 and eotaxin predict Hb negatively (favor profound anemia development) [62].

7. Pro-inflammatory (Th2) cytokines involvement in severe malarial anemia pathogenesis

By preventing over-production of pro-inflammatory mediators, anti-inflammatory cytokines like IL-10 render protection against SMA development. The later stages of the innate immune response in *P. falciparum* infection seek to downregulate the potentially pathogenic pro-inflammatory responses necessary for parasitemia eradication. Severity of malarial anemia can be predicted by the IL-10-TNF-α ration with low values associated low Hb concentration and hematocrit. Therefore, timing of the anti-inflammatory response relative to the proinflammatory cytokines activity and concentration has a strong influence on the malarial outcomes. Statistically significant positive association has been identified between IL-10 in the systemic circulation and malarial pigment containing leucocytes, indicating the regulatory role of *Pf*Hz in the development of systemic malarial pathology when it upregulated IL-10 production (**Figure 2**).

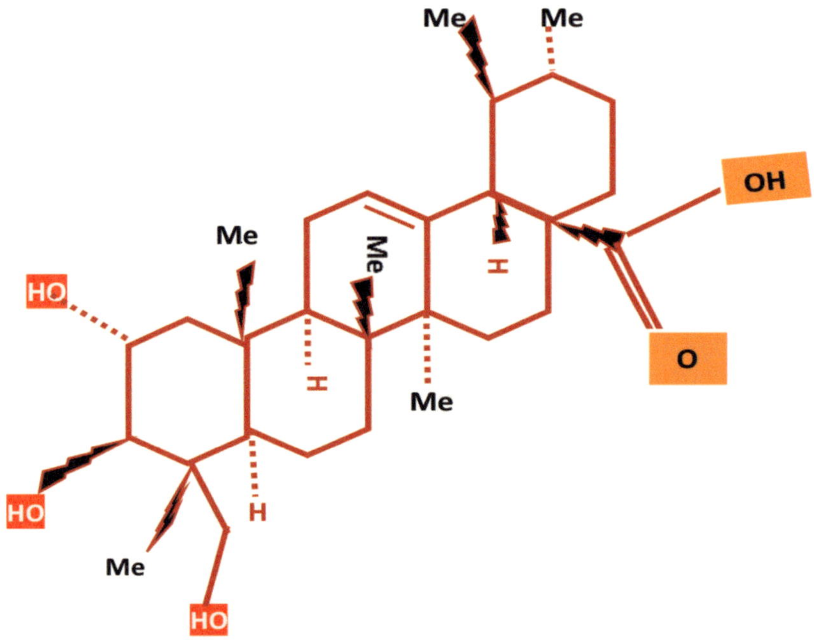

Figure 2. Chemical structure of asiatic acid. Formula $C_{30}H_{48}C_5$. MW: 488.69912. (G/mole). Redox characteristics: hydrogen bond donor (HBD) 7.1 and hydrogen bond acceptor (HBA) 4.176 [79].

Downregulation of TNF-α and IL-10, TGF-β1 (an anti-inflammatory and growth factor) tends to protect against severe malaria in mice. Importance of TGF-β in the pathogenesis of malaria is attributable to the cytokines that can influence the erythropoiesis either positively or negatively [63]. Serum concentration of the soluble form of TGF-β1 co-receptor, endoglin (sEng or CD105/TGF-βRIII), is elevated significantly in children with severe falciparum infection showing the importance of the cytokine in malarial pathogenesis and possibly SMA [64].

8. Severe malarial anemia pathogenesis and chemokines

Chemokines or chemotactic cytokines play a critical role in immune system activation, hematopoiesis, angiogenesis and antimicrobial activities. The chemokines' macrophage inflammatory protein 1α (MIP-1α)/CCL3 (C-C chemokine) and the C-X-C chemokine (IL-8/CXCL8) were the first to be investigated in acute *P. falciparum* malaria where a positive correlation with parasitemia was found with IL-8CXCL3. There is a much higher concentration of IL-8 in acute malaria that is necessary for the activation of neutrophils in severe nonfatal malaria that may be associated with slow cure rate after malarial chemotherapy. Chemokine production or suppression signal transduction depends on the phagocytosis of *Pf*Hz through oxidative stress-dependent and oxidative stress-independent mechanisms [65]. In both humans and PBMC, MIP-1α/CCL3, MIP-1β/CCL4 proteins and transcripts tend to be increased in production by the introduction of *Pf*Hz [66].

Normal T-cell expression, secretion (RANTES, CCL5) and regulated activation play a critical role in SMA pathogenesis. Secreted by monocytes, macrophages, fibroblasts, NK and T-cells, CD 34+ hematopoietic progenitors, RANTES protein is sequestered in platelets granules and is released by thrombin-stimulated platelets for both innate and adaptive immune response. Furthermore, RANTES stimulates hematopoiesis, angiogenesis, cell proliferation and development [67]. Through *Pf*Hz-induced suppression, both RANTES protein and transcripts tend to be decreased in malaria. Higher amount of RANTES tends to be protective against SMA [68]. Suppression of RANTES is closely associated with inefficient erythropoiesis and malaria-induced thrombocytopenia, which is promoted by *Pf*Hz through an IL-10-dependent mechanism. In this regard, thrombocytopenia appear to be the main cause of reduced RANTES which in turn tends to suppress erythropoiesis in SMA.

9. Role of growth factors in severe malarial anemia

Growth factors play a pivotal role in the erythropoiesis cascade. A longitudinal study of malaria has shown that serum concentrations of granulocyte-colony stimulating factor (G-CSF) were elevated at day 0 in complicated malaria followed by a decline to within reference interval on day 7. Significant correlation of G-CSF with procalcitonin, parasite density and erythropoietin is a common finding at the beginning of malaria [69]. G-CSF has a negative impact on erythropoiesis, and an increased concentration of the growth factor leads to SMA development. With high parasite density associated with elevated levels of G-CSF, the increased erythropoietin is a compensatory mechanism to protect against SMA development through a mechanism driven by both hypoxia and oxidative stress common in complicated malaria [70]. While G-CSF promotes erythropoiesis, it acts in synergy with TNF-α in increasing the eradication of parasites in erythrocytic cycle by neutrophils.

The genes/gene pathway that leads to the SMA pathogenesis has been human stem cell growth factor (SCGF, C-type lectin domain family member 11A-CLEC11A) which is up-regulated after *Pf*Hz stimulation of human PBMC's [71]. Primarily secreted by myeloid and fibroblasts possessing burst-promoting activity for human bone marrow erythroid progenitors, SCGF is a hematopoietic growth of 323-amino acid that is cleaved to a 245-amino acid SCGF-β active form. In children with SMA, SCGF tends to be suppressed and positively correlated with Hb concentration, erythropoietic response suppression and high concentrations of naturally acquired monocytic *Pf*Hz. Genetic polymorphism of the SCGF also tends to protect against SMA development and suppression of erythropoiesis in parasitized children [72].

10. Role of effector molecules in severe malarial anemia pathogenesis

Relative expression of inflammatory mediators largely determines the various clinical outcome of malaria. The relative concentrations and timing of release of pro-and anti-inflammatory cytokines, chemokines and growth factors have a direct effect on cellular response as well as on the down-stream effector molecule production. The most notable down-stream effectors include NO, reactive oxygen species (ROS) and prostaglandins E2 (PGE2).

The toxic free radical NO has an effect on SMA development. The catalysis of L-arginine by NO synthase (NOS) produces equimolar amounts of L-citrulline and NO and in malaria the inducible NOS (iNOS or NOS2) is responsible for most of the NO production from monocytes, macrophages and neutrophils [73]. Pro-inflammatory cytokines (IL-12, IFN-γ, TNF-α) upregulates iNOS-generated NO synthesis, whereas Th2 (anti-inflammatory) cytokines (IL-10, TGF-β) downregulates NOS2 expression in malaria. NO is both protective as it has potent parasiticidal properties limiting parasitemia and pathogenic effects as it sustained high level predispose to anemia through BM suppression, dyserythropoiesis and erythrophagocytosis.

ROS appear to be both protective and pathologic in *P. falciparum* malaria. Increased concentrations of the free radical have observed to accompany accelerated parasitaemia clearance in Gabonese children as well as controlling of peripheral parasitaemia in children with severe malaria [74]. In Kenyan children with severe malaria, ROS damaged the RBC membranes [74]. Severe malarial cases associated with significantly elevated markers of oxidative stress like high malondialdehyde concentrations, high protein carbonyl, high nitrite, low ascorbic acid and elevated plasma copper concentrations are suspected to have SMA [74]. The arachidonic acid product, PGE_2, has an inverse relationship with SMA development. Cyclooxygenase (COX) enzyme (prostaglandin-H_2 synthase) exists in two isoforms: COX-1 (PGH synthase-1) and COX-2 (PGH synthase-2). COX-1 catalyzes the immediate formation of PGE_2, whereas COX-2 catalyzes the delayed formation of PGE_2 involved in the regulation of the inflammatory response and immunity to invading pathogens. Acquisition of intraleukocytic *Pf*Hz in placental malaria reduces

http://dx.doi.org/10.5772/intechopen.70411

mononuclear cell PGE_2 production [75]. Furthermore, plasma bicycle-PGE_2 (stable end metabolite of PGE_2) and PBMC COX-2 ex vivo expression are significantly reduced in severe malaria. De novo COX-2 transcripts biosynthesis is inhibited when monocytes phagocytose *Pf*Hz [76]. Ingestion of *Pf*Hz by monocytes and the effects of antipyretics used to treat malarial fever promote overproduction of TNF-α and worsening of malarial pathophysiology like SMA when erythroid progenitors are targeted for apoptosis [76–78]. *Pf*Hz (in synergy with TNF-α) directly inhibits erythroid cell development by interfering with the erythropoietic cascade through induction of oxidative stress-driven erythroid precursor cell apoptosis and through cytokine-mediated inflammation effects on erythroid development leading to SMA.

11. Severe malarial anemia management

The only treatment that has been available for SMA has been largely blood transfusion in various forms. Erythropoietin supplementation has not been successful as most patients with SMA tend to have high concentrations of the hormone amidst a low reticulocyte count indicating a nonresponsive BM. Equally so has been the ferrous iron supplements that have proven to have worse outcomes and had to be prematurely stopped. As has been shown, SMA is a synergistic onslaught from the parasite producing *Pf*Hz, which is eventually taken up by activated leukocytes and breeds both pro-and anti-inflammatory mediators whose sustained synthesis results in malarial pathophysiology and derangements. Aiming the treatment at the parasite has been successful, to some extent. However, the continued harangue of the parasite among many populations is a tacit implication that more is required to eradicate or control the malarial pandemic. Aiming malarial treatment at the pathophysiology is an avenue currently being explored with commendable results.

Administration of the phytochemical triterpenes, asiatic acid and other triterpenoids has been shown to have antiparasitic effects and reduction of SMA development in murine malaria. Addressing the pathophysiology of malaria while eradicating parasitemia seems to provide a provocative approach that encompasses inflammation, immunoreactivity, glucose homeostasis, renal failure and other aspects, which commonly complicates malaria in humans.

11.1. Severe malarial anemia and asiatic acid administration in murine malaria

Hypothetically, drugs that may inhibit or reverse malarial pathophysiology or the disease components have a higher chance of controlling malaria even without parasite eradication. This may include targeting SMA, which is an independent malarial mortality predictor in pregnant women and children [80]. The concept of malarial pathophysiology being referred to as malarial disease and its management being denoted as antidisease in malaria is a novel term in malaria handling terminology introduced to differentiate this approach from the antiparasitic treatment [80].

Triterpenes with antidisease properties in other conditions similar to malaria, like inflammation in sepsis and hypoxia in anemia are able to eradicate the Plasmodium parasite as well as resolve the ensuing pathophysiology. Triterpenes with pleiotropic functions, sufficient to be antidisease as well as antiparasitic, have been reported. Betulinic acid (BA), ursolic acid (UA), maslinic acid (MA) and oleanolic acid [OA] have been shown to have moderate activity in vitro against the chloroquine-insensitive (K1) and chloroquine-sensitive (T9-96) *P. falciparum* parasites. MA, a possible multitargeting antimalarial, effectively inhibits proteolytic processing of the malarial merozoite surface protein [MSP1] complex, inhibits the metalloproteases and has several putative binding sites for the parasite antigens [81]. This multitarget phenomenon suppresses the parasitemia in more than one way. Furthermore, the age-old preoccupation with targeting single process of the parasite infective cycle (which is mutation prone) is avoided, and host-related responses potentiating antidisease and antiresistance outcomes are involved [80]. Asiatic acid (AA), an amphiphilic triterpene (**Figure 2**), has known for its antioxidant and pro-oxidant capacity, anti-inflammatory and antinociception activity in mice [82], calcium release-associated apoptosis induction [83, 84] and a potent immunomodulator. Asiatic acid shares structural and bioactivity properties with OA, MA, UA and BA. Targeting the pathophysiology of malaria, SMA, as well as the parasite provides new mechanisms for combating malaria. Noteworthy is that AA is known to attenuate, inhibit or ameliorate the above factors in other diseases, which formulate the bedrock of malarial disease and its sequelae.

11.2. Glycosylphosphatidylinositols (GPI) and severe malarial anemia

Immunity against severe malaria is partly antiparasitic and partly antitoxic (toxic effects in response to parasite factors) [85]. The majority of the adults in malarial endemic areas have resistance to severe malaria and subsequently to SMA.

The induction of innate pro-inflammatory cytokine responses is mediated by germline-encoded pattern-recognition receptors, such as toll-like receptors (TLR), which recognize conserved microbial structures, i.e., pathogen-associated molecular patterns (PAMP) [86]. Among the malarial PAMP, glycosylphosphatidylinositols (GPI) are considered the main pathogenicity factor [87]. While GPI structure is conserved among Plasmodium species, human and Plasmodium GPI differ considerably but provide potential therapeutic points [88]. Several functionally important parasite proteins, including MSP-1, MSP-2 and MSP-4, are anchored to the cell membranes through GPI moieties and are also abundantly present free of protein attachment in membranes of pathogenic protozoa [89]. *P. falciparum* GPI have been found to induce the production of NO, TNF, IL-1b in murine macrophages in vitro, and a synthetic malarial GPI glycan was demonstrated to be immunogenic in vivo [90].

AA modulates immunity by selective induction of mitochondria-dependent apoptosis of activated lymphocytes in the prevention of murine fulminant hepatitis [91], a mechanism that may be extendable to malaria. Using membrane DNA array technique, a wound-healing derivative of AA [2-Oxo-3, 23-isopropylidene-asiatate (AS2006A)] exerting anti-inflammatory effect was identified. The anti-inflammatory mechanism involved selective cytotoxicity to activated macrophage cell line (L-929). By upregulating the expression of apoptosis-inducing genes caspase-8, c-myc, inducible nitric oxide synthase (iNOS), mdm2, NF-k$\beta\alpha$, I-k$\beta\alpha$ and NF-kβ p105, the phytotherapeutics controlled inflammation [93]. This alludes to AA exerting anti-inflammatory effect by cytochrome c release, caspase 3 activation and poly (ADP-ribose) polymerase cleavage mechanism as did AS2006A [92].

In principle, GPI drives inflammation that leads to SMA and AA by curbing cytokine release and correcting dyserythropoiesis may be said to inhibit GPI effect.

11.3. Preservation of blood volume by asiatic acid through immune system modulation

The effect of AA in alleviating hemodynamic and metabolic alterations in metabolic syndrome is through restoration of endothelium nitric oxide synthase (eNOS)/iNOS expression [93]. Similar influence of AA in malaria may be anticipated where eNOS/iNOS ratio determines the bioavailability of NO necessary for vascular proliferation and angiogenesis. These are useful processes in the inhibition of SMA. By maintaining RBC's concentration in malaria, besides preventing SMA, AA also contributes toward modulation of hemodynamic systems.

The hematologic indices such as Hb concentration, RBC's volume and % hematocrit (%Hct) were depressed with increasing percentage of parasitemia, while oral administration of AA has been shown to preserve these parameters and ameliorated SMA. SMA has been shown to persist even when parasitemia has been resolved driven by an aberrant immune system and *Pf*Hz-induced oxidative stress, and the immune system modulation of AA may correct SMA, which is also relentless even after overt infection has dissipated. By suppressing parasitemia as well as having an effect on the retardation and correcting SMA, AA is a potential antidisease agent in malaria. Although not investigated, there is a possibility that other factors (including inflammatory mediator-impaired erythropoiesis) influencing SMA development are inhibited by AA. Destruction of pRBCs occurs when the schizonts mature and merozoites rapture cell membranes. pRBC's destruction is accompanied by the lysis of npRBCs at a ratio of 8.5 RBCs for each pRBCs hemolyzed through phagocytosis and increased oxidative stress. By selectively inducing apoptosis of activated macrophages and monocytes, AA may reduce the phagocytic activity of leukocytes in malaria as has been shown by SMA retardation. Also, the antioxidant facet of AA may preserve RBC's membrane deformability and reduce the trapping of the cells by the spleen.

SMA develops as the RBC mass is reduced rapidly without concurrent replacement as a result of ineffective erythropoiesis. This occurs when erythroid progenitor apoptosis is induced by oxidative stress. The high concentrations of EPO observed in SMA are at variance with the low degree of reticulocytosis present, indicating reduced BM response to anemia due to erythroid progenitor destruction. The antioxidant capacity of AA, by preserving erythroblast cells, corroborates with increasing EPO to alleviate SMA through increased reticulocytosis. Moreover, by reducing parasitemia, AA not only preserves erythroid precursor response in infection but also increases blood volume through normalizing reticulocytosis [94] that prevents overt SMA development.

11.4. Asiatic acid reduces oxidative stress and reduces red blood cell's destruction

The other mechanism by which npRBCs are destroyed in malaria involves increased erythrocytic oxidative stress and parasite antigens, which cause RBC's membrane to be less deformable and more fragile. This shortens RBC's life spans. These cells are trapped during splenic sequestration and destroyed through phagocytosis. AA has known for its antioxidant, anti-inflammatory and immunomodulatory properties that protects cell membranes from oxidative damage and rigidity, reduced erythrophagocytosis and reduced parasite proliferation. MA, a phytochemical similar in structure and polypharmacology with AA, has multitargeted inhibitory properties against malaria with possible blockade of parasite maturation from early ring to schizont stages [95]. BA and UA also share carbon skeleton with MA and AA. Analogs of these two triterpenes are antiplasmodial through disruption of parasite calcium homeostasis [96] and averting SMA through reduction in parasite densities. These together with AA inhibit parasitic proliferation limiting RBC's hemolysis and preserving hematologic indices. The pleiotropic biologic effects of AA influence host control of the parasite proliferation. By modulating the immune system and removing erythropoiesis-suppressive effect of parasitic infection, hematologic indices are corrected preventing the development of SMA.

11.5. Asiatic acid, hepcidin, iron homeostasis and severe malarial anemia

The resolution of SMA (normalized hematologic indices) indirectly indicates the abrogation of the immunologic and inflammatory processes by AA. The persistence of SMA beyond parasitemia eradication is orchestrated and sustained by immunologic sequelae, which upregulate hepcidin synthesis and modulation of iron metabolism, and the fact that SMA is inhibited by AA administration, suppression of hepcidin synthesis and continuation of normal iron metabolism is a factor that is associated with the beneficial effect of triterpenes in malaria [97].

12. Conclusion

The pathogenesis of SMA is largely driven by dysregulation and imbalance between pro- and anti-inflammatory cytokines, chemokines, growth factors, and effector molecules. Alterations in the phenotypic presentations of these innate inflammatory mediators is due, at least in part, to the phagocytosis of *Pf*Hz by monocytes, resident macrophages (including those in bone marrow), and neutrophils. The mechanisms that lead to the profoundly low Hb concentrations witnessed in children with SMA are due to hemolysis and phagocytosis of pRBCs and npRBCs, and to a large extent, by suppression of erythropoiesis that is driven by *Pf*Hz-generated dysregulation in innate inflammatory mediators.

One of the emerging novel methods for managing the malarial diseases is in aiming at ameliorating the disease aspects through utilization of antidisease initiatives. The administrations of triterpenes with known antidisease properties are indicating potential for averting SMA development through maintaining the hematologic indices in severe malaria. The use of AA, MA, OA and other phytochemicals holds potentials in eradication of SMA and pathophysiology of malaria through their antioxidant, anti-inflammatory and immunomodulation capabilities. This introduces a new era in the management of SMA.

http://dx.doi.org/10.5772/intechopen.70411

Acknowledgements

We like to thank the National University of Science and Technology (Zimbabwe) for providing an enabling environment for research and publications (Research Board initiatives) through which this work has been possible.

Conflict of interest

The authors declare no conflict of interest in this work.

Author details

Greanious Alfred Mavondo* and Mayibongwe Louis Mzingwane

*Address all correspondence to: greaniousa@gmail.com

National University of Science and Technology, Faculty of Medicine, Pathology Department, Ascot, Bulawayo, Zimbabwe

References

[1] WHO. World Malaria Report 2016 WHO. Geneva: WHO; 2016

[2] Pullan RL, Gitonga C, Mwandawiro C, et al. Estimating the relative contribution of parasitic infections and nutrition for anaemia among school-aged children in Kenya: A sub-national geostatistical analysis. BMJ Open. 2013;**3**:e001936

[3] Matangila JR, Doua JY, Linsuke S, et al. Malaria, schistosomiasis and soil transmitted helminth burden and their correlation with anaemia in children attending primary schools in Kinshasa, Democratic Republic of Congo. PloS One. 2014;**9**(11):e110789

[4] Matangila JR, Lufuluabo J, Ibalanky AL, et al. Asymptomatic *Plasmodium falciparum* infection is associated with anaemia in pregnancy and can be more cost-effectively detected by rapid diagnostic test than by microscopy in Kinshasa, Democratic Republic of the Congo. Malaria Journal. 2014;**13**:132

[5] Henning L, Schellenberg D, Smith T, et al. A prospective study of *Plasmodium falciparum* multiplicity of infection and morbidity in Tanzanian children. Transactions of the Royal Society of Tropical Medicine and Hygiene. 2004;**98**:687-694

[6] Lamikanra AA, Brown D, Potocnik A, et al. Malarial anemia of mice and men. Blood. 2007;**110**(1):18-28

[7] Kumar JK, Asha N, Murthy DS, et al. Maternal anaemia in various trimesters and its effect on newborn weight and maturity: An observational study. International Journal of Preventive Medicine. 2013;**4**(2):193-199

[8] Lelic M, Bogdanovic G, Ramic S, et al. Influence of maternal anaemia during pregnancy on placenta and newborns. Medicinski Arhiv. 2014;**68**(3):184-187

[9] de Sá SA, Willner E, Duraes Pereira TA, et al. Anemia in pregnancy: Impact on weight and in the development of anemia in newborn. Nutrición Hospitalaria. 2015;**32**(5):2071-2079

[10] Laflamme EM. Maternal hemoglobin concentration and pregnancy outcome: A study of the effects of elevation in el alto, Bolivia. McGill Journal of Medicine. 2012;**11**(1):47

[11] Lartey A. Maternal and child nutrition in sub-Saharan Africa: Challenges and interventions. The Proceedings of the Nutrition Society. 2008;**67**(1):105-108

[12] Ogetii GN, Akech S, Jemutai J, et al. Hypoglycaemia in severe malaria, clinical associations and relationship to quinine dosage. BMC Infectious Diseases. 2010;**10**:334

[13] Yau HK, Stacpoole PW. The pathophysiology of hypoglycemia and lactic acidosis in malaria. Encyclopedia of Malaria. 2014;**2014**:1-20

[14] Hemoglobin WHO. Concentrations for the Diagnosis of Anemia and Assessment of Severity. Vitamin and Mineral Nutrition Information System, Ed. WHO. Geneva: World Health Organization; 2011

[15] Quintero JP, Siqueira AM, Tobón A, et al. Malaria-related anaemia: A Latin American perspective. Memorias do Instituto Oswaldo Cruz. 2011;**106**(Suppl. I):91-104

[16] Vainieri ML, Blagborough AM, MacLean AL, et al. Systematic tracking of altered haematopoiesis during sporozoite-mediated malaria development reveals multiple response points. Open Biology. 2016;**6**(6):160038

[17] Wang W, Qian H, Jun Cao J. Stem cell therapy: A novel treatment option for cerebral malaria? Stem Cell Research & Therapy. 2015;**6**(1):141

[18] Geerligs PD, Brabin BJ, Eggelte TA. Analysis of the effects of malaria chemoprophylaxis in children on haematological responses, morbidity and mortality. Bulletin of the World Health Organization. 2003;**81**:205-216

[19] Mohandas N, An X. Malaria and human red blood cells. Medical Microbiology and Immunology. 2012;**201**(4):593-598

[20] Rowe JA, Claessens A, Corrigan RA, et al. Adhesion of *Plasmodium falciparum*-infected erythrocytes to human cells: Molecular mechanisms and therapeutic implications. Expert Reviews in Molecular Medicine. 2009;**e16**:11

[21] Moxon CA, Grau GE, Craig AG. Malaria: Modification of the red blood cell and consequences in the human host. The British Journal of Haematology. 2011;**154**:670-679

[22] Hiller NL, Bhattacharjee S, van Ooij C. A host-targeting signal in virulence proteins reveals a secretome in malarial infection. Science. 2004;**306**:1934-1937

[23] Marti M, Good RT, Rug M, et al. Targeting malaria virulence and remodeling proteins to the host erythrocyte. Science. 2004;**306**:1930-1933

[24] Sterkers Y, Scheidig C, da Rocha M, et al. Members of the low-molecular mass rhoptry protein complex of *Plasmodium falciparum* bind to the surface of normal erythrocytes. The Journal of Infectious Diseases. 2007;**196**:617-621

[25] Evans KJ, Hansen DS, van Rooijen N, et al. Severe malarial anemia of low parasite burden in rodent models results from accelerated clearance of uninfected erythrocytes. Blood. 2006;**107**:1192-1199

[26] Goka BQ, Kwarko H, Kurtzhals JA. Complement binding to erythrocytes is associated with macrophage activation and reduced haemoglobin in *Plasmodium falciparum* malaria. Transactions of the Royal Society of Tropical Medicine and Hygiene. 2001;**95**:545-549

[27] Perkins DJ, Were T, Davenport GC, et al. Severe malarial anemia: Innate immunity and pathogenesis. International Journal of Biological Sciences. 2011;**7**(9):1427-1442

[28] Layez C, Nogueira P, Combes V, et al. *Plasmodium falciparum* rhoptry protein RSP2 triggers destruction of the erythroid lineage. Blood. 2005;**106**(10):3632-3638

[29] Abdalla SH, Malaria GP. A Hematological Perspective, Ed. T Medicine. Vol. 4. London, River Edge, NJ: Imperial College Press; 2004 Distributed by World Scientific Pub

[30] Helleberg M, Goka BQ, Akanmori BD, et al. Bone marrow suppression and severe anaemia associated with persistent *Plasmodium falciparum* infection in African children with microscopically undetectable parasitaemia. Malaria Journal. 2005;**4**:56

[31] Chasis JA, Mohandas N. Erythroblastic islands: Niches for erythropoiesis. Blood. 2008;**112**:470-478

[32] Ohene SA, Perkins DJ, Were T, et al. Severe malarial anemia: Innate immunity and pathogenesis. International Journal of Biological Sciences. 2011;**7**(9):1427-1442

[33] Liu J, Istvan ES, Gluzman IY, et al. *Plasmodium falciparum* ensures its amino acid supply with multiple acquisition pathways and redundant proteolytic enzyme systems. Proceedings of the National Academy of Sciences of the United States of America. 2006;**103**(23):8840-8845

[34] Casals-Pascual C, Kai O, Cheung JOP, et al. Suppression of erythropoiesis in malarial anemia is associated with hemozoin in vitro and in vivo. Blood. 2006;**108**(8):2569-2577

[35] Awandare GA, Ouma Y, Ouma C, et al. Role of monocyte-acquired hemozoin in suppression of macrophage migration inhibitory factor in children with severe malarial anemia. Infection and Immunity. 2007;**75**(1):201-210

[36] Shio MT, Kassa FA, Bellemare MJ, et al. Innate inflammatory response to the malarial pigment hemozoin. Microbes and Infection. 2010;**12**(12-13):889-899

[37] Were T, Davenport GC, Yamo EO, et al. Naturally acquired hemozoin by monocytes promotes suppression of RANTES in children with malarial anemia through an IL-10-dependent mechanism. Microbes and Infection. 2009;**11**(8-9):811-819

[38] Clark IA, Budd AC, Alleva LM, et al. Human malarial disease: A consequence of inflammatory cytokine release. Malarial Journal. 2006;**5**:85

[39] Rockett KA, Awburn MM, Rockett EJ, et al. Tumor necrosis factor and interleukin-1 synergy in the context of malaria pathology. The American Journal of Tropical Medicine and Hygiene. 1994;**50**(6):735-742

[40] Hensmann M, Kwiatkowski D. Cellular basis of early cytokine response to *Plasmodium falciparum*. Infection and Immunity. 2001;**69**(4):2364-2371

[41] Artavanis-Tsakonas K, Riley EM. Innate immune response to malaria: Rapid induction of IFN-gamma from human NK cells by live *Plasmodium falciparum*-infected erythrocytes. The Journal of Immunology. 2002;**169**(6):2956-2963

[42] D'Ombrain MC, Hansen DS, Simpson KM, et al. Gammadelta-T cells expressing NK receptors predominate over cells NK and conventional T cells in the innate IFN-gamma response to *Plasmodium falciparum malaria*. European Journal of Immunology. 2007;**37**(7):1864-1873

[43] D'Ombrain MC, Robinson LJ, Stanisic DI, et al. Association of early interferon-gamma production with immunity to clinical malaria: A longitudinal study among Papua new Guinean children. Clinical Infectious Diseases. 2008;**47**(11):1380-1387

[44] Ong'echa JO, Lal AA, Terlouw DJ, et al. Association of interferon-gamma responses to pre-erythrocytic stage vaccine candidate antigens of *Plasmodium falciparum* in young Kenyan children with improved hemoglobin levels: XV. Asembo Bay Cohort Project. The American Journal of Tropical Medicine and Hygiene. 2003;**68**(5):590-597

[45] Clark IA, Cowden WB. The pathophysiology of *falciparum* malaria. Pharmacology & Therapeutics. 2003;**99**(2):221-260

[46] Dinarello CA. Infection, fever, and exogenous and endogenous pyrogens: Some concepts have changed. Journal of Endotoxin Research. 2004;**10**(4):201-222

[47] Pascual V, Allantaz F, Arce E, et al. Role of interleukin-1 (IL-1) in the pathogenesis of systemic onset juvenile idiopathic arthritis and clinical response to IL-1 blockade. The Journal of Experimental Medicine. 2005;**201**(9):1479-1486

[48] Dinarello CA. Blocking IL-1 in systemic inflammation. The Journal of Experimental Medicine. 2005;**201**(9):1355-1359

[49] Ouma C, Davenport GC, Awandare GA, et al. Polymorphic variability in the interleukin (IL)-1beta promoter conditions susceptibility to severe malarial anemia and functional changes in IL-1beta production. The Journal of Infectious Diseases. 2008;**198**(8):1219-1226

[50] Aubouy A, Deloron P, Migot-Nabias F. Plasma and in vitro levels of cytokines during and after a *Plasmodium falciparum* malaria attack in Gabon. Acta Tropica. 2002;**83**(3):195-203

[51] Krockenberger M, Dombrowski Y, Weidler C, et al. Macrophage migration inhibitory factor (MIF) contributes to the immune escape of ovarian cancer by downregulating NKG2D1. Journal of Immunology. 2008;**180**(11):7338-7348

[52] Vieira Ferro EA, Mineo JR, Ietta F, et al. Macrophage migration inhibitory factor is up-regulated in human first-trimester placenta stimulated by soluble antigen of *Toxoplasma gondii* resulting in increased monocyte adhesion on villous explants. The American Journal of Pathology. 2008;**172**(1):50-58

[53] Awandare GA, Hittner JB, Kremsner PG, et al. Decreased circulating macrophage migration inhibitory factor (MIF) protein and blood mononuclear cell MIF transcripts in children with *Plasmodium falciparum* malaria. Clinical Immunology. 2006;**119**(2):219-225

[54] Cua DJ, Sherlock J, Chen Y, et al. Interleukin-23 rather than interleukin-12 is the critical cytokine for autoimmune inflammation of the brain. Nature. 2003;**421**:774-748

[55] Wiekowski MT, Leach MW, Evans EW, et al. Ubiquitous transgenic expression of the IL-23 subunit p19 induces multiorgan inflammation, runting, infertility, and premature death. The Journal of Immunology. 2001;**166**(12):7563-7570

[56] Shimozato O, Ugai S-i, Chiyo M, et al. The secreted form of the p40 subunit of interleukin (IL)-12 inhibits IL-23 functions and abrogates IL-23-mediated antitumour effects. Immunology. 2006;**117**(1):22-28

[57] Ong'echa JM, Remo AM, Kristoff J, et al. Increased circulating interleukin (IL)-23 in children with malarial anemia: In vivo and in vitro relationship with co-regulatory cytokines IL-12 and IL-10. Clinical Immunology. 2008;**126**(2):211-221

[58] Keller CC, Yamo O, Ouma C, et al. Acquisition of hemozoin by monocytes down-regulates interleukin-12 p40 (IL-12p40) transcripts and circulating IL-12p70 through an IL-10-dependent mechanism: In vivo and in vitro findings in severe malarial anemia. Infection and Immunity. 2006;**74**(9):5249-5260

[59] Gao X, Lee H-Y, Lummertz da Rocha E, et al. TGF-β inhibitors stimulate red blood cell production by enhancing self-renewal of BFU-E erythroid progenitors. Blood. 2016;**128**(23): 2637-2641

[60] Ouma C, Davenport GC, Were T. Haplotypes of IL-10 promoter variants are associated with susceptibility to severe malarial anemia and functional changes in IL-10 production. Human Genetics. 2008;**124**:515-524

[61] Davenport GC, Hittner J, Were T, et al. Relationship between inflammatory mediator patterns and anemia in HIV-1 positive and exposed children with *Plasmodium falciparum* malaria. American Journal of Hematology. 2012;**87**:652-658

[62] Ong'echa JM, Davenport GC, Vulule JM, et al. Identification of inflammatory biomarkers for pediatric malarial anemia severity using novel statistical methods. Infection and Immunity. 2011;**79**(11):4674-4680

[63] Prakash D, Fesel C, Jain R, et al. Clusters of cytokines determine malaria severity in *Plasmodium falciparum*-infected patients from endemic areas of Central India. The Journal of Infectious Diseases. 2006;**194**(2):198-207

[64] Dietmann A, Helbok R, Lackner P, et al. Endoglin in African children with *Plasmodium falciparum* malaria: A novel player in severe malaria pathogenesis. The Journal of Infectious Diseases. 2009;**200**(12):1842-1848

[65] Jaramillo M, Godbout M, Olivier M. Hemozoin induces macrophage chemokine expression through oxidative stress-dependent and -independent mechanisms. The Journal of Immunology. 2005;**174**(1):475-484

[66] Ochiel DO, Awandare GA, Kelle CC, et al. Differential regulation of beta-chemokines in children with *Plasmodium falciparum* malaria. Infection and Immunity. 2005;**73**(7): 4190-4197

[67] Luster AD. The role of chemokines in linking innate and adaptive immunity. Current Opinion in Immunology. 2002;**14**(1):129-135

[68] Were T, Ouma C, Otieno RO. Suppression of RANTES in children with *Plasmodium falciparum* malaria. Haematologica. 2006;**91**(10):1396-1399

[69] Stoiser B, Looareesuwan S, Thalhammer F, et al. Serum concentrations of granulocyte-colony stimulating factor in complicated *Plasmodium falciparum* ma-Aria. European Cytokine Network. 2000;**11**(1):75-80

[70] Dang C, Hudis C. Can granulocyte-colony stimulating factor worsen anemia? Journal of Clinical Oncology. 2006;**24**:2985-2986

[71] Keller CC, Ouma C, Ouma Y, et al. Suppression of a novel hematopoietic mediator in children with severe malarial anemia. Infection and Immunity. 2009;**77**(9):3864-3871

[72] Collins Ouma C, Keller CC, Davenport GC, et al. A novel functional variant in the stem cell growth factor promoter protects against severe malarial anemia. Infection and Immunity. 2010;**78**(1):453-460

[73] Keller CC, Kremsner PG, Hittner JB, et al. Elevated nitric oxide production in children with malarial anemia: Hemozoin-induced nitric oxide synthase type 2 transcripts and nitric oxide in blood mononuclear cells. Infection and Immunity. 2004;**72**(8):4868-4873

[74] Narsaria N, Mohanty C, Das BK, et al. Oxidative stress in children with severe malaria. Journal of Tropical Pediatrics. 2012;**58**(2):147-150

[75] Perkins DJ, Moore J, Otieno J, et al. In vivo acquisition of hemozoin by placental blood mononuclear cells suppresses PGE2, TNF-alpha, and IL-10. Biochemical and Biophysical Research Communications. 2003;**311**(4):839-846

[76] Keller CC, Davenport GC, Dickman KR, et al. Suppression of prostaglandin E2 by malaria parasite products and antipyretics promotes overproduction of tumor necrosis factor-alpha: Association with the pathogenesis of childhood malarial anemia. The Journal of Infectious Diseases. 2006;**193**(10):1384-1393

[77] Lamikanra AA, Theron M, Kooij TWA, et al. Hemozoin (malarial pigment) directly promotes apoptosis of erythroid precursors. PloS One. 2009;**4**(12):e8446

[78] Awandare GA, Kempaiah P, Ochiel DO, et al. Mechanisms of erythropoiesis inhibition by malarial pigment and malaria-induced proinflammatory mediators in an in vitro model. American Journal of Hematology. 2011;**86**(2):155-162

[79] Patel H, Dhangar K, Sonawane Y, et al. In search of selective 11 beta-HSD type 1 inhibitors without nephrotoxicity: An approach to resolve the metabolic syndrome by virtual based screening. Arabian Journal of Chemistry. 2015; In press DOI: org/10.1016/j.arabjc.2016.08.003

[80] Mavondo GA, Mkhwanazi BN, Mabandla MV, et al. Asiatic Acid Influences Parasitaemia Reduction and Ameliorate Malaria Anaemia in P. berghei Infected Sprague Dawley Male Rats. BMC CAM 2016;**16**:357 DOI: 10.1186/s12906-016-1338-z

[81] Moneriz C, Mestres J, Bautista JM, et al. Multi-targeted activity of maslinic acid as an antimalarial natural compound. The FEBS Journal. 2011;**278**:2951-2961

[82] Huang S-S, Chiu C-S, Chen H-J, et al. Antinociceptive activities and the mechanisms of anti-inflammation of Asiatic acid in mice. Evidence-Based Complementary and Alternative Medicine. 2011;10 pages. Article ID 895857, DOI:10.1155/2011/895857

[83] Lee YS, Jin DQ, Beak SM, et al. Inhibition of ultraviolet-A-modulated signaling pathways by asiatic acid and ursolic acid in HaCaT human keratinocytes. European Journal of Pharmacology. 2003;**476**:173-178

[84] Looareesuwan S, Merry AH, Phillips RE. Reduced erythrocyte survival following clearance of malarial parasitaemia in Thai patients. British Journal of Haematology. 1987;**67**(4):473-478

[85] Dunst J, Azzouz N, Liu X, et al. Interaction between *Plasmodium* glycosylphosphatidylinositol and the host protein moesin has no implication in malaria pathology. Frontiers in Cellular and Infection Microbiology. 2017;**7**:183

[86] Kawai T, Akira S. Toll-like receptors and their crosstalk with other innate receptors in infection and immunity. Immunity. 2011;**34**:637-650

[87] Gowda DC. TLR-mediated cell signaling by malaria GPIs. Trends in Parasitology. 2007;**23**:596-604

[88] Boutlis CS, Riley EM, Anstey NM, et al. Glycosylphosphatidylinositols in malaria pathogenesis and immunity: Potential for therapeutic inhibition and vaccination. Current Topics in Microbiology and Immunology. 2005;**297**:145-185

[89] Gazzinelli RT, Kalantari P, Fitzgerald KA, et al. Innate sensing of malaria parasites. Nature Reviews. Immunology. 2014;**14**:744-757

[90] Schofield L, Hewitt MC, Evans K, et al. Synthetic GPI as a candidate anti-toxic vaccine in a model of malaria. Nature. 2002;**418**:785-789

[91] Guo W, Liu W, Hong S, et al. Mitochondria-dependent apoptosis of con A-activated T lymphocytes induced by Asiatic acid for preventing murine fulminant hepatitis. PloS One. 2012;**7**(9):e46018

[92] Cho MK, Sung M-A, Kim DS, et al. 2-Oxo-3, 23-isopropylidene-asiatate (AS2006A): A wound-healing asiatate derivative, exerts anti-inflammatory effect by apoptosis of macrophages. International Immunopharmacology. 2003;**3**:1429-1437

[93] Pakdeechote P, Bunbupha S, Kukongviriyapan U, et al. Asiatic acid alleviates hemodynamic and metabolic alterations via restoring eNOS/iNOS expression, oxidative stress, and inflammation in diet-induced metabolic syndrome rats. Nutrients. 2014;**6**(1):355-370

[94] Chang K-H, Tam M, Stevenson MM. Erythropoietin-induced reticulocytosis significantly modulates the course and outcome of blood-stage malaria. The Journal of Infectious Diseases. 2004;**189**:735-743

[95] Siewert B, Csuk R. Membrane damaging activity of a maslinic acid analog. European Journal of Medicinal Chemistry. 2014;**74**:1-6

[96] Innocente AM, Silva GNS, Cruz LN, et al. Synthesis and antiplasmodial activity of betulinic acid and ursolic acid analogues. Molecules. 2012;**17**:12003-12014

[97] Howard CT, McKakpo US, Quakyi IA, et al. Relationship of hepcidin with parasitemia and anemia among patients with uncomplicated *Plasmodium falciparum* malaria in Ghana. The American Journal of Tropical Medicine and Hygiene. 2007;**77**:623-626

Section 4

Hepcidin and Anemia

Chapter 11

Influence of Hepcidin in the Development of Anemia

Cadiele Oliana Reichert, Filomena Marafon,
Débora Levy, Luciana Morganti Ferreira Maselli,
Margarete Dulce Bagatini, Solange Lúcia Blatt,
Sérgio Paulo Bydlowski and Celso Spada

Additional information is available at the end of the chapter

http://dx.doi.org/10.5772/intechopen.71476

Abstract

Anemia presents a global public health problem. It is related to several factors, ranging from deficiency in nutrients from food to genetic alterations in iron absorption and metabolism. In this context, hepcidin is a peptide molecule that regulates iron homeostasis. Hepcidin is synthesized, in part, by hepatocytes. In physiological conditions, increased serum transferrin, serum iron, inflammation, and erythropoiesis trigger stimuli that promote hepcidin antimicrobial peptide (HAMP) gene transcription and hepcidin synthesis. However, in pathological situations, an overexpression of hepcidin occurs, an increase in the plasma concentration that damages the organism. Hepcidin contributes to the pathogenesis of iron deficiency anemia, anemia of inflammation, in hemoglobinopathies. Then, there is a restriction of the availability of iron to the tissues and the formation of new erythroid precursors, with the consequent development of anemia.

Keywords: anemia, chronic disease anemia, ferroportin, hepcidin, HAMP gene, iron deficiency, iron deficiency anemia, IRIDA, iron homeostasis, sickle cell, thalassemia

1. Introduction

The World Health Organization (WHO) characterizes anemia as a condition in which the concentration of hemoglobin is below 13 g/L for males and 12 g/L for females. Anemia is a condition in which the number of red blood cells or their oxygen carrying capacity is insufficient to meet physiological needs, which vary according to the age, gender, altitude, smoking status, and pregnancy status. Iron deficiency (ID) is considered to be the most common cause of anemia, although there are other conditions such as folate deficiency, vitamin B12 and vitamin A, chronic inflammation, parasitic infections, and hereditary disorders related to iron metabolism and the formation of hemoglobin [1]. Iron deficiency impairs erythroid cell formation and decreases hemoglobin synthesis. Iron has functions vital to the body, requiring daily intake through food and the constant recycling of senescent erythrocytes by macrophages to maintain adequate concentration. In view of this, the control of iron uptake and movement in the form of ferritin occur through the plasma hepcidin concentration, a peptidic hormone, which regulates iron metabolism through the negative modulation of ferroportin [2–4].

Iron deficiency and/or hypoferremia involve(s) changes in hepcidin concentration and iron metabolism markers (serum iron, transferrin and ferritin). Hepcidin has been shown to act in the direct inhibition of food absorption of iron in the duodenum, in blocking the release of iron recycled by macrophages and in controlling the movement of iron stores contained in hepatocytes, enterocytes, and macrophages [5–7]. However, the serum concentration of hepcidin assists in the prognosis of the main hematological alterations involving the iron metabolism with the development of anemia, influencing the severity of iron deficiency anemia, iron-refractory iron deficiency anemia, anemia of chronic disease, hemoglobinopathies, mainly HbS, thalassemias, and hemolytic anemia, among others.

2. Hepcidin: function and structure

The hepcidin molecule ("hep" hepatic origin, "cidin" antimicrobial activity) was described in the year 2000; it is an antimicrobial peptide that acts in parts in innate immunity and iron metabolism. It was isolated from human blood and urine [3, 4]. The relationship between hepcidin and its action on iron homeostasis was demonstrated in knockout animals for the gene encoding hepcidin, the HAMP gene, in a clinical condition compatible with hemochromatosis. However, transgenic animals with increased hepcidin expression had decreased serum iron, erythropoiesis deficiency with severe microcytic-hypochromic anemia [8, 9].

Extrahepatic production of hepcidin occurs to a lesser extent, and it is believed that at these sites it acts as an antimicrobial peptide. In the kidney, hepcidin modulates the defense barriers against urinary tract infections. In the heart, hepcidin maintains iron homeostasis in cardiac tissue by an autocrine regulation of the expression of ferroprotein on the surface of cardiomyocytes [10, 11]. Hepcidin is encoded in a molecule containing 84 amino acids, a prehepcidin, which undergoes proteolytic cleavage in one region and gives prohepcidin, composed of 64 amino acids. Prohepcidin is biologically inactive and is cleaved subsequently by the enzyme furin in a specific NH_2 region, resulting in biologically active hepcidin composed of 8 cysteine residues, bound by 4 bisulfide bridges containing 25 amino acids [3, 4, 8].

2.1. Iron

Iron is an integral constituent of several metalloproteins; being essential for oxygen transport, it acts on the transfer of electrons from the respiratory chain and in various catalytic reactions. The biological versatility of iron is based on its ability to act as electron donor and receptor. Thus, iron can easily convert between its oxidized state, ferric iron (Fe^{+3}), and reduced state, ferrous iron (Fe^{+2}). Spontaneous aerobic oxidation of Fe^{+2} to Fe^{+3} is practically insoluble at physiological pH, which hinders the acquisition of iron by cells and tissues, requiring other proteins and enzymes that facilitate the conversion of $Fe^{+3} \rightarrow Fe^{+2}$ [12].

An adult human body contains approximately 3–5 g of iron, with men presenting approximately 55 mg/kg and women 44 mg/kg. Approximately 70% of body iron is stored as heme in hemoglobin present in erythroblasts and erythrocytes. Muscle contains about 2.5% iron in the form of myoglobin; iron reserve in the macrophages corresponds to 5% and in the hepatocytes to 20%. Diet maintains the iron stores, and a diet rich in red meat provides approximately 10–15 mg iron/day as heme (Fe^{+2}) present in myoglobin and hemoglobin. Around 20–40% of heme and 10–20% of nonheme iron (Fe^{+3}) are available for absorption. This turnover maintains the iron stores for the physiological needs, since the quantities of iron required by the organism vary according to the age group and gender of each individual [12, 13].

2.1.1. *Iron homeostasis*

Iron in both ferrous and ferric forms is absorbed in the duodenum in different ways. In order for ferric iron to be absorbed more efficiently, it must undergo an oxidation of its state from Fe^{+3} to Fe^{+2}. However, some factors influence the absorption of iron Fe^{+3}, such as a diet rich in polyphenols and phytic acid, since these molecules bind to iron from vegetables and cereals, as well as deficiency of vitamin C and antioxidant substances, gastritis caused by *Helicobacter pylori*, and bariatric surgery, among other factors [14].

The oxidation reaction, $Fe^{+3} \rightarrow Fe^{+2}$, is performed by the enzyme cytochrome b duodenal (dCytB), present on the plasma membrane of enterocytes. Thereafter, ferrous iron is mobilized via the divalent metal-1 type metal transporter (DMT-1) to the intracellular medium. However, heme iron from the diet is internalized by the heme-1 carrier protein (HCP-1) into the cells. Both forms of iron derived from the diet may be stored as ferritin or transported to different tissues and organs (**Figure 1**) [15, 16].

2.1.2. *Transport and delivery of iron to the cells*

Transferrin transports iron into tissues. It is necessary that the iron in its iron state be oxidized to ferric iron through the oxidizing action of the enzymes hephaestin and ceruloplasmin [17]. Transferrin is a beta-globulin, which has an ellipsoidal shape, with two iron-binding sites. Transferrin saturation (TS) determines its functional status. In healthy subjects, about 30% of transferrin is saturated with iron. When the two iron-binding sites are occupied, it is termed diferric transferrin; when only one site is connected to iron, it is called monoferric transferrin; and when no site contains iron, it is called apotransferrin [18].

Under physiological conditions, transferrin saturation determines its affinity to cells and cell receptors; the less saturated and/or iron-bound, the greater the affinity of apotransferrin to enterocytes. On the other hand, the diferric transferrin has a greater affinity to the transferrin receptors (TfR1 and TfR2) than the monoferric transferrin receptors. The ability of apotransferrin is to prevent the accumulation of free iron not bound to transferrin (NTBI), which is a redox-active and toxic [12, 18].

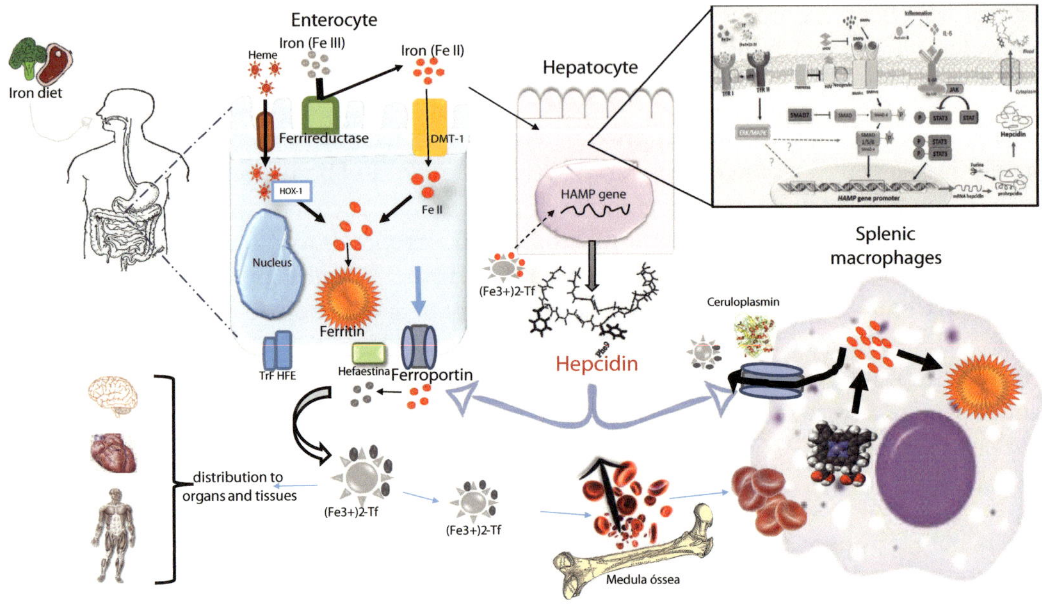

Figure 1. Iron homeostasis [29].

Transferrin binds the TfR1 and TfR2 receptor subunits on the cell surface to form a ferro-carbonate-transferrin complex. The cell internalizes this complex by endocytosis. After the internalization of the complex, the acidic pH present in the intracellular medium favors the release of Fe^{+3}, and then it is reduced to Fe^{+2} by the ferroreductase, Steap3 (six-transmembrane epithelial antigen of prostate 3) and transported in the intracellular medium by DMT1. The receptor-transferrin complex returns to the cell surface and the apotransferrin is released to a new cycle. Replenishment of transferrin occurs through iron stored in macrophages [12, 18–20].

2.1.3. Recycling and storage of iron

Each erythrocyte contains approximately 1.2×10^9 molecules of the heme group associated with hemoglobin, with approximately 200 billion erythrocytes reaching senescence and intravascular hemolysis each day. Hemoglobin released from senescent erythrocytes can be easily oxidized, releasing the heme group, which can promote protein oxidation, generate lipid peroxides, and damage DNA through the formation of reactive oxygen species [21]. The heme group is metabolized within the splenic macrophages by the activity of heme oxygenase (HO-1 and HO-2). The intracellular concentration of HO-1 increases after heme phagocytosis. The breakdown of heme by HO-1 gives rise to Fe^{+2} and the remaining portion is biliverdin, which after the action of the enzyme biliverdin reductase gives rise to bilirubin. About 70% of body bilirubin comes from erythrophagocytosis [15].

Iron is stored in the body in the form of ferritin. All the cells of the organisms have reserves of irons. Ferritin is a complete molecule composed of a protein, apoferritin, and iron. Apoferritin has a shell shape of 24 subunits, which stores about 4000 iron atoms. Three different genes encode apoferritin: the heavy chain (H) is encoded by the FTH gene, located on chromosome 11; the light chain (L) is encoded by the FTL gene located on chromosome 19; and the mitochondrial apoferritin is encoded by the FTMT gene and is on chromosome 5. In situations that decrease serum iron and erythropoietic activity, stored iron is mobilized from the interior of ferritin by the action of natural chelating and reducing agents such as glutathione and cysteine, into the intracellular medium, into the cell's cytosol and then exported to the extracellular medium through the ferroportin [22].

2.1.4. *Export of stored iron to the extracellular medium*

Ferroportin is a transmembrane protein that mediates the stored iron efflux of macrophages, enterocytes, and hepatocytes into plasma, maintaining systemic iron homeostasis. Through stimuli originated by the increase of serum iron, serum transferrin, erythropoiesis, and proinflammatory cytokines, the HAMP gene transcription occurs, increasing the plasma concentration of hepcidin, which binds to ferroportin in the extracellular medium through its portion N-terminal, promoting its phosphorylation, internalization, and ubiquitination in lysosomal endosomes. As with other receptors that undergo ligand-induced endocytosis, the interaction of hepcidin with ferroportin causes a conformational change in ferroportin and covalent modifications of one or more cytoplasmic segments to initiate endocytosis. The specific interaction between hepcidin and ferroportin, when altered, favors the iron accumulation of the organism [23, 24].

2.2. Regulation of hepcidin expression

Serum hepcidin concentration is regulated by several factors that may increase or decrease its serum concentration. Among the main factors that increase the serum concentration of hepcidin are infections and chronic diseases, hepatic diseases, alcohol abuse, genetic alterations in the TMPRSS6 gene, blood transfusion, dialysis in renal disease, and administration of iron by orally or intravenously. The factors that decrease the serum concentration of hepcidin are erythropoiesis, erythropoietin, and erythropoietin-stimulating agents in order to allow the movement and delivery of iron in the bone marrow. Genetic alterations are related to the development of hemochromatosis, hypoxia, and steroid hormones, among others [25–29].

These factors activate the HAMP gene, located on chromosome 19q13 to transcribe the hepcidin mRNA. Literatures have described several HAMP signaling pathways, without much evidence. However, two pathways are described as the main ways of regulating and activating the HAMP gene. These pathways are related to increased serum iron and the production of inflammatory cytokines. The first signaling pathway occurs through the induction of the pathway related to bone morphogenetic proteins (BMPs), being activated by the concentration of circulating iron. Second, the Janus kinase (JAK)/signal transducer and activator of transcription (STAT) signaling pathway is activated by inflammatory stimuli. Increased transferrin saturation and its binding to the TfR1 and TfR2 receptors cause a displacement of the HFE protein to its receptor, TfR2, where activation of hemojuvelin (HJV), a BMP coreceptor occurs. Then, intracellular signaling proceeds until the activation of HAMP gene [30].

The BMP cytokines are proteins that are part of the great family transforming growth factor-β (TGF-β). Activation of the BMP path requires interaction with its BMP-r receptor and with the BMP-R receptor coreceptor, the HJV protein. The integration between HIV-BMP-R induces phosphorylation of the BMP receptor, thus activating it. This activation generates an intracellular signaling cascade through the binding of a threonine/serine kinase type I and type II receptor complex [31–33].

The activated receptor type II activates the type I receptor. This action may activate other receptors and other intracellular proteins, such as the R-SMAD protein, which regulates the phosphorylation of SMAD-1/5/8 proteins, leaving them active. However, these proteins cannot promote the transcription of the HAMP gene but are necessary for union with the SMAD-4 factor. After formation of the SMAD1/5/8/–SMAD4 complex, migration to the nucleus commences. These proteins bind to the promoter region of the HAMP gene by initiating its transcription. The negative intracellular feedback of the SMAD pathway is performed by the SMAD-7 protein, which prevents phosphorylation and formation of the SMAD-1/5/8/SMAD-4 complex. Currently, it has been thought to use SMAD-7 as a therapeutic target to suppress hepcidin mRNA in diseases where hepcidin overexpression occurs. The BMP/SMAD pathway has shown promise in the development of candidate hepcidin suppressors [34–37].

Inflammatory mediators influence the expression of HAMP gene through the JAK/STAT signaling pathway. Initially, a conformation shift on the subunits of the JAK receptors is required. JAK receptors are present in the intracellular medium coupled with other transmembrane receptors. When the inflammatory cytokines, interleukin-6 (IL-6), IL-1β, IL-22, activin-B, and interferon-α bind to their receptors, they activate the cytoplasmic JAK. As an example, IL-6 binds to its receptor, which is formed by two subunits: one alpha subunit (IL-6-R) and another beta subunit (GP130). When IL-6 binds to IL-6-R, a dimerization of gp130 occurs, which recruits the cytoplasmic JAK to phosphorylate the gp130 protein. After phosphorylation, the STAT-1 and STAT-3 proteins bind to gp130 and autophosphorylate soon after the formation of a complex that migrates to the nucleus and induces the transcription of the HAMP gene (**Figure 2**) [38–43].

2.3. Hepcidin and anemia

2.3.1. Iron deficiency and iron deficiency anemia

Iron deficiency (ID) and iron deficiency anemia (IDA) are distinct forms, even though they are often used as synonyms. Capellini et al. [44] define "iron deficiency is a health-related condition in which iron availability is insufficient to meet the body's needs and which can be presented with or without anemia."

ID defines a condition in which iron stores are reduced (ferritin <12 μg/L) in the absence of anemia, but the supply of iron to erythropoiesis is maintained. IDA occurs when there is no iron available for erythropoiesis, characterizing a decrease in hemoglobin synthesis. When IDA is the result of progressive ID, it usually develops slowly and can be well tolerated by organisms, making its diagnosis difficult. The diagnosis of IDA requires laboratory tests, since the symptoms may be present, but they are nonspecific and often ignored [45].

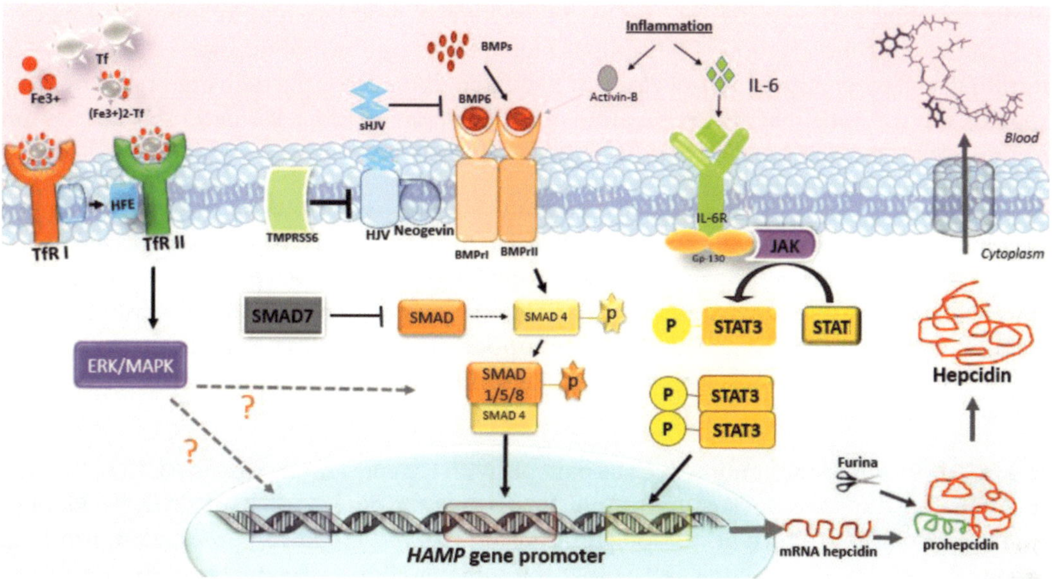

Figure 2. Hepcidin expression [29].

The treatment for ID/IDA is done with oral iron replacement; however, when the serum concentration of hepcidin is increased, this iron is not absorbed in the duodenum and it is necessary to use injectable iron. ID is commonly reported in obese individuals due to their elevated serum concentration of hepcidin and reduction of iron absorption due to inflammation developed by adipose tissue [46, 47]. Serum hepcidin, ferritin, and iron content in hepatic and skeletal muscle are increased in obese individuals, and after weight loss, values tend to normalize [48].

2.3.2. Chronic disease anemia

Chronic disease anemia (CDA) or anemia of inflammation (AI) refers to the impaired production of erythrocytes associated with chronic inflammatory conditions, including cancer, chronic infection, or autoimmune diseases. Recent data indicate that anemia can also occur in situations of severe and acute inflammation, or with persistent inflammatory signs that occur in obesity, aging, and renal failure. Anemia of inflammation is defined by low concentration of serum iron (<60 μg/dL) with normal or elevated serum ferritin (>12 ng/mL) and saturation of transferrin around 15% [49].

The clinical picture of anemia, established in the AI, is due to the production of cytokines as IL-1β, INF-γ, and TNF-α, which influence negatively on erythropoiesis, by inhibiting the production of erythropoietin (EPO). In addition, when the erythropoietin concentration is decreased, there is an increase in hepatic synthesis of hepcidin. Other factors that influence the alteration of iron metabolism through modulation of hepcidin expression are interleukin IL-6, IL-1β, IL-22, INF-γ, and TNF-α. These cytokines act on the HAMP gene through the activation of the signaling pathway JAK-STAT. Due to the intense production of inflammatory mediators, the serum concentration of hepcidin is high, restricting the mobilization of iron stores of ferritin in enterocytes and hepatocytes and making it difficult for the delivery of iron by macrophages in the bone marrow to generate new precursors erythroid. Due to this fact, serum ferritin is elevated and transferrin is decreased [49, 50].

Morbid obesity is considered a chronic inflammatory state with altered iron metabolism. ID may initially occur due to malabsorption of iron in the duodenum, as well as increased hepcidin due to the chronic inflammatory process. Most obese individuals present serum transferrin saturation below 20%, and after weight loss, markers of iron metabolism normalize over a period of up to 4–6 months. This evidence supports the hypothesis that obesity favors iron sequestration with the development of anemia of inflammation, but AI in obesity may or may not be preceded by ID [50, 51].

In some more serious situations, such as patients with chronic kidney disease (CKD), the anemia is mainly due to the lack of erythropoietin. During the development of CKD, the kidneys lose the ability to produce erythropoietin, causing less red blood cell production, resulting in anemia. Another interesting fact is that the inflammation generated by CKD stimulates the synthesis of hepcidin, which prevents the mobilization of iron stores in the macrophages present in the marrow. These facts alone or together contribute to the development of anemia in CKD. Besides that, the renal function plays a role in clearance of hepcidin. Renal dysfunction results in decreased clearance of hepcidin and consequent storage of hepcidin with development of anemia. As CKD progresses, the serum concentration of hepcidin increases independent of the inflammatory state. In this clinical context, it is common to develop an anemia of inflammatory disease with ID anemia, since several compartments involved in the metabolism and maintenance of iron stores are compromised [50, 52–54].

2.3.3. Iron-refractory iron deficiency anemia

Iron-refractory iron deficiency anemia (IRIDA OMIM # 206200) is an autosomal recessive disease characterized clinically by microcytic and hypochromic congenital anemia, unresponsive to treatment with oral iron and partial response to treatment with parenteral iron, and has low transferrin saturation, low iron concentration, high serum ferritin, and excess hepcidin. Mutations present in the TMPRSS6 gene, which encodes the matriptase-2 protein, confer the pathogenesis of IRIDA. The matriptase-2 protein is a type II transmembrane serine protease, expressed in hepatocytes, enterocytes, and other cells. The biological function of matriptase-2 is to regulate hepcidin expression in liver cells [55–57].

The polymorphism of rs855791 (p.Ala736Val) of the single nucleotide polymorphism (SNP) type is the most frequent underlying pathology. In this genetic alteration, the amino acid alanine is replaced by a valine at position 736, in the serine protease domain of matriptase-2. Thus, the protein matriptase-2 does not undergo proteolytic cleavage, losing its function of negatively regulating the action of hepcidin. Another variant is T287N, which inactivates hemojuvelin cleavage. Cleavage of the hemojuvelin is required so that it binds to the BMP receptors inactivating the signaling pathways of the HAMP gene [58–60].

The appearance of anemia in IRIDA occurs in early childhood; there are reports that the process of instituting anemia begins in the intrauterine life. The most serious cases of IRIDA reported are in children. The clinical-laboratorial picture presents as characteristics of the disease congenital hypochromia, microcytic anemia with very low MCV, low transferrin saturation (<15–5%), and abnormal iron absorption with the use of defective iron. IRIDA can develop with varying degrees of anemia, ranging from severe to moderate or mild; the common feature among all is resistance to oral iron therapy and genetic inheritance with changes in the TMPRSS6 gene. Initially, the concentration of hepcidin in mild and moderate IDA and IRIDA is high, restricting the iron absorption in the duodenum and making it impossible to mobilize the iron stores. However, in the treatment of IDA with iron replacement, the serum concentration of hepcidin decreases rapidly, facilitating the absorption and replacement of the iron stores [61, 62].

2.3.4. *Sickle cell anemia*

Hemoglobinopathies are hereditary changes that affect hemoglobin. These changes may be structural or deficient synthesis. In structural hemoglobinopathies, the change in one or more hemoglobin chains occurs. In the vast majority of cases, such changes are caused by point mutations, which determine the exchange of one amino acid by another. Among structural hemoglobinopathies, hemoglobin S is the most common inherited hematological abnormality in human being. Its etiology is genetic, with an autosomal recessive pattern and due to mutation in the beta globin gene, producing a structural alteration in the molecule. Approximately 300,000 infants are born per year with sickle cell anemia globally [63].

In its homozygous form, it is called sickle cell anemia and, where at least one gene is HbS, is called sickle cell disease. The hemoglobin S (HbS) variant results from the substitution of valine for glutamic acid in the sixth amino acid of β-globin. Sickle cell disease or anemia is characterized by reduced blood hemoglobin concentration, susceptibility to infections, recurrent vaso-occlusion, tissue infarction, and complications such as stroke, avascular necrosis of the joints, or nephropathy. Tissue hypoxia of vessel obstruction facilitates the deoxygenation of HbS, its crystallization, hepatic eruption, and chronic hemolysis. The iron overload present in sickle cell anemia is due to blood transfusions, requiring the use of oral chelants, since free iron is toxic. The high concentration of inflammatory cytokines increases the retention of cellular iron stores and in the endothelial reticulum, due to the high serum hepcidin. Use of iron chelators in the treatment of sickle cell anemia lowers the serum concentration of hepcidin and mobilizes iron stores for erythropoiesis [64–66].

2.3.5. *Thalassemias*

The thalassemias are derived from partial or total deficiency in the synthesis of one or more types of globin chains, leading to defective production of hemoglobin. Thalassemia is an autosomal recessive genetic disorder. In the literature, alpha thalassemia, thalassemia intermediary, and beta-thalassemias have been described. Mediterranean population is most affected by the disease. Among the main symptoms are fatigue and weakness, due to the development of anemia; pale or yellowish skin; increased direct bilirubin; facial bone deformities and slow growth; lack of iron in hemopoiesis; abdominal bloating, due to the increase of blood and iron deposition in the organs of abdominal cavity; and dark urine, due to the presence of hemoglobin, urobilinogen, and iron. Individuals with thalassemia also develop serious heart problems. Thalassemia is an anemia with iron overload. The iron overload results from the blood transfusions patients often receive and the hemolysis of the red blood cells [67].

The relationship between thalassemia and hepcidin was initially observed in mice with thalassemia. These animals had a low expression of hepcidin and severe anemia. Decreased serum hepcidin concentration favors increased iron uptake from diet and iron overload. Anemia, tissue hypoxia, and increased erythropoietin production observed in beta-thalassemia promote suppression of hepcidin. Another mitigating factor in the thalassemia clinical framework is the overexpression of the erythroid hormone erythroferrone (ERFE). ERFE regulates the synthesis of hepcidin, together with erythropoietin, during erythropoiesis [68, 69].

3. Conclusion

The development of anemia is complex and requires better understanding and studies related to iron metabolism. Hepcidin controls the metabolism of iron, but when an imbalance occurs in its serum concentration, it causes serious damage to the organism, it is necessary to consider hepcidin level for the laboratory diagnosis of anemias, a practice that is not performed, and to establish a reference value for hepcidin.

Conflict of interests

The authors state that there are no conflicts of interest.

Author details

Cadiele Oliana Reichert[1*], Filomena Marafon[1,4], Débora Levy[2], Luciana Morganti Ferreira Maselli[2,3], Margarete Dulce Bagatini[4], Solange Lúcia Blatt[1], Sérgio Paulo Bydlowski[2,3] and Celso Spada[1]

*Address all correspondence to: kadielli@hotmail.com

1 Laboratory of Clinical Hematology, Clinical Analysis Department, Health Sciences Center, Federal University of Santa Catarina (FUSC), Florianópolis, Brazil

2 Laboratory of Genetics and Molecular Hematology (LIM31), University of São Paulo School of Medicine (USPSM), São Paulo, Brazil

3 Research Division, Pro-Blood Hemocenter, São Paulo Foundation, São Paulo, Brazil

4 Laboratory of Microbiology, Immunology and Parasitology, Federal University Southern Frontier (FUSF), Campus Chapecó, Brazil

References

[1] World Health Organization. Anemia. WHO; 2017 [Available]: http://www.who.int/topics/anaemia/en/

[2] Brugnara C. Iron deficiency and erythropoiesis: New diagnostic approaches. Clinical Chemistry. 2003;**49**(10):1573-1578. DOI: 10.1373/49.10.1573

[3] Krause A, Neitz S, Mägert HJ, Schulz A, Forssmann WG, Schulz-Knappe P, et al. LEAP-1, a novel highly disulfide-bonded human peptide, exhibits antimicrobial activity. FEBS Letters. 2000;**480**(2-3):147-150

[4] Park CH, Valore EV, Waring AJ, Ganz T. Hepcidin, a urinary antimicrobial peptide synthesized in the liver. The Journal of Biological Chemistry. 2001;**276**(11):7806-7810. DOI: 10.1074/jbc.M008922200

[5] Nemeth E, Ganz T. Anemia of inflammation. Hematology/Oncology Clinics of North America. 2014;**28**(4):671-681. DOI: 10.1016/j.hoc.2014.04.005

[6] Fleming MD. The regulation of hepcidin and its effects on systemic and cellular iron metabolism. Hematology. American Society of Hematology Education Program. 2008:151-158. DOI: 10.1182/asheducation-2008.1.151

[7] Ganz T. Hepcidin and iron regulation, 10 years later. Blood. 2011;**117**(17):4425-4433. DOI: 10.1182 /blood-2011-01-258467

[8] Pigeon C, Ilyin G, Courselaud B, Leroyer P, Turlin B, Brissot P, et al. A new mouse liver-specific gene, encoding a protein homologous to human antimicrobial peptide hepcidin, is over-expressed during iron overload. The Journal of Biological Chemistry. 2001;**276**(11):7811-7819. DOI: 10.1074/jbc.M008923200

[9] Nicolas G, Bennoun M, Porteu A, Mativet S, Beaumont C, Grandchamp B, et al. Severe iron deficiency anemia in transgenic mice expressing liver hepcidin. Proceedings of the National Academy of Sciences of the United States of America. 2002;**99**(7):4596-4601. DOI: 10.1073/pnas.072632499

[10] Michels K, Nemeth E, Ganz T, Mehrad B. Hepcidin and host defense against infectious diseases. PLoS Pathogens. 2015;**11**(8):e1004998. DOI: 10.1371/journal.ppat.1004998

[11] Daher R, Karim Z. Iron metabolism: State of the art. Transfusion Clinique et Biologique. 2017;**24**(3):115-119. DOI: 10.1016/j.tracli.2017.06.015

[12] Papanikolaou G, Pantopoulos K. Systemic iron homeostasis and erythropoiesis. IUBMB Life. 2017;**69**(6):399-413. DOI: 10.1002/iub.1629

[13] Markova V, Norgaard A, Jørgensen KJ, Langhoff-Roos J. Treatment for women with postpartum iron deficiency anaemia. Cochrane Database of Systematic Reviews. 2015;**8**:CD010861. DOI: 10.1002/14651858

[14] Evstatiev R, Gasche C. Iron sensing and signalling. Gut. 2012;**61**(6):933-952. DOI: 10.1136/gut.2010.214312

[15] Krishnamurthy P, Xie T, Schuetz JD. The role of transporters in cellular heme and porphyrin homeostasis. Pharmacology & Therapeutics. 2007;**114**(3):345-358. DOI: 10.1016/j.pharmthera.2007.02.001

[16] Knutson MD. Iron transport proteins: Gateways of cellular and systemic iron homeostasis. The Journal of Biological Chemistry. 2017;**292**(31):12735-12743. DOI: 10.1074/jbc.R117.786632

[17] Musci G, Polticelli F, Bonaccorsi di Patti MC. Ceruloplasmin-ferroportin system of iron traffic in vertebrates. World Journal of Biological Chemistry. 2014;**5**(2):204-215. DOI: 10.4331/wjbc.v5.i2.204

[18] Harris WR. Anion binding properties of the transferrins. Implications for function. Biochimica et Biophysica Acta. 2012;**1820**(3):348-361. DOI: 10.1016/j.bbagen.2011.07.017

[19] Wang J, Pantopoulos K. Regulation of cellular iron metabolism. The Biochemical Journal. 2011;**434**(3):365-381. DOI: 10.1042/BJ20101825

[20] Vashchenko G, MacGillivray RT. Multi-copper oxidases and human iron metabolism. Nutrients. 2013;**5**(7):2289-2313. DOI: 10.3390/nu5072289

[21] Alam MZ, Devalaraja S, Haldar M. The heme connection: Linking erythrocytes and macrophage biology. Frontiers in Immunology. 2017;**8**:33. DOI: 10.3389/fimmu.2017.00033

[22] Arosio P, Levi S. Cytosolic and mitochondrial ferritins in the regulation of cellular iron homeostasis and oxidative damage. Biochimica et Biophysica Acta. 2010;**1800**(8):783-792. DOI: 10.1016/j.bbagen.2010.02.005

[23] Nemeth E, Tuttle MS, Powelson J, Vaughn MB, Donovan A, Ward DM, et al. Hepcidin regulates cellular iron efflux by binding to ferroportin and inducing its internalization. Science. 2004;**306**(5704):2090-2093. DOI: 10.1126/science.1104742

[24] Drakesmith H, Nemeth E, Ganz T. Ironing out ferroportin. Cell Metabolism. 2015;**22**(5):777-787. DOI: 10.1016/j.cmet.2015.09.006

[25] Girelli D, Nemeth E, Swinkels DW. Hepcidin in the diagnosis of iron disorders. Blood. 2016;**127**(23):2809-2813. DOI: 10.1182/blood-2015-12-639112

[26] Pak M, Lopez MA, Gabayan V, Ganz T, Rivera S. Suppression of hepcidin during anemia requires erythropoietic activity. Blood. 2006;**108**(12):3730-3735. DOI: 10.1182/blood-2006-06-028787

[27] Kautz L, Jung G, Valore EV, Rivella S, Nemeth E, Ganz T. Identification of erythroferrone as an erythroid regulator of iron metabolism. Nature Genetics. 2014;**46**(**7**):678-684. DOI: 10.1038/ng.2996

[28] Kautz L, Jung G, Du X, Gabayan V, Chapman J, Nasoff M, et al. Erythroferrone contributes to hepcidin suppression and iron overload in a mouse model of β-thalassemia. Blood. 2015;**126**(**17**):2031-2037. DOI: 10.1182/blood-2015-07-658419

[29] Reichert CO, da Cunha J, Levy D, Maselli LMF, Bydlowski SP, Spada C. Hepcidin: Homeostasis and diseases related to iron metabolism. Acta Haematologica. 2017;**137**(4): 220-236. DOI: 10.1159/000471838.

[30] Schmidt PJ. Regulation of iron metabolism by hepcidin under conditions of inflammation. The Journal of Biological Chemistry. 2015;**290**(31):18975-18983. DOI: 10.1074/jbc.R115.650150

[31] Miyazawa K, Shinozaki M, Hara T, Furuya T, Miyazono K. Two major Smad pathways in TGF-beta superfamily signalling. Genes to Cells. 2002;**7**(12):1191-1204

[32] Chen S, Feng T, Vujić Spasić M, Altamura S, Breitkopf-Heinlein K, Altenöder J, Weiss TS, et al. Transforming growth factor β1 (TGF-β1) activates Hepcidin mRNA expression in hepatocytes. The Journal of Biological Chemistry. 2016 Jun 17;**291**(25):13160-13174. DOI: 10.1074/jbc.M115.691543

[33] Babitt JL, Huang FW, Xia Y, Sidis Y, Andrews NC, Lin HY. Modulation of boné morphogenetic protein signaling in vivo regulates systemic iron balance. The Journal of Clinical Investigation. 2007;**117**(7):1933-1939. DOI: 10.1172/JCI31342

[34] Lin L, Valore EV, Nemeth E, Goodnough JB, Gabayan V, Ganz T. Iron transferrin regulates hepcidin synthesis in primary hepatocyte culture through hemojuvelin and BMP2/4. Blood. 2007;**110**(6):2182-2189. DOI: 10.1182/blood-2007-04-087593

[35] Mleczko-Sanecka K, Casanovas G, Ragab A, Breitkopf K, Müller A, Boutros M, et al. SMAD7 controls iron metabolism as a potent inhibitor of hepcidin expression. Blood. 2010;**115**(13):2657-2665. DOI: 10.1182/blood-2009-09-238105

[36] Canali S, Vecchi C, Garuti C, Montosi G, Babitt JL, Pietrangelo A. The SMAD pathway is required for hepcidin response during endoplasmic reticulum stress. Endocrinology. 2016;**157**(10):3935-3945. DOI: 10.1210/en.2016-1258

[37] Poli M, Asperti M, Ruzzenenti P, Regoni M, Arosio P. Hepcidin antagonists for potential treatments of disorders with hepcidin excess. Frontiers in Pharmacology. 2014;**5**:86. DOI: 10.3389/fphar.2014.00086

[38] Wang CY, Babitt JL. Hepcidin regulation in the anemia of inflammation. Current Opinion in Hematology. 2016;**23**(3):189-197. DOI: 10.1097/MOH.0000000000000236

[39] Canali S, Core AB, Zumbrennen-Bullough KB, Merkulova M, Wang CY, Schneyer AL, et al. Activin B induces noncanonical SMAD1/5/8 signaling via BMP type I receptors in hepatocytes: Evidence for a role in hepcidin induction by inflammation in male mice. Endocrinology. 2016;**157**(3):1146-1162. DOI: 10.1210/en.2015-1747

[40] Rawlings JS, Rosler KM, Harrison DA. The JAK/STAT signaling pathway. Journal of Cell Science. 2004;**117**(8):1281-1283. DOI: 10.1242/jcs.00963

[41] Fleming RE. Hepcidin activation during inflammation: Make it STAT. Gastroenterology. 2007;**132**(1):447-449. DOI: 10.1053/j.gastro.2006.11.049

[42] Pietrangelo A, Dierssen U, Valli L, Garuti C, Rump A, Corradini E, et al. STAT3 is required for IL-6-gp130-dependent activation of hepcidin in vivo. Gastroenterology. 2007;**132**(1):294-300. DOI: 10.1053/j.gastro.2006.10.018

[43] Bartnikas TB, Fleming MDA. Tincture of hepcidin cures all: The potential for hepcidin therapeutics. The Journal of Clinical Investigation. 2010;**120**(12):4187-4190. DOI: 10.1172/JCI45043.

[44] Cappellini MD, Comin-Colet J, de Francisco A, Dignass A, Doehner W.S.P, Lam C, et al. Iron deficiency across chronic inflammatory conditions: International expert opinion on definition, diagnosis, and management. American Journal of Hematology. 2017;**92**(10):1068-1078. DOI:10.1002/ajh.24820

[45] Hamza RT, Hamed AI, Kharshoum RR. Iron homeostasis and serum hepcidin-25 levels in obese children and adolescents: Relation to body mass index. Hormone Research in Paediatrics. 2013;**80**(1):11-17. DOI: 10.1159/000351941

[46] Stroh C, Manger T, Benedix F. Metabolic surgery and nutritional deficiencies. Minerva Chirurgica. 2017;**72**(5):432-441. DOI: 10.23736/S0026-4733.17.07408-9

[47] Moreno-Navarrete JM, Moreno M, Puig J, Blasco G, Ortega F, Xifra G, et al. Hepatic iron content is independently associated with sérum hepcidin levels in subjects with obesity. Clinical Nutrition. 2017;**36**(5):1434-1439. DOI: 10.1016/j.clnu.2016.09.022

[48] Moreno-Navarrete JM, Blasco G, Xifra G, Karczewska-Kupczewska M, Stefanowicz M, Matulewicz N, et al. Obesity is associated with gene expression and imaging markers of iron accumulation in skeletal muscle. The Journal of Clinical Endocrinology and Metabolism. 2016;**101**(3):1282-1289. DOI: 10.1210/jc.2015-3303

[49] Cheng PP, Jiao XY, Wang XH, Lin JH, Cai YM. Hepcidin expression in anemia of chronic disease and concomitant iron-deficiency anemia. Clinical and Experimental Medicine. 2011;**11**(1):33-42. DOI: 10.1007/s10238-010-0102-9

[50] D'Angelo G. Role of hepcidin in the pathophysiology and diagnosis of anemia. Blood Research. 2013;**48**(1):10-15. DOI: 10.5045/br.2013.48.1.10

[51] Fraenkel PG. Anemia of inflammation: A review. Medical Clinics of North America. 2017;**101**(2):285-296. DOI: 10.1016/j.mcna.2016.09.005

[52] Fraenkel PG. Understanding anemia of chronic disease. Hematology. American Society of Hematology. Education Program. 2015;**2015**:14-18. DOI: 10.1182/asheducation-2015.1.14

[53] Malyszko J, Mysliwiec M. Hepcidin in anemia and inflammation in chronic kidney disease. Kidney & Blood Pressure Research. 2007;**30**(1):15-30. DOI: 10.1159/000098522

[54] Mercadal L, Metzger M, Haymann JP, Thervet E, Boffa JJ, Flamant M, et al. The relation of hepcidin to iron disorders, inflammation and hemoglobin in chronic kidney disease. PLoS One. 2014;**9**(6):e99781. DOI: 10.1371/journal.pone.0099781

[55] Finberg KE, Heeney MM, Campagna DR, Aydinok Y, Pearson HA, Hartman KR, et al. Mutations in TMPRSS6 cause iron-refractory iron deficiency anemia (IRIDA). Nature Genetics. 2008;**40**(5):569-571. DOI: 10.1038/ng.130

[56] Finberg KE. Iron-refractory iron deficiency anemia. Seminars in Hematology. 2009;**46**(4): 378-386. DOI: 10.1053/j.seminhematol.2009.06.006

[57] Ramsay AJ, Hooper JD, Folgueras AR, Velasco G, López-Otín C. Matriptase-2 (TMPRSS6): A proteolytic regulator of iron homeostasis. Haematologica. 2009;**94**(6):840-849. DOI: 10.3324/haematol.2008.001867

[58] Heeney MM, Finberg KE. Iron-refractory iron deficiency anemia (IRIDA). Hematology/ Oncology Clinics of North America. 2014;**28**(4):637-652. DOI: 10.1016/j.hoc.2014.04.009

[59] Folgueras AR, de Lara FM, Pendás AM, Garabaya C, Rodríguez F, Astudillo A, et al. Membrane-bound serine protease matriptase-2 (Tmprss6) is an essential regulator of iron homeostasis. Blood 2008;**112**(6):2539-2545. DOI: 10.1182/blood-2008-04-149773

[60] De Falco L, Sanchez M, Silvestri L, Kannengiesser C, Muckenthaler MU, Iolascon A, et al. Iron refractory iron deficiency anemia. Haematologica. 2013;**98**(6):845-853. DOI: 10.3324/haematol.2012.075515

[61] Capra AP, Ferro E, Cannavò L, La Rosa MA, Zirilli G. A child with severe iron-deficiency anemia and a complex TMPRSS6 genotype. Hematology. 2017;**22**(9):559-564. DOI: 10.1080/10245332.2017.1317990

[62] Sal E, Keskin EY, Yenicesu I, Bruno M, De Falco L. Iron-refractory iron deficiency anemia (IRIDA) cases with 2 novel TMPRSS6 mutations. Pediatric Hematology and Oncology. 2016;**33**(3):226-232. DOI: 10.3109/08880018.2016.1157229

[63] Azar S, Wong TE. Sickle cell disease: A brief update. Medical Clinics of North America. 2017;**101**(2):375-393. DOI: 10.1016/j.mcna.2016.09.009

[64] Ngo D, Steinberg M. Hematology clinic. Sickle cell disease. Hematology. 2014;**19**(4):244-245. DOI: 10.1179/1024533214Z.000000000276

[65] Walter PB, Harmatz P, Vichinsky E. Iron metabolism and iron chelation in sickle cell disease. Acta Haematologica. 2009;**122**(2-3):174-183. DOI: 10.1159/000243802

[66] Kroot JJ, Laarakkers CM, Kemna EH, Biemond BJ, Swinkels DW. Regulation of serum hepcidin levels in sickle cell disease. Haematologica. 2009;**94**(6):885-887. DOI: 10.3324/haematol.2008.003152

[67] Gardenghi S, Grady RW, Rivella S. Anemia, ineffective erythropoiesis, and hepcidin: Interacting factors in abnormal iron metabolism leading to iron overload in β-thalassemia. Hematology/Oncology Clinics of North America. 2010;**24**(6):1089-1107. DOI: 10.1016/j.hoc.2010.08.003

[68] Leecharoenkiat K, Lithanatudom P, Sornjai W, Smith DR. Iron dysregulation in beta-thalassemia. Asian Pacific Journal of Tropical Medicine. 2016;**9**(11):1035-1043. DOI: 10.1016/j.apjtm.2016.07.035

[69] Schmidt PJ, Fleming MD. Modulation of hepcidin as therapy for primary and secondary iron overload disorders: Preclinical models and approaches. Hematology/Oncology Clinics of North America. 2014;**28**(2):387-401. DOI: 10.1016/j.hoc.2013.11.004

Section 5

Laboratory Approach to Anemia

Chapter 12

Laboratory Approach to Anemia

Ebru Dündar Yenilmez and Abdullah Tuli

Additional information is available at the end of the chapter

http://dx.doi.org/10.5772/intechopen.70359

Abstract

Anemia is a major cause of morbidity and mortality worldwide and can be defined as a decreased quantity of circulating red blood cells (RBCs). The epidemiological studies suggested that one-third of the world's population is affected with anemia. Anemia is not a disease, but it is instead the sign of an underlying basic pathological process. However, the sign may function as a compass in the search for the cause. Therefore, the prediagnosis revealed by thorough investigation of this sign should be supported by laboratory parameters according to the underlying pathological process. We expect that this review will provide guidance to clinicians with findings and laboratory tests that can be followed from the initial stage in the anemia search.

Keywords: anemia, complete blood count, red blood cell indices, reticulocyte

1. Introduction

Anemia, the meaning of which in Greek is "without blood," is a relatively common sign and symptom of various medical conditions. Anemia is defined as a significant decrease in the count of total erythrocyte [red blood cell (RBC)] mass, although this definition is rarely used in clinical settings. According to the World Health Organization, anemia is a condition in which the number of red blood cells (RBCs, and consequently their oxygen-carrying capacity) is insufficient to meet the body's physiologic needs [1, 2]. The individual variation such as a person's age, gender, residential elevation above sea level (altitude), and different stages of pregnancy changes the specific physiologic requirements of the body. Anemia is not a disease, but is instead the sign of an underlying basic pathological process. Nonetheless, the sign may function as a compass in the search for the cause, as well as function as a road marker in the investigation of underlying pathological process [3]. Hence, the diagnosis according to the symptoms obtained by history and physical examination of patients with anemia should be supported by laboratory parameters related to the underlying pathological cause. The first step in the diagnosis of anemia is detection with predictive, accurate tests so that important clues to underlying disease are not missed and patients are not subjected to unnecessary tests for and treatment of nonexistent anemia. Instead, clinicians rely on several other measures to identify the degree and the cause of anemia in a given patient.

The purpose of this chapter is to discuss the clinical approaches with which a practicing physician is able to evaluate a patient with underlying anemia.

2. Classification of anemia

Based on determination of the red blood cell mass, anemia can be classified as either relative or absolute. Relative anemia is characterized by a normal total red blood cell mass in an increased plasma volume, resulting in a dilution anemia, a disturbance in plasma volume regulation. However, dilution anemia is of clinical and differential diagnostic importance for the hematologist [4]. Classification of the absolute anemias with decreased red blood cell mass is difficult because the classification has to consider kinetic, morphologic, and pathophysiologic interacting criteria. Anemia of acute hemorrhage is not a diagnostic problem and is usually a genitourinary or gastrointestinal event, not a hematologic consideration.

Initially, anemias should be classified into two groups as diminished production and increased destruction of RBCs. The number of reticulocytes is a remarkable parameter in the materialization of this classification. Then, diagnostic analysis is able to be based upon both morphologic and pathophysiological hallmarks.

Anemias can morphologically be classified into three subgroups as macrocytic, normocytic, and microcytic hypochromic anemias. This classification is based on mean corpuscular volume (MCV) and mean corpuscular hemoglobin concentration (MCHC) of complete blood count (CBC) and aids the physician to the diagnosis and monitoring of anemias that can be easily cured, such as deficiency of vitamin B_{12}, folic acid, and iron.

Pathophysiologic classification is best suited for relating disease processes to potential treatment (**Figure 1**). In addition, anemia resulting from vitamin- or iron-deficiency states occurs in a significant proportion of patients with normal red blood cell indices.

Each step indicated in **Figure 1** can be disrupted and cause anemia. Identifying the affected step is important for therapeutic intervention and specific treatment. The limitation of pathophysiologic classification is that pathogenesis involves several steps in most anemias. Therefore, the provided chapter is a guideline for the practical understanding of the processes underlying the production and destruction of RBCs. Despite all these morphological classification is more useful in terms of convenience and clinical usage. Hence, morphological classification serves to support the diagnosis and indirectly treatment in connection with the laboratory and clinic. The major limitation of such a classification is that it tells nothing about the etiology or reason for the anemia [5].

http://dx.doi.org/10.5772/intechopen.70359

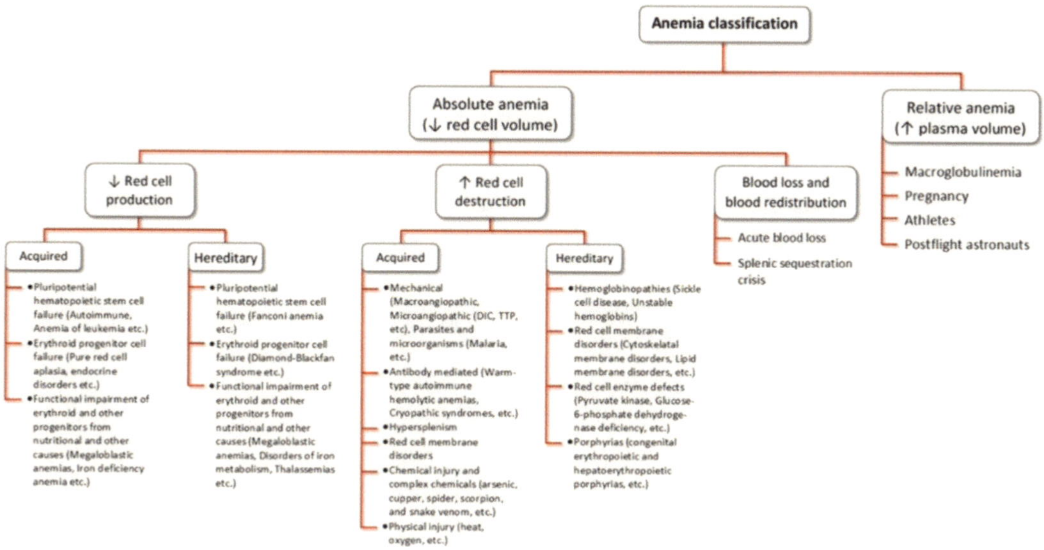

Figure 1. Classification of anemia according to pathophysiologic characteristics (figure has been modified from Ref. [4]).

3. Laboratory evaluation

A comprehensive laboratory evaluation is required for definitive diagnosis and treatment for any anemia, although the anamnesis (history of patient) and physical examination of the patient may indicate the presence of anemia and propose its cause. As appropriate to this aim, the various tests for the diagnosis of anemia are done with routine hematological tests such as CBC and reticulocyte counts as well as studies of iron status that serve as a leaping point to the diagnosis (**Figure 2**). When the diagnosis of specific anemic conditions is confirmed, a large number of other specific tests are used [6]. Laboratory tests used in the diagnosis of anemia are roughly summarized in **Figure 2**. The laboratory investigation of anemias involves the quantitative and semiquantitative measurements of RBCs and supplementary testing of blood and body fluids. The laboratory results obtained from these parameters are important arguments in the diagnosis, treatment, and monitoring of the anemias.

3.1. Complete blood count

Prior to the development of modern hematology blood analyzers, blood counts included hemoglobin (Hb) concentration, white blood cell (WBC) count, and manual platelet count. The other parameters like mean corpuscular volume (MCV) had to be mathematically calculated by using the measured parameters such as Hb, RBC count, and hematocrit (Hct). Modern analyzers provide CBC indices by using various physical and chemical methods such as electronic impedance, laser light scattering, light absorption, and staining properties [7].

How will CBC parameters such as Hb concentration, Hct, RBC count, MCV, MCHC, WBC count, platelet count, and other parameters related to formed elements of blood measured by modern blood analyzers help the diagnosis or management of the patient? CBC identifies

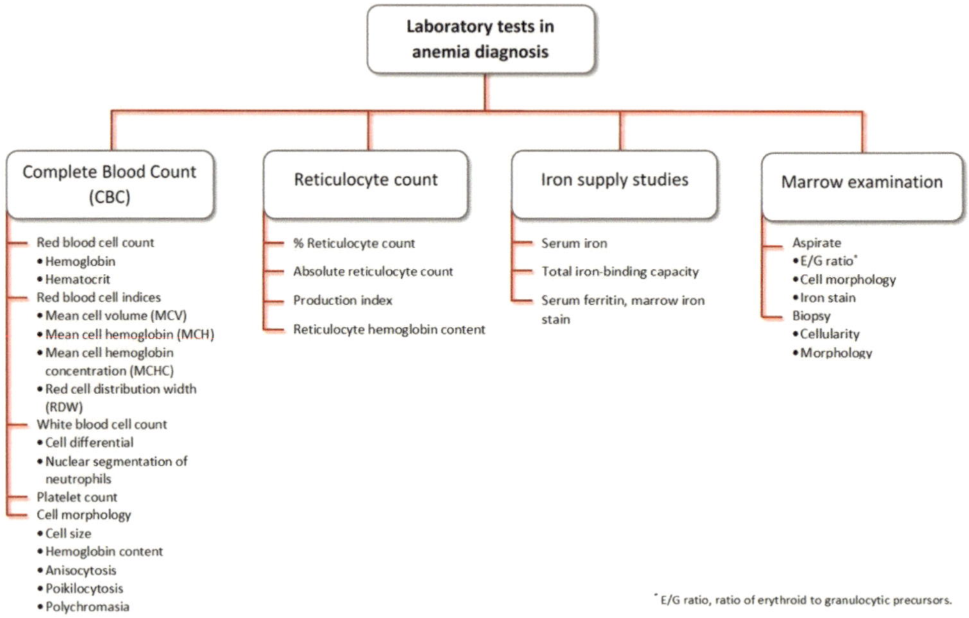

Figure 2. Laboratory tests used in anemia diagnosis (figure has been modified from Ref. [4]).

several different parameters and can provide a great deal of information. Hematologic and biochemical variations of red blood cells determine whether the patient is anemic or not. If anemia is present, MCV is likely to provide clues about the cause of anemia. While an infection can lead to increased WBC, lymphocytosis can be seen in viral infections (but not always so). Abnormal size or number of platelets may be either due to the direct effect of any underlying blood disease or may simply be the reflection of the presence of some other underlying pathologies. Because of all these, CBC parameters obtained as a result of clinical evaluation should be reassessed more carefully and curiously [7]. Therefore, the fundamental parameters of CBC such as Hb concentration, RBC, Hct, MCV, mean corpuscular hemoglobin (MCH), MCHC, and red blood cell distribution width (RDW) which plays an important role in the diagnosis, treatment, and monitoring of the anemic patient will be explained below.

3.2. Hemoglobin concentration

Determination of Hb is a part of CBC. Hemoglobin is intensely colored, and this property has been used in methods for estimating its concentration in the blood. Erythrocytes contain a mixture of hemoglobin, oxyhemoglobin, carboxyhemoglobin, methemoglobin, and minor amounts of other forms of hemoglobin [4].

Monitoring the response to treatment of anemia and to evaluate polycythemia, Hb concentration is used to screen for diseases associated with anemia and to determine the severity of anemia [6]. Finding an **increased Hb concentration** requires a systematic clinical approach for differential diagnosis and further investigation. The conditions such as polycythemia vera, congestive heart failure, chronic obstructive pulmonary disease, etc., can cause Hb levels to rise.

Decreased Hb levels are found in anemia. Hb must be evaluated along with the RBC and Hct. In iron deficiency, hemoglobinopathies, pernicious anemia, liver disease, hypothyroidism, hemorrhage (chronic or acute), hemolytic anemia (caused by transfusions, reactions to chemical or drugs, infectious and physical agents), and various systemic diseases (e.g., Hodgkin's disease, leukemia, etc.), decrease in Hb levels can be observed.

Variations in Hb levels occur after hemorrhages, transfusions, and burns (Hb and Hct are both high during and immediately after hemorrhage). Hb and Hct supply valuable information in an emergency situation [8].

Excessive fluid intake, pregnancy, and drugs, etc., which cause increase in plasma volume and decrease the Hb values, are interfering factors. Drugs such as methyldopa and extreme physical exercise can give rise to increased Hb levels. In addition, people living in high altitudes have increased Hb concentration, Hct, and RBC count [8].

3.3. Red blood cell count

The quantification of the percentage of microcytic and hypochromic RBCs has proved its clinical usefulness in the differential diagnosis of microcytic anemia [9]. RBC count has been recognized as the most efficient single classical measurement in the differential diagnosis of microcytic anemia [10]. Iron-deficient erythropoiesis is characterized by the production of RBC with a **decrease in Hb content**, so a high percentage of hypochromic cells are present.

In β-thalassemia cases, increased RBC count is a characteristic as a result of chronic increase in erythropoiesis. Therefore, MCV and MCH are lower in beta thalassemia than in iron deficiency anemia [11].

3.4. Hematocrit

The word hematocrit, also called packed cell volume (PCV), means "to separate blood," which underscores the mechanism of the test, because the plasma and blood cells are separated by centrifugation [6].

Decreased Hct values are an indicator of anemia, in which there is a reduction in the Hct. An Hct ≤30% means that the patient is severely anemic. Decreased values also occur in leukemias, lymphomas, Hodgkin's disease, adrenal insufficiency, chronic diseases, acute and chronic blood loss, and hemolytic reactions (transfusions, chemical, drug reactions, etc.).

Increased Hct values are observed in erythrocytosis, polycythemia vera, and shock (when hemoconcentration rise) [4].

Interfering factors such as pregnancy, age, sex, and dehydration have different effects in Hct. People living in high altitudes have increased Hct values and RBC count. Hct decreases in the physiologic hydremia of pregnancy. Hct varies with age and gender. Hct levels are lower in men and women older than 60 years of age. Severe dehydration from any cause falsely increases the Hct value [8, 12].

4. Red blood cell indices

The size and hemoglobin content of erythrocytes (red blood cell indices), based on population averages, have traditionally been used to assist in the differential diagnosis of anemia [13]. Some red blood cell parameters (for instance, RBC count, Hb concentration, MCV, RDW) are directly measured, while the others (e.g., Hct, MCV, MCHC) are derived from these primary measurements [14]. These measurements are provided by any of the common automated instruments. Instruments vary somewhat in their technologies. The most commonly used method is either a combination of a highly focused light source, an electric field, and a laser-based flow cytometry or a radiofrequency wave to discriminate between cells. Automated instruments are not only fast but extremely accurate. The coefficient of variation (measurement error) of an automated counter is usually less than 2%, and each of the major measurements, including the hemoglobin level, red blood cell count, and mean corpuscular volume, can be standardized independently with commercial red blood cell and hemoglobin standards [4, 6, 12].

4.1. Mean corpuscular volume (MCV)

MCV has been used to guide the diagnosis of anemia in patients, for example, testing patients with microcytic anemia for iron deficiency or thalassemia and those with macrocytic anemia for deficiency of folate or vitamin B_{12} [4, 15].

The reference value of MCV ± 2 SD is 90 ± 9 fL and generally coincides with the peak of the Gaussian distribution of RBC size. Although MCV is both accurate and highly reproducible, errors may be introduced by RBC agglutination, distortions in cell shape, the presence of very high numbers of WBCs, and sudden osmotic swelling [8]. MCV results are the basis of the classification system used to evaluate an anemia (**Table 1**, **Figure 3**).

Increased reticulocytes and marked leukocytosis can also increase MCV [8]. The mixed population of microcytes and macrocytes results in normal MCV values and is an **interfering factor** in evaluating MCV.

4.2. Mean corpuscular hemoglobin (MCH)

MCH, the amount of hemoglobin per red blood cell, increases or decreases in parallel with MCV and generally provides similar diagnostic information. Because this parameter is affected by both hypochromia and microcytosis, it is least sensitive as MCV in detecting iron deficiency states [16].

The reference value of MCH is 32 ± 2 pg. This is an excellent measure of the amount of hemoglobin in individual red blood cell. Patients with iron deficiency or thalassemia who are unable to synthesize normal amounts of hemoglobin show significant reductions in the MCH [8, 17].

An **increase of MCH** is associated with macrocytic anemia; a **decrease of MCH** is associated with microcytic anemia.

http://dx.doi.org/10.5772/intechopen.70359

Microcytic anemias (MCV 50–79 fL)	
• Disorders of iron metabolism	Iron deficiency anemia, anemia of chronic disease, congenital hypochromic-microcytic anemia with iron overload
• Disorders of porphyrin and heme synthesis	Acquired sideroblastic anemias, idiopathic refractory sideroblastic anemia
• Disorders of globin synthesis	Thalassemias, hemoglobinopathies, characterized by unstable hemoglobins
Normocytic normochromic anemia (MCV 80–98 fL)	
• Anemia with appropriate bone marrow response	Acute posthemorrhagic anemia, hemolytic anemia
• Anemia with impaired marrow response	Aplastic anemia, pure red blood cell aplasia, myelofibrosis
Macrocytic anemias (MCV 99–150 fL)	
• Cobalamin (B_{12}) deficiency	Lack of animal products, intrinsic factor deficiency, pernicious anemia, hyperthyroidism, pregnancy, enzyme deficiencies
• Folate deficiency	Lack of vegetables, celiac disease, hypothyroidism, folic acid antagonists, hemodialysis
• Unresponsive to cobalamin or folate	Metabolic inhibitors (i.e., 6-mercaptopurine), inborn errors (Lesch-Nyhan syndrome)

Table 1. Classification and possible diagnosis of anemia according to MCV in clinical use [8].

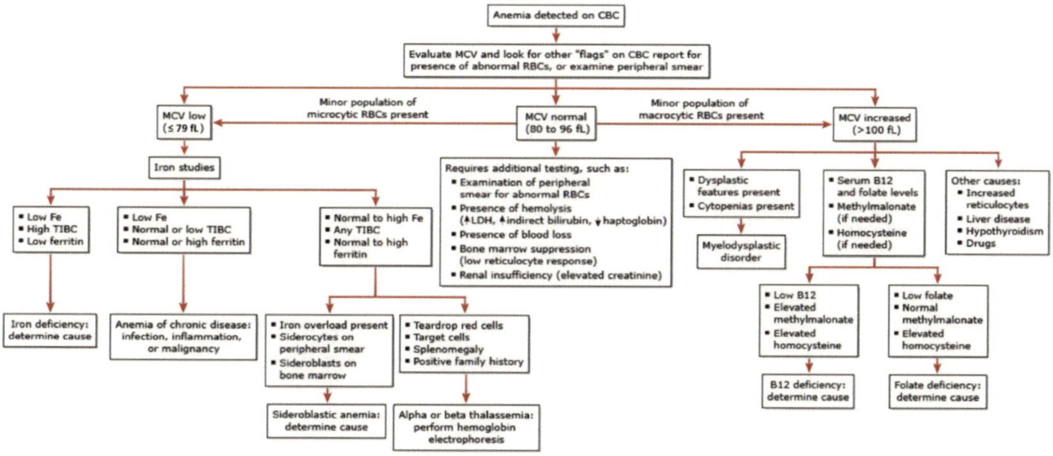

* CBC: complete blood count; MCV: mean corpuscular volume: RBCs: red blood cells; Fe: iron; TIBC: total iron-binding capacity (trasferrin); LDH: lactate dehydrogenase

Figure 3. Flowchart to follow in the diagnosis of anemia according to MCV [4].

Hyperlipidemia is one of the **interfering factors** of MCH because it falsely increases MCH values. WBC counts >50,000/mm^3 also falsely provide increased level for MCV as well as for Hb. In addition, high heparin concentrations also falsely elevate MCH value [8].

4.3. Mean corpuscular hemoglobin concentration (MCHC)

MCHC is not used frequently for diagnostic purpose, but is primarily useful for quality control purposes, such as detecting sample turbidity. Because MCHCs are average quantities in the blood with mixed-cell populations, it is difficult for these red blood cell indices to detect abnormalities in the blood [4].

The reference value of MCHC is 33 ± 3 g/dL. The principal purpose of MCHC is to detect patients with hereditary spherocytosis who has very small, dense spherocytes in the circulation. These spherocytes represent cells that have lost considerable intracellular fluid because of a membrane defect. In situations such as sideroblastic anemia, recently transfused patients, patients with severe pernicious anemia with red blood cell fragmentation, and in conditions where both folate and iron deficiency are present, both large and small red blood cells are observed, which compromise the value of MCV. When present in significant numbers, they will cause MCHC to increase to levels in excess of 36 g/dL [4, 6, 15].

Decreased MCHC indicates that packed RBCs (a unit volume) contain less Hb than normal. MCHC is decreased in hypochromic anemia (MCHC < 30 g/dL) observed in iron deficiency, microcytic anemias, chronic blood loss anemia, and some thalassemias.

Increased MCHC levels (RBCs cannot accommodate more than 37 g/dL Hb) occur in spherocytosis, in newborns and infants.

Because of falsely elevating MCHC, lipemia, cold agglutinins or rouleaux, and high heparin concentrations may be among the **interfering factors**. MCHC cannot be greater than 37 g/dL because the RBC cannot accommodate more than 37 g/dL Hb [8].

4.4. Red blood cell distribution width (RDW)

RDW is an estimate of the variance in the volume within the population of red blood cells [4]. RDW, provided by automated counters, is an index of the distribution of RBC volumes. RDW is derived from pulse height analysis and can be expressed as an SD (fL) or as a coefficient of variation (%) of the red cell volume. Automated counters use two methods to calculate RDW [6]. The first is referred to as **RDW-CV**. RDW-CV is the ratio of the width of the red blood cell distribution curve at 1 SD divided by MCV (normal RDW-CV = 13 ± 1%) (**Figure 4**). Since it is a ratio, changes in either the width of the curve or MCV will influence the result. In microcytosis, any changes in the RDW-CV simply reduce the denominator of the ratio. Conversely, in macrocytosis the change in the width of the curve will minimize the change in RDW-CV. A second method of measuring the RDW is **RDW-SD** and is independent of MCV. RDW-SD is measured by calculating the width at the 20% height level of the red blood cell size distribution histogram (normal RDW-SD = 42 ± 5 fL) [6, 8, 15].

http://dx.doi.org/10.5772/intechopen.70359

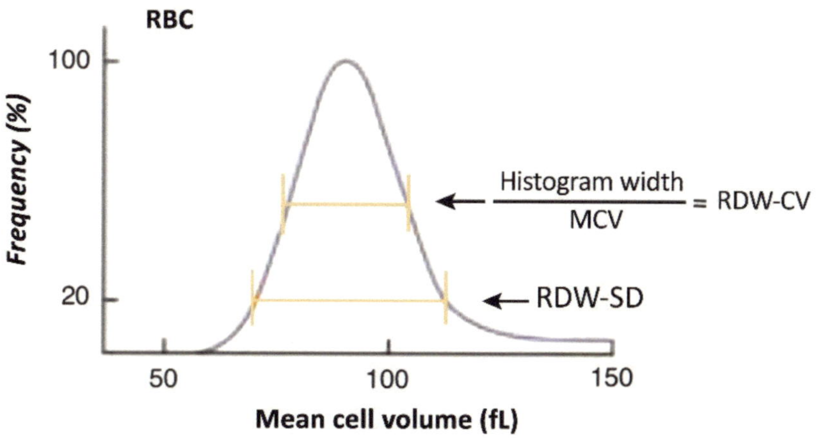

Figure 4. Red blood cell distribution width. Automated counters provide measurements of the width of the red blood cell distribution curve. RDW-CV is calculated from the width of the histogram at 1 SD from the mean divided by MCV [6].

Both measurements of RDW are essentially mathematical statement of anisocytosis. **Increases in the RDW** suggest the presence of a mixed population of cells. Double populations, whether microcytic cells mixed with normal cells or macrocytic cells mixed with normal cells, will widen the curve and increase the RDW. The RDW-SD is more sensitive to the appearance of minor populations of macrocytes or microcytes since it is measured lower on the red blood cell volume-distribution curve (**Figure 4**) [4, 8].

The RDW can be used to distinguish thalassemia (normal RDW) from iron deficiency anemia (high RDW). Also, it can be used to distinguish chronic disease anemia (normal RDW) from early iron deficiency anemia (elevated RDW). RDW increases in iron deficiency anemia, vitamin B_{12} or folate deficiency (pernicious anemia), abnormal Hb (S, S-C, or H), S-β thalassemia, immune hemolytic anemia, marked reticulocytosis, and posthemorrhagic anemia.

The RDW may be an alternate marker for systemic inflammation and/or oxidative stress; however, the predictive value of RDW is independent of other inflammatory markers. This suggests that this biomarker also follows other nonempirical processes [8, 17]. The determination of the physiological and biological mechanisms that associate RDW to adverse clinical results is important in using these prognostic biomarkers to therapeutic decisions [18].

4.5. Stained peripheral blood smear

Peripheral blood smears can provide important additional information about RBC morphology in anemia and are easily prepared manually using glass slides. The hematology laboratory usually examines a peripheral blood smear if the patient's indices are abnormal (unless there has been no major change from previous CBCs). If an underlying blood disorder is suspected, a film should be requested. Automated instruments ensure accurate RBC counts and indices and WBC counts and differentials in both healthy and diseased individuals [8, 19].

The peripheral blood smear complements the automated countermeasurements of MCV and MCH. Visible changes in cell diameter, shape, and hemoglobin content can be used to distinguish both microcytic and macrocytic cells from normocytic/normochromic RBCs (**Table 2**) [6].

In clinical cases, the variation such as staining, color, shape, and inclusion bodies in the blood smear of RBCs is not only an indication of RBC abnormalities but also a diagnosis of diseases.

4.6. Reticulocyte count

Reticulocyte count is an essential component of CBC and has a substantial role in initially classifying any anemia. Reticulocytes are newly formed red blood cells with residual strands of nuclear material called "reticulin" that remain following extrusion of the nucleus from bone marrow normoblasts [20]. The reticulocyte is a young red blood cell containing residual ribosomal RNA that can be stained with a supravital dye such as acridine orange or new methylene blue [4]. The reticulocyte count can be used in differentiation of the patients with a functionally normal marrow response to anemia/hypoxia and those with a failed marrow response. Whenever the reticulocyte production index (RPI) increases to levels greater than three times normal in response to an anemia (hematocrit <30%), it can be assumed that the patient has normal renal function with an appropriate erythropoietin response and a normal erythroid marrow with an adequate supply of key nutrients (iron, folic acid, and vitamin B_{12}) [6, 15].

The patterns of some abnormal RBCs	Comment
Macrocyte	Larger than normal (>8.5 μm diameter)
Microcyte	Smaller than normal (<7 μm diameter)
Hypochromic	Less hemoglobin in the cell. Enlarged area of central pallor
Spherocyte	Loss of central pallor, stains more densely, often microcytic. Hereditary spherocytosis and certain acquired hemolytic anemias
Target cell	Hypochromic with central "target" of hemoglobin. Liver disease, thalassemia, Hb D, and postsplenectomy
Leptocyte	Hypochromic cell with a normal diameter and decreased MCV. Thalassemia
Elliptocyte	Oval to cigar shaped. Hereditary elliptocytosis, certain anemias (particularly vitamin B_{12} and folate deficiency)
Stomatocyte	Slit-like area of central pallor in erythrocyte. Liver disease, acute alcoholism, malignancies, hereditary stomatocytosis, and artifact
Acanthocyte	Five to ten spicules of various lengths and at irregular intervals on surface of RBCs
Echinocyte	Evenly distributed spicules on surface of RBCs, usually 10–30. Uremia, peptic ulcer, gastric carcinoma, pyruvate kinase deficiency, and preparative artifact
Sickle cell	Elongated cell with pointed ends. Hb S and certain types of Hb C

Table 2. Various forms and interpretations of RBCs observed in the peripheral blood smear examination [31].

Reticulocytosis, increased RBC production, occurs when the bone marrow is replaced, is lost, or has prematurely destroyed cells. Identifying reticulocytosis is important for the recognition of other clinic conditions such as hidden chronic hemorrhage or unrecognized hemolysis (e.g., thalassemia, sickle cell anemia). Reticulocyte levels increase in hemolytic anemia, immune hemolytic anemia, primary RBC membrane problems, hemoglobinopathy, RBC enzyme deficits, and malaria.

Increased reticulocyte count after hemorrhage (3–4 days) or after treatment of anemias can be used as an index for an effective treatment. In iron deficiency anemia, reticulocytes may increase to more than 20% after sufficient doses of iron. A proportional increase in reticulocytes can also be seen when pernicious anemia is treated by transfusion or vitamin B_{12} therapy.

If there is not enough erythrocyte production in the bone marrow, the reticulocyte count decreases in untreated iron deficiency anemia and aplastic anemia, untreated pernicious anemia, anemia of chronic disease, radiation therapy, endocrine problems, tumor in the marrow (bone marrow failure), myelodysplastic syndromes, and alcoholism.

Interfering factors: Reticulocytes are normally increased in infants and during pregnancy. Recently transfused patients have a lower count because of the dilution effect. The presence of Howell-Jolly bodies falsely elevates reticulocyte count when automated methods are used.

Some other laboratory tests are useful to define the physiologic defects responsible for anemia. Indirect serum bilirubin and lactic dehydrogenase (LDH) levels increase in patients with increased hemolysis and in ineffective erythropoiesis. Indirect bilirubin levels correlate with RBC turnover rate. Serum LDH is exceedingly responsive to increased rates of RBC destruction (because of the excess levels of LDH 1 in RBCs) [8, 21].

Reticulocyte hemoglobin content (CHr or Ret-He) measurement demonstrates Hb synthesis in marrow precursors. Ret-He also reflects the early stages of iron deficiency. Ret-He is defined as an auxiliary parameter in the differential diagnosis of anemias.

5. Additional new red blood cell and reticulocyte indices

Current high-end automated cell counters measure unique properties of mature red blood cells and reticulocytes on a cell-by-cell basis, not just as population averages. This results a plethora of new indices that are in many cases specific to an instrument manufacturer, presenting diagnostic opportunities but also a confusing nomenclature and a potential lack of comparability. Some examples of parameters that have been studied include hypochromic erythrocytes (**HypoHe%**), percentage microcytic red blood cells (**MicroR%**), reticulocyte hemoglobin equivalent (**Ret-He**), reticulocyte hemoglobin content (**CHr**), red blood cell size factor (**RSf**), low hemoglobin density (**LHD%**), and fragmented red blood cells (**FRCs**) [22–24].

Ret-He demonstrates the real-time information on the synthesis of young RBCs in the bone marrow. Other available parameters are the percentage of RBCs with Hb content equivalent ≤17 pg (HypoHe%) and the percentage of RBCs with a volume of <60 fL (MicroR%), which reflects the subpopulation of mature RBCs exhibiting evidence of insufficient iron content [6, 8].

Estimates of reticulocyte-specific hemoglobin content (which are comparable) by light-scatter measurements of reticulocytes are closely related to adequacy of iron availability to erythroid precursors during the preceding 24–48 hours and have been described as diagnostically useful in detecting functional iron deficiency [8, 22].

The CHr may be a better predictor of depleted marrow iron stores than traditional serum iron parameters in nonmacrocytic patients and is a more sensitive predictor of iron deficiency than hemoglobin for screening infants and adolescents for iron deficiency [25, 26].

Schistocytes or FRC is also used as new red blood cell indices. Nevertheless only a few studies have been published on this parameter, but concerns have been expressed for false positivity in the presence of hypochromic samples. Schistocytes are elevated in thrombotic microangiopathies [1].

5.1. Marrow examination

Bone marrow examination has a special place in the cause of anemia since it is the organ of blood production [20]. The marrow examination is of greatest value in patients who fail to show an appropriate increase in the reticulocyte production index in response to anemia. A sample of the marrow can easily be obtained by needle aspirate or biopsy to evaluate overall cellularity, the ratio of erythroid to granulocytic precursors (E/G ratio), and cellular morphology. In these patients defects in erythroid precursor proliferation or maturation play a major role. Examination of any marrow aspirate should include a careful assessment for evidence of a red blood cell maturation abnormality, especially changes in cell size, nuclear morphology, and hemoglobin production. A number of anemias are characterized by distinct abnormalities in the maturation sequence and the morphology at each stage of maturation [6]. The assessment of the bone marrow is the gold standard in iron deficiency. The presence of the mineral in reticuloendothelial cells is the key to the diagnosis [20].

5.2. Tests of iron

Iron supply tests (serum iron level, transferrin iron-binding capacity, and serum ferritin level) play an important role in the initial differential diagnosis of an anemia. They are essential components to the marrow iron stain whenever a marrow aspirate is performed [8, 22, 25].

1. Serum iron levels. This is serum iron (SI) measurement which reflects an amount of iron bound to transferrin. The reference range of SI level is 50–150 μg/dL for an individual. The proliferative capacity of the erythroid marrow and its ability to synthesize hemoglobin are assessed by serum iron level [6].

2. Total iron-binding capacity (TIBC). The amount of iron which is bound to transferrin is called TIBC. Actually, it is equivalent to measuring the level of transferrin. The reference value of TIBC is 300–360 μg/dL. TIBC increases in excess of 360 μg/dL in patients with severe iron deficiency.

3. Serum ferritin level. Ferritin is a spherical protein and is used clinically to evaluate total body storage iron (body iron stores). A normal adult male has a serum ferritin level of between 50 and 150 μg/L, reflecting iron stores of 600–1000 mg. Serum ferritin levels decrease when the

iron stores are depleted. Levels below 10–15 μg/L indicate iron deficiency due to exhaustion of iron store [6].

5.3. Other measurements

For the diagnosis of specific hematopoietic disorders, there are some other laboratory tests. **Table 3** demonstrates some of the special assays for such disorders [1, 4].

The flowchart that follows is intended as a first approach for the diagnosis of anemia and is a supplement to this chapter to demonstrate how the steps might be placed in a logical order (**Figure 3**).

5.4. Evaluation and investigation of the patient with anemia according to laboratory parameters

A CBC and differential and reticulocyte counts together with stained peripheral blood smear examination should be the starting point of investigations. These confirm the clinical suspicion of anemia and direct further investigation [5].

Hypoproliferative anemias	Maturation disorders	Hemolytic anemias
*Cytometric assay of CD59/CD55 levels (paroxymal nocturnal hemoglobinuria) *Chromosomal analysis (leukemias) *Marrow aspirate/biopsy special stains • Trichrom stain, silver stain for reticulin (myelofibrosis)	*Serum vitamin B_{12} level (vitamin B_{12} deficiency) *Serum RBC folate level (folic acid deficiency) *Hb electrophoresis (abnormal hemoglobins) *Hb A_2 level-HPLC (β-thal) *Hb F level-HPLC (β-thal) RBC protoporphyrin level (iron deficiency) Brillant aresyl blue stain	*Hb electrophoresis and HPLC (hemoglobinopathies) *Coombs test (autoimmune hemolytic anemia) *Cold aglutinin titer (autoimmune hemolytic anemia) *Haptoglobin level (hemolysis) *G6PD screen (G6PD deficiency)

Table 3. Specific hematopoietic disorders and the associated laboratory tests [6].

The points to be followed in **Figure 5** (A–F) may help to begin anemia investigation:

A. Check **RBC status** of the patient.

The RBC performs some functions such as transportation of O_2 and CO_2. An increase in RBC is referred as polycythemia. Patient may have α- or β-thalassemia. Confirm abnormal hemoglobins with electrophoresis, Hb A_2 value in β-thalassemia will be >3.5%, check if there are target cells, etc. A decrease in RBC accounts for less hemoglobin. If RBC count is low, patient iron status should be checked (iron, TIBC, Sat%, ferritin, etc.).

B. If **red blood cell morphology** demonstrates schistocytes.

1. Red blood cell fragmentation can be investigated. Fragmented red blood cells (FRCs) and hemolysis occur when RBCs get stressed through partial vascular occlusions or over

abnormal vascular surfaces. "Split" RBCs, or schistocytes, are considered on peripheral blood smears under these conditions; significant quantities of lactate dehydrogenase are released into the blood from injured RBCs [4].

2. The ethnicity of the patient is important for this situation.

Check the patient for sickle cell disease (SCD). If the patient is normal for SCD, investigate iron deficiency anemia.

C. Screen for uncorrected **reticulocyte count**.

Reticulocyte count and indices: Reticulocytes are stained by supravital staining. Typical normal range is 0.5–1.5%. The count depends on total RBC count [12]. For both the pathophysiological classification of anemia and to monitor marrow response after therapeutic interventions, reticulocyte count is clinically important [11, 19].

Reticulocyte count was used in the clinical and laboratory practice for a long time due to three main factors: technical limitations in the detection of cell, the imprecision of manual microscopic method, and high coefficient of variations in counts [28, 29]. The index is the corrected value in relation to total red blood cell mass and Hb%. Increased count indicates increased red blood cell turnover. Reticulocyte count can be used as a measure of red blood cell production by correcting red blood cell count for both changes in hematocrit. The result of correction reflects the effect of erythropoietin on reticulocyte release from the marrow [6].

Obtain single correction reticulocyte count (reticulocyte index) (S):

$$S = \text{Reticulocyte count} \times (\text{Patient Hct}/0.45) \quad (1)$$

Double-corrected reticulocyte count or reticulocyte production index (RPI) is calculated by dividing the single correction reticulocyte count by the maturation index.

In situations where the reticulocyte count is elevated, other possibilities should be investigated, for example, serum haptoglobin and hemopexin, which are degraded hemoglobin-bound complexes, are impaired and can't be monitored in acute intravascular hemolysis. Unconjugated bilirubin in serum and urobilinogen in urine should be also measured. Unconjugated hyperbilirubinemia in the absence of urobilirubinogen in urine is a marker of hemolysis [12].

If reticulocyte production index (**RPI**) **is ≥3,** peripheral blood smear should be examined for abnormal morphology, and the values of bilirubin, LDH, serum-free Hb, urine Hb, urine hemosiderin, and haptoglobin should be evaluated.

If **Haptoglobin** is **>40 mg/dL**, the patient probably has/had an acute hemorrhage or is responding to hematinic. Patient should be evaluated for external or internal bleeding.

If **Haptoglobin** is **<30 mg/dL,** probably the patient has hemolytic anemia. Bilirubin is usually between 1.0 and 5.0 mg/dL. Mostly indirect bilirubin is present.

Screen for uncorrected reticulocyte count if the patient has any morphological abnormalities screen for uncorrected reticulocyte count.

Often, the etiology of a patient's anemia can be determined if the shape or size of RBCs is altered or if they include inclusion bodies (**Table 2**). *Plasmodium falciparum* malaria is suggested by the presence of more than one ring form in an RBC, and the infection produces pan-hemolysis of RBCs of all ages [30].

D. If **normocytic, heterogeneous anemia** is present.

The levels of ferritin and RBC folate/vitamin B_{12} should be examined to confirm/exclude the possible early diagnosis of iron deficiency anemia, sideroblastic or megaloblastic anemia, mixed deficiency, and myeloproliferative disorder. Serum transferrin receptor, homocysteine, and methylmalonic acid levels can be also considered.

E. Check **pyruvate kinase** and **glucose-6-phosphate dehydrogenase (G6PD)** enzyme.

In severe hemolytic anemia, spherocytosis and RBC fragmentation may be seen in the stained film. Although drug-induced hemolysis may indicate "bite cells" in the blood of patients with G6PD deficiency, this may not always be associated with G6PD deficiency because such cells are generally not found in patients with acute hemolytic conditions of chronic G6PD variants or patients with chronic hemolytic G6PD deficiency [4]. Repeat the history and physical examination for splenomegaly.

F. If **macrocytic, heterogeneous anemia** is present.

The pattern of folate or vitamin B_{12} of the patient should be checked. The homocysteine, methylmalonic acid, LDH, and indirect bilirubin values can be investigated. It is necessary to evaluate the intrinsic factor and parietal cell antibody to confirm or exclude pernicious anemia.

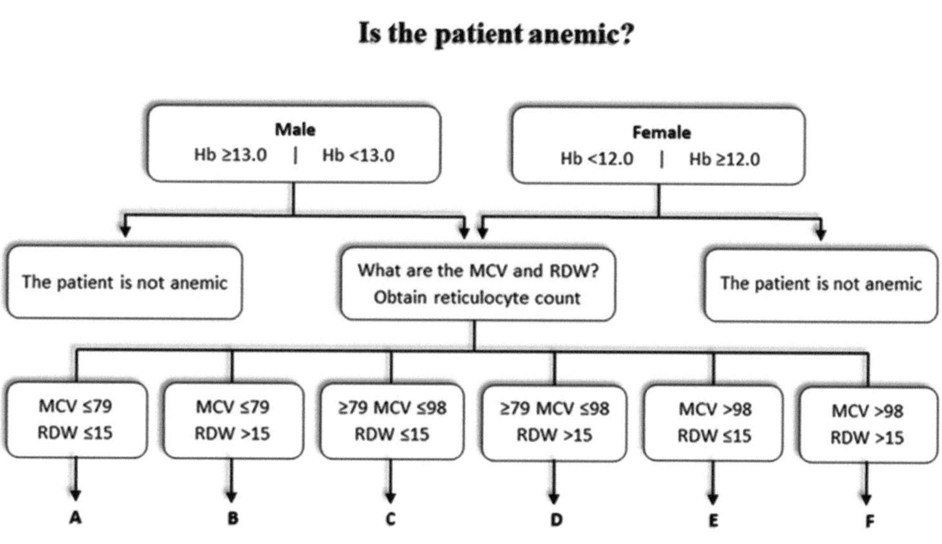

Figure 5. Flowchart as a first approach to diagnose anemia. In anemic patients, approaches should follow according to MCV and RDW because of their comprehensibility and simplicity [27].

The proper use and interpretation of laboratory tests are important in the diagnosis and treatment of anemia. Whether the patient is anemic can be determined by using Hb, Hct, or RBC count and the reference intervals for age and sex or the patient's previous values [31]. Routine examination of the blood includes CBC and examination of a stained peripheral blood smear. The values could be normal in mild anemia with RBC count in normal range [32].

6. Conclusion

There is no single optimal marker or test combination in the differential diagnosis of anemias [33]. The knowledge and experience of the physician who demands appropriate hematological and biochemical tests related to preliminary diagnosis have the important role in the diagnosis of anemias. It is recommended to use algorithms as a tool in determination of anemias in order to reduce the laboratory tests and accurately diagnose the underlying cause(s) in patients.

For the past decade, remarkable progress has been made in the procedures and algorithms in the differential diagnosis of anemias. CBC is the main procedure for investigating anemia. The percentage of microcytic RBCs is considered in the first step. In the second step, MCV, RDW, and RBC count should be examined. It is advocated that innovative algorithms, including parameters reflecting hemoglobinization of RBCs and reticulocytes, are integrated to improve the differentiation between anemias. Subsequently, new algorithms, including conventional as well as innovative hematological parameters, were assessed for subgroups with microcytic erythropoiesis. Nowadays automated reticulocyte counts provide new parameters to evaluate marrow activity [29]. It is therefore important to establish accurate and reliable criteria for both identifying the specific causes of anemia and evaluating the impact of intervention strategies. These should be followed by laboratory tests that are mandatory and simple to perform.

7. Key points of this chapter

CBC is the most sensitive measure in the routine use to obtain the information about the presence and severity of anemia.

For the evaluation of anemia, there are some essential basic laboratory tests such as CBC, reticulocyte count, blood smear morphology changes, iron balance studies, and bone marrow morphology reports.

Severity of the hematocrit/hemoglobin changes in MCV, RDW, and blood smear morphology are the first parameters to evaluate anemia. These help to define the anemia as normocytic, microcytic, or macrocytic.

Reticulocyte index defines the adequacy of the erythropoietin and red blood cell production response.

Bone marrow examination can also provide information about proliferative response and whether there is any defect in precursor maturation.

Iron studies should also be included in the investigation of anemia.

In conclusion, identification of the cause of anemia by the clinician with the support of laboratory data is an important step to diagnose, treat, and monitor the underlying pathological process.

Author details

Ebru Dündar Yenilmez* and Abdullah Tuli

*Address all correspondence to: edundar@cu.edu.tr

Department of Medical Biochemistry, Faculty of Medicine, Çukurova University, Adana, Turkey

References

[1] Brugnara C, Mohandas N. Red cell indices in classification and treatment of anemias: From M.M. Wintrobes's original 1934 classification to the third millennium. Current Opinion of Hematology. 2013;**20**(3):222-230

[2] WHO Scientific Group. Nutritional anemias. In: WHO Meeting; 13-17 March 1967; Geneva. Switzerland: WHO; 1968. pp. 1-28

[3] Bridges KP, Howard A. Principles of anemia evaluation. In: Bridges KP, Howard A, editors. Anemias and Other Cell Disorders. 1st ed. USA: The McGraw-Hill; 2008. pp. 4-18. DOI: 10.1036/0071419403

[4] Narla M. The erythrocyte. In: Kenneth K, Marshall A, Lichtman JT, Marcel L, Oliver W, Caligiuri MA, editors. Williams Hematology. 9th ed. USA: McGraw-Hill Education; 2016. pp. 461-915. DOI: 978-0-07-183301-1

[5] Alli N, Vaughan J, Patel M. Anaemia: Approach to diagnosis. South African Medical Journal. 2016;**107**(1):23-27. DOI: 10.7196/SAMJ.2017.v107i1.12148

[6] Hillman R, Ault K, Leporrier M. Red blood cell disorders. In: Hillman R, editor. Hematology in Clinical Practice. 5th ed. USA: McGraw-Hill Education; 2010. pp. 10-26. DOI: 978001766531

[7] Provan D, Singer CRJ, Baglin T, Inderjeet D. Oxford Handbook of Clinical Haematology. UK: Oxford University Press; 2009. DOI: 019922739X

[8] Fischbach FT, Dunning MB. A Manual of Laboratory and Diagnostic Tests. 8th ed. China: Wolters KluwerHealth/Lippincott W&W; 2009. 1064 p. DOI: 978-0-7817-7194-8

[9] Urrechaga E. Discriminant value of microcytic/hypochromic ratio in the differential diagnosis of microcytic anemia. Clinical Chemistry and Laboratory Medicine. 2008;**46**(12):1752-1758

[10] Urrechaga E. Red blood cell microcytosis and hypochromia in the differential diagnosis of iron deficiency and β-thalassaemia trait. International Journal of Laboratory Hematology. 2009;**31**(5):528-534

[11] Urrechaga E, Borque L, Escanero JF. Erythrocyte and reticulocyte parameters in iron deficiency and thalassemia. Journal of Clinical Laboratory Analysis. 2011;**25**(3):223-228. DOI: 10.1002/jcla.20462

[12] Mukherjee N. A Clinical Approach. In: Anemia. India: CME; 2004. pp. 358-363

[13] Wintrobe M. Anemia: Classification and treatment on the basis of differences in the average volume and hemoglobin content of red corpuscles. Archives of Internal Medicine. 1934;**54**(2):256-280

[14] Ryan DH. Clinical evaluation of the patient. In: Kaushansky K, editor. Williams Hematology. 9th ed. USA: McGraw-Hill Education; 2016. pp. 11-26. DOI: 978-0-07-183301-1

[15] Coyer SM. Anemia: Diagnosis and management. Journal of Pediatric Health Care. 2005;**19**(6): 380-385

[16] Jolobe OM. Mean corpuscular haemoglobin, referenced and resurrected. Journal of Clinical Pathology. 2011;**64**(9):833-834

[17] Wang F, Pan W, Pan S, Ge J, Wang S, Chen M. Red cell distribution width as a novel predictor of mortality in ICU patients. Annals of Medicine. 2011;**43**(1):40-46

[18] Patel A, Brett SJ. Identifying future risk from routine tests? Cricical Care Medicine. 2014;**42**(4):999-1000

[19] Buttarello M. Laboratory diagnosis of anemia: Are the old and new red cell parameters useful in classification and treatment, how? International Journal of Laboratory Hematology. 2016;**38**(S1):123-132

[20] Bridges KP, Howard A. Principles of anemia evaluation. In: Bridges KP, Howard A, editors. Anemias and Other Red Cell Disorders. 1st ed. United States of America: The McGraw-Hill Companies, Inc.; 2008. p. 374. DOI: 10.1036/0071419403

[21] Buttarello M, Plebani M. Automated blood cell counts: State of art. American Journal of Clinical Pathology. 2008;**130**(1):104-116

[22] Prchal JT. Clinical manifestations and classification of erythrocyte disorders. In: Kaushansky K, editor. Wiliams Hematology. 9th ed. United States: McGraw-Hill Education; 2016. pp. 503-511. DOI: 978-0-07-183301-1

[23] Torino ABB, Gilberti MFP, de Costa E, de Lima GAF, Grotto HZW. Evaluation of red cell and reticulocyte parameters as indicative of iron deficiency in patients with anemia of chronic disease. Revista Brasileira de Hematologia e Hemoterapia. 2014;**36**(6):424-429

[24] Chabot-Richards D, Zhang Q-Y, George TI. Automated hematology. In: Rifai N, Horvath AR, Wittwer CT, editors. Tietz Textbook of Clinical Chemistry and Molecular Diagnostics. 6th ed. St. Louis, Missouri, USA: Elsevier; 2017. p. e1734. DOI: 978032335921

[25] Mast AE, Blinder MA, Lu Q, Flax S, Dietzen DJ. Clinical utility of the reticulocyte hemoglobin content in the diagnosis of iron deficiency. Blood. 2002;**99**(4):1489-1491

[26] Ullrich C, Wu A, Armsby C, Rieber S, Wingerter S, Brugnara C, et al. Screening healthy infants for iron deficiency using reticulocyte hemoglobin content. Jama. 2005;**294**(8):924-930

[27] DeMott WR, Skikne BS. Hematology. In: Jacobs DS, Oxley DK, editors. Laboratory Test Handbook. 5th ed. USA: Lexi Comp Inc.; 2001. pp. 391-399

[28] Grotto HZW. Platelet and reticulocyte new parameters: Why and how to use them?. Revista Brasileira de Hematologia e Hemoterapia. 2016;**38**(4):283-284

[29] Cortellazzi LC, Teixeira SM, Borba R, Gervásio S, Cintra CS, Grotto HZ. Reticulocyte parameters in hemoglobinopathies and iron deficiency anemia. Revista Brasileira de Hematologia e Hemoterapia. 2003;**25**(2):97-102

[30] Medscape. Anemia Workup [Internet]. 2016 [Updated: September 24, 2016]. Available from: http://emedicine.medscape.com/article/198475-workup#showall [Accessed: April 15, 2017]

[31] McPherson RA, Pincus MR, Henry JB. Henry's Clinical Diagnosis and Management by Laboratory Methods. 22nd ed. China: Elsevier; 2011. 1513 p

[32] Baker RD, Greer FR. Diagnosis and prevention of iron deficiency and iron-deficiency anemia in infants and young children (0-3 years of age). Pediatrics. 2010;**126**(5):1040-1050

[33] Schoorl M, Linssen J, Villanueva MM, NoGuera JA, Martinez PH, et al. Efficacy of advanced discriminating algorithms for screening on iron-deficiency anemia and beta-thalassemia trait: A multicenter evaluation. American Journal of Clinical Pathology. 2012;**138**(2):300-304

Section 6

Management of Anemia by a Novel Food Product

Foods Produced with Cowpea Flour as a Strategy to Control Iron Deficiency Anemia in Children

Regilda Saraiva dos Reis Moreira-Araújo and
Amanda de Castro Amorim Serpa Brandão

Additional information is available at the end of the chapter

http://dx.doi.org/10.5772/intechopen.69892

Abstract

Cowpeas (*Vigna unguiculata* L. *Walp*) are widely distributed throughout the world, being a relatively cheap source of protein and energy, but underutilized in most countries. The World Health Organization (WHO) estimated that about 1.62 billion people are affected by anemia and that preschool children are the most affected, with a prevalence of 47.4%. Several countries have stepped up efforts to reduce iron deficiency anemia by supplementing iron, as well as universal fortification of foods with iron and other micronutrients and vitamins. Parallel to these programs, several intervention studies were carried out with the same objective, using various forms of food fortification/enrichment aimed at the control of anemia. Fortification/food enrichment has contributed to the reduction of the prevalence of anemia. The biofortification of foods, such as cowpea, produced in countries of Africa and Latin America, including Brazil, where the prevalence of anemia is high, deserves attention because can be used in the usual form of ingestion and also in the form of flour in the preparation of products for children, with greater acceptance by them, constituting a new and promising strategy to reduce the levels of iron deficiency anemia.

Keywords: cowpea, iron deficiency anemia, cowpea flour, children, enrichment, food fortified

1. Introduction

Among the various legumes, cowpea (*Vigna unguiculata* (L.) *Walp*) is present in tropical and subtropical regions, being widely distributed throughout the world. It is considered a relatively inexpensive source of protein and energy, but is still underutilized in most countries [1].

The World Health Organization (WHO) estimates a high prevalence of anemia in worldwide, with children being the most affected, especially at preschool age, leading to several injuries ranging from the reduction of physical capacity to the increase in propensity to infections and mortality [2].

In an attempt to reduce this problem, several countries have intensified actions directed to reduce this lack by iron supplementation as well as through the universal food fortification with iron and other micronutrients and vitamins [3, 4]. Cowpea tree genetic improvement programs, such as HarvestPlus, aim to obtain cultivars with high productivity, resistance to diseases, and biofortification with micronutrients, also improving the nutritional quality of the beans [5]. Concomitant to this process, studies have been carried out and enriched/fortified products have been developed in an attempt to help in the fight against iron deficiency anemia. In this sense, cowpea flour is a raw material with great potential to be used in the development of products aimed at children as a strategy to reduce and/or control iron deficiency anemia.

2. Cowpea

The cowpea (*V. unguiculata* L. *Walp*) is a legume found in several countries, from Africa to other developing and developed countries, such as the United States of America. For a large part of the population in several countries is the main source of protein, calories, dietary fiber, minerals, and vitamins [1, 6, 7]. It also has bioactive compounds, highlighting the phenolic compounds [8], which makes it potentially important for the human diet from the nutritional point of view. It is mainly consumed in the form of dry beans, and may also be eaten as a vegetable, in the form of fresh beans and pods, or in the form of flours obtained from dry beans, weighing 16.5 g (weight of 100 grains). The plant has a semipruned size, with flourishing of 40–45 days after sowing and cycle of 65–75 days after seeding [9–11]. Despite being a relatively inexpensive source of protein and energy, it is underutilized in many countries, especially the developed ones, while it has been incorporated as an important staple food of poor communities in developing countries [9].

In Brazil, it is one of the most important crops in the North and Northeast regions and in great expansion in the Midwest region of the country, which is adapted to the heat conditions and water deficiency present in these regions due to its rusticity and precocity [10, 12, 13]. Specifically in the Northeast, according to a survey by the Brazilian Institute of Geography and Statistics—IBGE, the production and the productivity yield around 258,187 t and 250 kg/ha, respectively, and the largest producing states of this region are the states of Bahia (106,653 t), Ceará (52,721 t), Maranhão (34,837 t), and Piauí (26,520 t) [14]. In this sense, the cultivation of cowpea in much of the country is held by family-based farmers; however, it has been incorporated into a production system of small, medium, and large companies, using modern technologies [15]. The growing interest in its cultivation has led to the production of several cultivars with good nutritional, culinary, and agronomic characteristic such as the Brazilian (BRS) cultivars BRS-Xiquexique, BRS-Aracê, BRS-Tumucumaque, BRS17-Gurguéia, BRS-Marataúã, among others [15, 16].

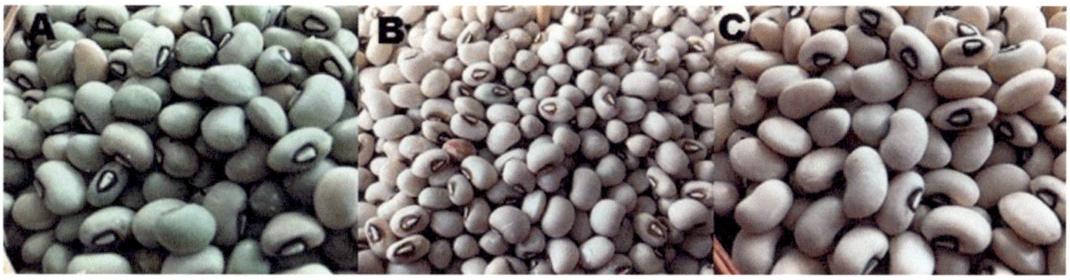

Figure 1. Cowpea cultivars: (A) BRS-Aracê, (B) BRS-Xiquexique, and (C) BRS-Tumucumaque.

The HarvestPlus program is developing genetic improvement research of various foods around the world in an attempt to counter the most varied micronutrient deficiencies. Among the researches developed are of bean (*Phaseolus vulgaris*) and the cowpea (*Vigna unguiculata*), because these are the most common legumes in Latin America and Africa (East and southern regions), regions of high prevalence of iron deficiency anemia [5]. The Food and Agricultural Organization (FAO) presents estimates of cowpea production in 35 countries. In Brazil, the Empresa Brasileira de Pesquisa Agropecuária (EMBRAPA) also develops biofortified agricultural products, one of which involves the cowpea (*V. unguiculata* (L). *Walp*), a species rich in iron (61.3 mg/kg), zinc (44.7 mg/kg), and protein (24 g/100 g), with several cultivars, among them, BRS-Aracê, BRS-Xiquexique, and BRS-Tumucumaque (**Figure 1**) [17].

In order to increase the efforts on complementary interventions to numerous nutritional deficiencies, biofortification has emerged as an option, in order to reduce the problems of deficiencies of several micronutrients, including iron, and is characterized by the increase of nutrient content in foods, through conventional breeding or genetic engineering [18, 19].

The biofortification of cowpea combined with the positive results obtained in intervention studies boosted research using cowpea flour in the development and improvement of commonly consumed products, sensorially accepted with nutritional characteristics superior to the standard formulation, such as cheese breads [20], blends containing cowpea flour for the production of fortified maize snack [21].

3. Nutritional and iron deficiency anemia

Nutritional anemia is defined as a pathological process in which the hemoglobin concentration in erythrocytes is abnormally low, with respect to the variation of age and sex, which is due to the lack of one or more essential nutrients such as iron, folic acid, and/or vitamins A, whatever the cause, with iron deficiency being the most common [22, 23]. Although different nutrients and cofactors are involved in the maintenance of normal hemoglobin synthesis, iron deficiency anemia has been the most widespread and frequent nutritional deficiency in the world, both in industrialized and developing countries, the prevalence being four times higher in the latter [23, 24].

The iron deficiency anemia, in turn, is characterized by the reduction or absence of iron reserves, low iron concentration in the serum, low transferrin saturation, low hemoglobin concentration, and hematocrit reduction. Initially, the forms of iron, ferritin, and hemosiderin, reserve decreased, with hematocrit and hemoglobin levels remaining normal. Furthermore, the serum iron level decreases and, concomitantly, the iron-binding capacity in transferrin increases, resulting in a decrease of the percentage of iron saturation in transferrin. Consequently, there is a slight decrease in red cells circulation. This stage can be called iron deficiency without anemia. The iron deficiency anemia represents the most advanced stage of hyposiderosis, characterized by the reduction of hemoglobin and hematocrit, which is reflected in changes in erythrocyte cytomorphology, presenting microcytosis and hypochromy and causing disturbance in the mechanism of oxygen transport, leading to inadequate supply of iron to the tissues and possible functional damage to the organism [24–26].

The World Health Organization (WHO), in a global analysis of anemia, estimated that about 1.62 billion people are affected by this condition across the world and that the preschool age children are most affected, with prevalence of 47.4% [2].

Some of the most varied injuries triggered by the installation of anemia in the infant population are the deficit of cognitive development, the reduction of physical capacity, the commitment of the work activity, the physical and psychomotor development retardation, depression of the immune system with a greater propensity to infections, and increased mortality [27]. These negative implications lead to severe damage in school performance, which means that this deficiency is considered a major public health problem in both developing and developed countries. Its consequences affect not only the population health but also the social and economic development of the world [2, 28, 29].

A serious and frequent problem in childhood anemia is the fact that many children are born to mothers who have iron deficiency anemia and therefore start in life with iron deficiency. This congenital iron deficiency can be further aggravated by nutritional insufficiency both qualitatively and quantitatively, further exacerbating the problem [30].

The highest susceptibility of anemia in children occurs at the preschool age, especially in children 24 months of age, strengthening the hypothesis that the disease is significantly more prevalent in younger children. This greater vulnerability can be attributed to the accelerated growth accompanied by a consequent increase in iron requirements in the first year of life. Low iron reserve at birth can also be an important factor in the onset of anemia, since the intrauterine mineral storage and exclusive maternal breastfeeding ensure that the needs of the infant are met only until the first 6 years of life [31].

Table 1 shows the studies performed in the period from 2014 to 2016 by different authors in the international scope that evaluated the prevalence of anemia in children. The results show that the prevalence of anemia is moderate to severe in several countries, including in Europe. This study was carried out in 19 European countries, highlighting the importance of interventions for the control, as it is a serious public health problem.

In Brazil, there is no national survey of prevalence of anemia; there are only studies in different regions of the country, showing a high notoriety, being considered an important public health problem, since it is not restricted to poor malnourished populations [39]. **Table 2** shows the prevalence of anemia in children from 2010 to 2016 in Brazil, according to different authors.

Location	Sample number/age	Anemia (%)	Year	References
Ghana	2168/<5 years	78.4	2014	[32]
China	1290/6–23 months	49.5	2015	[33]
Peru	1372/<5 years		2015	[34]
	Indigenous	51.3		
	No indigenous	40.9		
Armenia	729/0–59 months	32.4	2015	[35]
Europe	7297/6–12 months	2–25	2015	[36]
	12–36 months	3–48		
Brazil	1210/2–6 years	26.3	2016	[37]
United States	1437/1–5 years	1.1	2016	[38]

Table 1. Prevalence of anemia in children in studies published between 2014 and 2016.

Region	Anemia (%)	Year	References
North	57.3	2011	[40]
North	30.6	2011	[41]
North	13.6	2012	[42]
North	51.8	2012	[43]
Northeast	92.4	2010	[44]
Northeast	32.8	2011	[45]
Northeast	36.5	2012	[46]
Northeast	35.0	2013	[47]
Northeast	36.0	2014	[48]
Northeast	26.3	2016	[37]
South	63.7 (12–16 months) 38.1 (3–4 years)	2010	[49]
South	29.7	2011	[50]
South	58.5	2011	[51]
Southeast	26.0	2011	[52]
Southeast	30.8	2012	[53]

Table 2. Prevalence of anemia in children by region of Brazil, studies published between 2010 and 2016.

4. Strategies for control of anemia

According to Stevens et al. [54], world awareness about anemia and its consequences for the health and development of women and children has increased in recent decades. In 2012, the 65th World Health Assembly adopted a plan of action and strategies for mothers and children with the goal of halving the prevalence of anemia in reproductive age until 2025, from 2011 levels, thus increasing attention to nutritional intervention initiatives [54].

Among the measures for the prevention and control of iron deficiency anemia, several countries have intensified actions directed to reduce this lack by iron supplementation as well as through the universal food fortification with iron and other micronutrients and vitamins [3, 4]. The most frequently used target vehicles for fortification are cereals [4]. In this sense, as other countries, Brazil instituted the universal mandatory fortification of wheat and maize flour with iron and folic acid in the last decade [55]. In parallel to these programs, several intervention studies have also been carried out in order to contribute to the control of this deficiency, through the development of interventional researches that use various forms of food fortification/enrichment aiming the anemia control.

The iron supplementation, according to WHO guidelines for direct daily iron supplementation, it should be considered a first-line intervention in high-risk or high-prevalence groups. In endemic regions, the empirical administration of anthelmintic medications may also be justified [2]. However, studies highlight the low adherence to supplementation with iron salts. Even when the supplements are available, and mothers are instructed to supplement their children, they often do not administer the correct dosage and long enough to get benefits in hemoglobin levels due to side effects such as diarrhea, cramps, among others [56, 57].

As a successful example of this type of intervention, we have the intervention performed by Moreira-Araújo et al. [58], who performed a nutritional intervention with a snack developed with chickpea, bovine lung, and corn, rich in iron for 60 days, three times a week, to control anemia in preschool children, decreasing the prevalence of anemia from 61.5 to 11.5% [58]. Other studies used iron-fortified cowpea in the interventions. Adom et al. [59] investigated the effect of iron-fortified maize-cowpea blend (ferrous fumarate added) in controlling iron deficiency anemia in Ghana's high-risk population. Fifty-six children aged 6–18 months were randomly assigned (i) iron-fortified food or (ii) noniron-fortified food, fed daily for 6 months. Significant differences were observed in hemoglobin concentration (1.08 ± 1.43 compared with 0.40 ± 1.72 g/dL, $p = 0.0009$), and the risk of developing anemia was about three times less likely among this group compared to the nonfortified group [59]. Another study conducted in Ghana with children aged 5–12 years with cowpea meal fortified with iron (NaFeEDTA) and nonfortified cowpea showed a reduction of 30 and 47% in the prevalence of iron deficiency and iron deficiency anemia, respectively, with the use cowpea meal fortified with iron (NaFeEDTA) indicating that when used for targeted school-based interventions, fortification of cowpea flour is effective in improving iron status and consequently reducing the prevalence of iron deficiency anemia [60].

On the other hand, Paganini et al. [61] warn of the risks of fortification of complementary foods at home by adding micronutrient powders, widely used in African countries. It also shows that, in controlled studies, these micronutrient powders containing iron significantly increase the risk of diarrhea in infants, with an increase in the number of hospitalization. These foods decrease the number of beneficial intestinal bacteria, increasing the ratio of enterobacteria to bifidobacteria, contributing to an increase in the number of opportunistic pathogens and inducing intestinal inflammation in school-age children [61].

5. Product development with cowpea flour with potential to be used in interventions in children

The development of foods enriched/fortified has great importance not only for the food industry but also to raise the quality of food and nutrition of the population, since it is possible to create new products or improve existing ones with balanced compositions in relation to some nutrients, thus improving the nutritional value of various foods available in the market. Many of these products have been developed using unconventional raw materials selected to produce naturally enriched foods which are a means of substantially improve their nutritional quality [62]. Often these raw materials are not included in consumers' habits and can contribute to improve the intake of important nutrients that are not usually found in conventional foods [58, 63, 64]. Flour production has been outstanding for this purpose, as they are rich in starch and mineral salts and present great variability for the food industry, especially in bakery products, dietetic products, and baby foods [65]. In this sense, studies have been carried out using cowpea bean flour (**Figure 2**).

In 2010, Frota et al. [66] have developed a work whose objective was to enrich bakery products, such as cookie and *rocambole roulade* with cowpea flour, to evaluate their acceptance and chemical composition, including the mineral content (iron, zinc, magnesium, potassium, and phosphorus) and vitamins (thiamine and pyridoxine). For this, three cookie formulations containing 10, 20, and 30% of cowpea flour and two *rocambole* formulations containing 10 and 20% of the flour were developed. It was observed an increase in the protein content of the cookie with 30% and of the *rocambole* with 20% of cowpea flour and the amount of

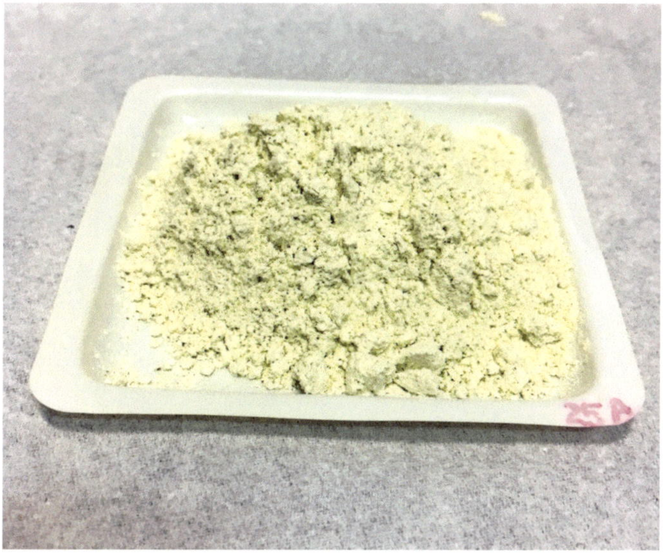

Figure 2. Cowpea flour.

ashes of the cookies with 20 and 30% and rocambole with 20% of cowpea flour, when compared to the standard formulations. The content of the analyzed minerals and pyridoxine has increased as the cowpea flour was added, while the thiamine concentration increased only in the *rocambole* with 20% of the flour. The cookie with 10% of cowpea flour was the most sensorially accepted (84.4%) by means of the nine-point Hedonic scale sensory test, ranging from 1 "extremely disliked" to 9 "extremely liked," among the cookies formulated with the flour, in addition, the rocambole with 10 and 20% of the flour had good acceptance (86.7 and 77.8%, respectively). Thus, all formulations containing cowpea flour had scores higher than 6, showing that the products were sensorially accepted. Thereby, the study showed that the addition of cowpea flour improved the nutritive value of cereal-based formulations and that this practice is feasible [66].

Cavalcante et al. [20] developed a cheese bread enriched with whole grain biofortified cowpea flour and evaluated their acceptance and chemical composition (**Figure 3A**). For this, two formulations of cheese bread, F1 and F2, containing 5.6 and 8% of cowpea flour in substitution of flour, respectively. To check the acceptance, three sensorial tests (Hedonic scale, purchase intention, and matched comparison) were used, and F1 was sensorially viable, according to the assessors, being chemically analyzed. The addition of cowpea increased the levels of copper, iron, phosphorus, magnesium, manganese, and zinc, as well as the levels related to proteins and carbohydrates. On the other hand, the moisture contents, lipids, and total caloric content decreased when compared to the standard formulation. Therefore, it was concluded that cowpea, a raw material in evidence in the national market, presents itself as an option for the enrichment of gluten-free bakery foods, such as cheese bread, including improving the technological quality of this product in relation to the growth and expansion of the mass, providing a better texture, due to its chemical composition [20]. Shakpo and Osundahunsi

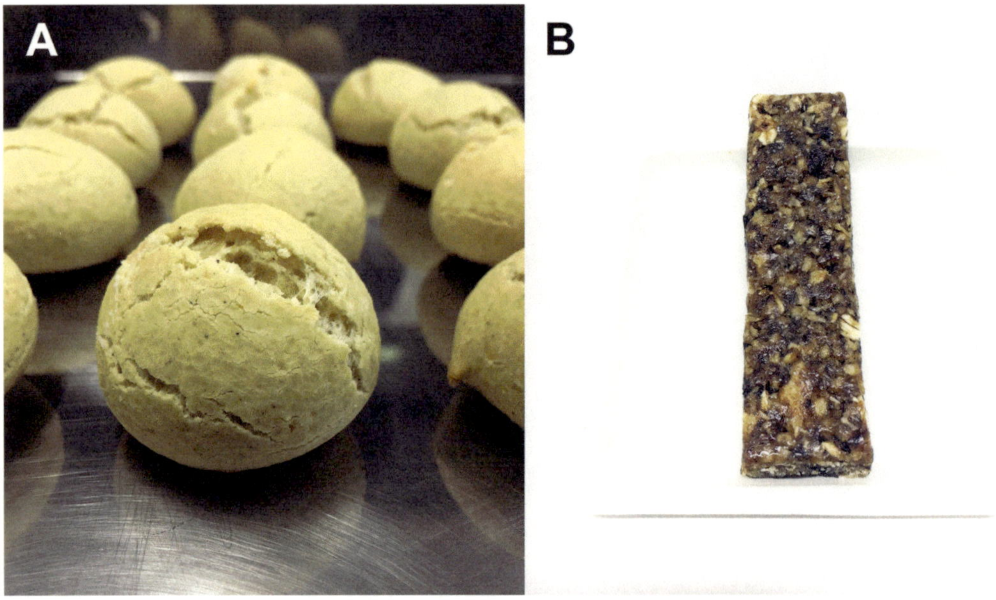

Figure 3. (A) Cheese bread and (B) cereal bar enriched with cowpea flour.

[21] studied the effect of the addition of cowpea on corn flour. Flour mixtures were produced from corn and cowpea flours in the following proportions of corn:cowpea 90:10, 80:20, 70:30, and 100% corn as a control, and the overall result showed that 20% of cowpea substitution was the most adequate percentage to produce a mixture of nutritious and acceptable corn and cowpea flour, which can be useful for pastry and confectionery [21].

Other products fortified with cowpea have been developed, such as cereal bars in technological innovation projects. A patent application filing of a cereal bar enriched with cowpea, cashew fiber, honey, and cashew nuts was made, registration number: BR1020140169873 [67] and a cereal bar enriched with cowpea flour (**Figure 3B**), registration number: BR1020140169792 [68]. These products were accepted by more than 90% of the sensory assessors, which attributed grades between 8 (I really liked) and 9 (I liked very much), demonstrating the potential of acceptance of the products for nutritional interventions in population, both adults and children, to control endemic deficiencies such as iron deficiency anemia.

6. Nutritional interventions with cowpea flour to control iron deficiency anemia

Most studies with nutritional interventions using cowpea flour to control iron deficiency anemia were developed with cowpea fortified with elemental iron, as in the studies of Adom et al. and Abizari et al. [59, 60], but satisfactory results were also obtained with the use of cowpea flour without addition of elemental iron in the control of anemia in children. This can be observed in this same study carried out by Abizari et al. [60], in which an intervention was performed with cowpea meal fortified with iron (NaFeEDTA) and nonfortified cowpea (control group), and it was observed that the group that ingested nonfortified cowpea flour also presented reduction in the prevalence of anemia, iron deficiency, and iron deficiency anemia at the end of the study, showing that the use of cowpea flour alone may be a good strategy in the control of this endemic disease.

In Brazil, Landim et al. [69] conducted an intervention study with 262 preschool children aged 2–5 years attended at municipal Childhood Educational Centers in Teresina, Piauí. One group received cookies prepared with wheat flour fortified with iron and folic acid. The other group received cookies prepared with cowpea flour biofortified with iron and zinc in addition to wheat flour enriched with iron and folic acid (**Figure 4A** and **B**) and noted that both cookies reduced the prevalence of anemia with a larger reduction in the latter group. In addition, a higher increase in hemoglobin levels (12.4–14.7) was observed in the group receiving the cookie prepared with cowpea flour fortified with iron and zinc ($p = 0.003$), whereas the group that received cookies prepared with wheat flour fortified with iron and folic acid showed hemoglobin levels of 12.6 and 12.7 ($p = 0.0754$) before and after the intervention, respectively. The study showed that the use of cookie based on cowpea flour of the biofortified BRS Xiquexique cultivar, as a nutritional intervention proposal, is a viable option because it contains a low cost ingredient, from the habit of the population and that resulted in a product with adequate composition and acceptance by the studied population [69].

The high prevalence of anemia worldwide has warned government institutions and researchers to develop several research studies in an attempt to reduce the numbers and damage, especially

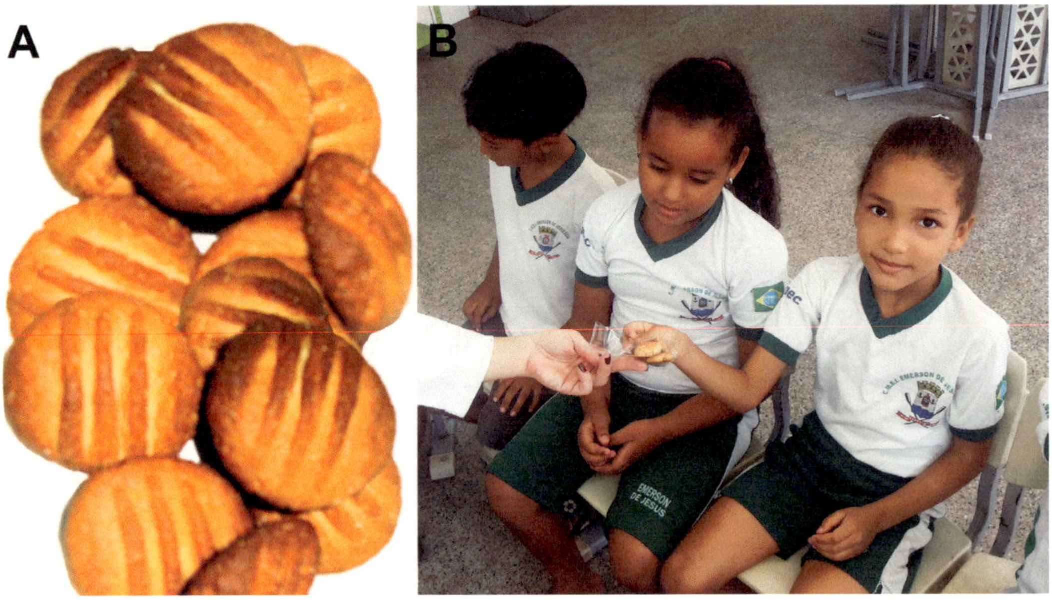

Figure 4. Cookie enriched with cowpea flour of the biofortified BRS Xiquexique cultivar and intervention with preschool children.

to the most vulnerable groups such as children. Drug supplementation has been shown to be effective, but still presents a considerable degree of resistance to the use by children and mothers. Food fortification/enrichment is routinely practiced in several countries and has contributed to reduce the prevalence of anemia, but the biofortification of food as the cowpea, which is produced in countries in Africa and Latin America, including Brazil, where the prevalence of anemia is high, deserves attention because it can be used in the usual form of ingestion (in the form of grains), can be used in the form of flour in the preparation of products for children, with greater acceptance by them, constituting a new and promising strategy to reduce the levels of iron deficiency anemia.

Cowpea is a food that can assist to reduce nutritional endemics, such as iron deficiency anemia, and also improve the quality of the population's diet. It can be used as a raw material in formulations such as snacks, cereal bars, cookies, pizza dough, and various bakery products, in addition to its use in the traditional may as a cooked legume, because it contains nutrients such as proteins, minerals, vitamins, and bioactive compounds.

Author details

Regilda Saraiva dos Reis Moreira-Araújo[1*] and Amanda de Castro Amorim Serpa Brandão[2]

*Address all correspondence to: regilda@ufpi.edu.br

1 Department of Nutrition, Federal University of Piauí, Teresina, Piauí, Brazil

2 Postgraduate Program in Food and Nutrition (PPGAN), Federal University of Piauí, Teresina, Piauí, Brazil

References

[1] Phillips RD, McWatters KH, Chinnan MS, Hung, Y, Beuchat LR, Sefa-dedeh S, Sakiy-Dawson E, Ngoddoy P, Nnanyelugo D, Enwere J, Komey NS, Liu K, Mensa-Wilmot Y, Nnanna IA, Okeke C, Prinnyawiwatkul W, Saalia FK. Utilization of cowpeas for human food. Field Crops Research. 2003;**82**(2-3):193

[2] World Health Organization, Centers for Disease Control and Prevention. Worldwide prevalence of anaemia 1993-2005: WHO global database on anaemia. Geneva: WHO, 2008. Available from http://whqlibdoc.who.int/publications/2008/9789241596657_eng.pdf

[3] Najafi TF, Roudsari RL, Hejazi M. Iron supplementation protocols for iron deficiency anemia: A comparative review of iron regimens in Three Countries of India, Iran and England. Journal of Midwifery and Reproductive Health. 2013;**1**(2):89. DOI: 10.22038/jmrh.2013.2088

[4] World Health Organization, Food and Agricultural Organization of the United Nations. Guidelines on Food Fortification with Micronutrients. Geneva: World Health Organization; 2006

[5] HarvestPlus. Biofortification Progress Briefs. Washington DC: Harvest; 2014. p. 82

[6] Singh BB, Ajeigbe HA, Tarawali SA, Fernandez-Rivera S, Abubakar M. Improving the production and utilization of cowpea as food and fodder. Field Crops Research. 2003;**84**(1-2):169-177

[7] Carvalho AFU, Sousa NM, Farias DF, Rocha-Bezerra LCB, Silva RMP, Viana MP, Gouveia ST, Sampaio SS, Sousa MB, Lima GPG, Morais SM, Barros CC, Filho FRF. Nutritional ranking of 30 Brazilian genotypes of cowpeas including determination of antioxidant capacity and vitamins. Journal of Food Composition and Analysis. 2012;**26**(1-2):81

[8] Moreira-Araújo RSR, Sampaio GR, Soares RAM, Araújo MAM, Arêas JAG. Identificação e Quantificação de Compostos Fenólicos no Feijão-caupi, cultivar BRS XiqueXique. Revista Caatinga. 2017

[9] Prinyawiwatkul W, McWatters KH, Beuchat LR, Phillips RD, Uebersak MA. Cowpea flour: A potential ingredient in food products. Critical Reviews in Food Science and Nutrition. 1996;**36**(5):413-416

[10] EMBRAPA Meio-Norte. Cultivares de feijão-caupi ricas em ferro e zinco. 2010. Available from: http://www.alice.cnptia.embrapa.br [Accessed: 2017/02/12]

[11] EMBRAPA Meio-Norte. BRS-Guaribas, BRS-Nova Era e BRS-Xiquexique-Novas Cultivares de Feijão-caupi para o Amazonas. 2009. Available from: http://www.alice.cnptia.embrapa.br/r [Accessed: 2017/02/12]

[12] Dantas JP, Marinho FJL, Ferreira MMM, Amorim MSN, Andrade SIO, Sales AL. Avaliação de genótipos de caupi sob sanilidade. Revista Brasileira de Engenharia Agrícola e Ambiental. 2002;**6**(3):425

[13] EMBRAPA Meio-Norte. Cultivo de feijão-caupi. Teresina, 2003

[14] BRASIL. Ministério do Planejamento, Orçamento e Gestão. Instituto Brasileiro de Geografia e Estatística – IBGE. Levantamento Sistemático da Produção Agrícola. Rio de Janeiro: IBGE. 2013;**26**(8)

[15] EMBRAPA Meio-Norte. BRS-Xiquexique: Cultivar de feijão-caupi rica em ferro e zinco para cultivo em Roraima. Comunicado Técnico. 2008

[16] Moura JO. Potencial de populações segregantes de feijão-caupi para biofortificação de grãos [Thesis]. Teresina: Universidade Federal do Piauí; 2011

[17] Freire-filho FR, Ribeiro VQ, Rocha MM, Silva KJD, Nogueira MSR, Rodrigues EV. Production, Breeding and Potential of Cowpea Crop in Brazil. Embrapa Mid-North. 2012

[18] Pfeiffer WH, Mcclafferty B. HarvestPlus: Breeding crops for better nutrition. Crop Science. 2007;**47**:S88-S105

[19] Rios AS, Alves KR, Costa NMB, Martino HSD. Biofortificação: culturas enriquecidas com micronutrientes pelo melhoramento genético. Revista Ceres. 2009;**56**(6):713-718

[20] Cavalcante RBM, Morgano MA, Silva KJD, Rocha MM, Araújo MAM, Moreira-Araújo RS. Cheese bread enriched with biofortified cowpea flour. Ciênc Agrotec. 2016;**40**(1):97-103

[21] Shakpo IO, Osundahunsi OF. Effect of cowpea enrichment on the physico-chemical, mineral and microbiological properties of maize: Cowpea flour blends. Research Journal of Food Science and Nutrition. 2016;**1**:35-41

[22] Cappellini MD, Motta I. Anemia in clinical practice-definition and classification: Does hemoglobin change with aging? Seminars in Hematology. 2015;**52**(4):161-169

[23] World Health Organization. Leaning from Large-scale Community-Based Programmes to Improve Breastfeeding Practices. Geneva: World Health Organization, United Nations Children's Fund/UNICEF, Academy for Educational Development/EAD; 2008

[24] Capanema FD, Lamounier JA, Norton RC, Jacome AAA, Rodrigues DA, Coutinho RL. Anemia ferropriva na infância: novas estratégias de prevenção, intervenção e tratamento. Revista de Medica de Minas Gerais. 2003;**13**(4):30-34

[25] Lopez A, Cacoub P, Macdougall I, Peyrin-Biroulet L. Iron deficiency anaemia. Lancet. 2016;**387**:907-916

[26] Camaschella C. Iron-deficiency anemia. New England Journal of Medicine. 2015;**372**: 1832-1843

[27] World Health Organization. Iron Deficiency Anaemia: Assessment, Prevention and Control: A Guide for Programme Managers. Geneva: World Health Organization; 2001. p. 114

[28] Silva FCD, Vitalle MSS, Quaglia EC, Braga JAP, Medeiros HGR. Anemia proportion according to pubertal stage using two diagnostic criteria. The Revista de Nutrição. 2007;**20**(3):297-306. DOI: 10.1007/s11046-011-9473-z

[29] Ribeiro LC, Sigulem DM. Treatment of iron deficiency anemia with iron bis-glycinate chelate and growth of young children. The Revista de Nutrição. 2008;**1**(5):483-490. DOI: 10.1590/S1415-52732008000500001

[30] Milman N. Anaemia—still a major health problem in many parts of the world! Annals of Hematology. 2011;**90**(4):369-377

[31] Braga JAP, Vitalle MSS. Deficiência de ferro na criança. Revista Brasileira Hematologia e Hemoterapia. 2010;**32**(2):38-44

[32] Ewusie JE, Ahiadeke C, Beyene J, Hamid JS. Prevalence of anemia among under-5 children in the Ghanaian population: Estimates from the Ghana demographic and health survey. BMC Public Health. 2014;**14**:626. DOI: 10.1186/1471-2458-14-626

[33] Huo J, Sun J, Fang Z, Chang S, Zhao L, Fu P, et al. Effect of home-based complementary food fortification on prevalence of anemia among infants and young children aged 6 to 23 months in poor rural regions of China. Food and Nutrition Bulletin. 2015;**36**:405-414

[34] Calderón TA, Martin H, Volpicelli K, Diaz C, Gozzer E, Buttenheim AM. Formative evaluation of a proposed mHealth program for childhood illness management in a resource-limited setting in Peru. Revista Panamericana de Salud Pública. 2015;**38**(2):144-151

[35] Demirchyan A, Petrosyan V, Sargsyan V, Hekimian K. Prevalence and determinants of anaemia among children aged 0-59 months in a rural region of Armenia: A case-control study. Public Health Nutrition. 2016;**19**:1260-1269

[36] Eussen S, Alles M, Uijterschout L, Brus F, van der Horst-Graat J. Iron intake and status of children aged 6-36 months in Europe: A systematic review. Annals of Nutrition and Metabolism. 2015;**66**:80-92

[37] Costa FV. Diagnóstico nutricional de pré-escolaresno município de Teresina [Thesis]. Teresina: Universidade Federal do Piauí; 2016

[38] Côrtes MH, Vasconcelos IAL, Coitinho DC. Prevalence of iron-deficiency anemia in Brazilian pregnant women: A review of the last 40 years. The Revista de Nutrição. 2009;**22**(3):409-418

[39] Oliveira CSM, Cardoso MA, Araújo TS, Muniz PT. Anemia em crianças de 6 a 59 meses e fatores associados no município de Jordão, Estado do Acre, Brasil. Caderno de Saúde Pública. 2011;**27**(5):1008-1020

[40] Castro TG, Silva-Nunes M, Conde WL, Muniz PT, Cardoso MA. Anemia e deficiência de ferro em pré-escolares da Amazônia Ocidental: Prevalência e fatores associados. Caderno de Saúde Pública. 2011;**27**(1):131-142

[41] Cardoso MA, Scopel KK, Muniz PT, Villamor E, Ferreira MU. Underlying factors associated with anemia in Amazonian children: A population-based, cross-sectional study. PLoS ONE. 2012;**7**(5):e3634

[42] Souza OF, Macedo LF, Oliveira CSM, Araujo TS, Muniz PT. Prevalence and Associated Factors to Anaemia in Children. Journal of Human Growth and Development. 2012;**22**(3):307-313

[43] Carvalho AGC, Lira PIC, Barros MFA, Aléssio MLM, Lima MC, Carbonneau MA et al. Diagnosis of iron deficiency anemia in children of Northeast Brazil. Revista de Saúde Pública. 2010;**44**(3):513-519

[44] Leal LP, Batista-Filho M, Lira PIC, Figueroa JN, Osório MM. Prevalência da anemia e fatores associados em crianças de seis a 59 meses de Pernambuco. Revista de Saúde Pública. 2011;**45**(3):457-466

[45] Gondim SSR, Diniz AS, Souto RA, Bezerra GRS, Albuquerque EC, Paiva AA. Magnitude, tendência temporal e fatores associados à anemia em crianças do Estado da Paraíba. Revista de Saúde Pública. 2012;**46**(4):649-656

[46] Paula WKAS, Caminha MFC, Figueirôa JN, Batista Filho M. Anemia e deficiência de vitamina A em crianças menores de cinco anos assistidas pela Estratégia Saúde da Família no Estado de Pernambuco, Brasil. Ciênc. saúde coletiva. 2014;**19**(4):1209-1222

[47] Pessoa MLSB. Anemia Ferropriva, Antropometria e Consumo Alimentar em Pré-Escolares do Município de Teresina [Thesis]. Teresina: Universidade Federal do Piauí; 2014.

[48] Bortolini GA, Vitolo MR. Importância das práticas alimentares no primeiro ano de vida na prevenção da deficiência de ferro. Revista de Nutrição. 2010;**23**(6):1051-1062

[49] Bortolini GA, Vitolo MR. Relationship between iron deficiency and anemia in children younger than 4 years. Journal of Pediatrics. 2010;**86**(6):488-492

[50] Rodrigues VC, Mendes BD, Gozz A, Sandrini F, Santana RG. Deficiência de ferro, prevalência de anemia e fatores associados em crianças de creches públicas do oeste do Paraná, Brasil. Revista de Nutrição. 2011;**24**(3):407-420

[51] Silva EB, Villani MS, Jahn AC, Coco M. Prevalência da anemia em crianças avaliada pela palidez palmar e exame laboratorial: Implicações para enfermagem. Esc. Anna Nery. 2011;**5**(3):497-506

[52] Netto MP, Rocha DS, Franceschini SCC, Lamounier JA. Fatores associados à anemia em lactentes nascidos a termo e sem baixo peso. Revista da Associação Médica Brasileira. 2011;**57**(5):550-558

[53] Rocha DS, Capanema FD, Netto MP, Franceschini SCC, Lamounier JA. Prevalência e fatores determinantes da anemia em crianças assistidas em creches de Belo Horizonte-MG. Revista Brasileira de Epidemiologia. 2012;**15**(3):675-684

[54] Stevens GA, Fincane MM, De-Regil LM, Paciorek CJ, Flaxman SR, Branca F, Peña-Rosas JP, Bhutta ZA, Ezzati M and on behalf of Nutrition Impact Model Study Group (Anaemia). Global, regional, and national trends in haemoglobin concentration and prevalence of total and severe anaemia in children and pregnant and nonpregnant women for 1995-2011: A systematic analysis of population-representative data. Lancet Global Health. 2013;**1**(1):16-25. DOI: 10.1016/S2214-109X(13)70001-9

[55] Brasil. Ministério da Saúde, Agência Nacional de Vigilância Sanitária. Resolução – RDC n° 344 de 13 de Dezembro de 2002. Aprova o Regulamento Técnico para a Fortificação das Farinhas de Trigo e das Farinhas de Milho com Ferro e Ácido Fólico. Diário Oficial da União 2002

[56] Panamá. Ministerio de Salud (MS). Direccion General de Salud. Departamento de Nutricion. Fondo de las Naciones Unidas para la Infancia (UNICEF). Organización Panamericana de la Salud. Situación de deficiencia de hierro y anemia. Panamá: MS; 2006

[57] Azeredo CM, Cotta RMM, Silva LS, Franceschini SCC, Sant Ana LFR, Lamounier JA. A problemática da adesão na prevenção da anemia ferropriva e suplementação com sais de ferro no município de Viçosa (MG). Ciênc. Saúde Coletiva. 2013;**18**(3):827-836

[58] Moreira-Araújo RSR, Araújo MAM, Arêas JA. Fortified food made by extrusion of a mixture of chickpea corn and bovine lung controls iron-deficiency anaemia in preschool children. Food Chemistry. 2008;**107**(1):158-164. DOI: 10.1016/j.foodchem.2007.07.074

[59] Adom T, Steiner-Asiedu, M, Sakyi-Dawson E, Anderson AK. Effect of fortification of maize with cowpea and iron on growth and anaemia status of children. African Journal of Food Science. 2010;**4**(4):136-142

[60] Abizari AR, Moretti D, Zimmermann MB, Armar-Klemesu M, Brouwer ID. Whole cowpea meal fortified with NaFeEDTA reduces iron deficiency among Ghanaian school children in a malaria endemic area. Journal of Nutrition. 2012;**142**(10):1836-1842

[61] Paganini D, Uyoga MA, Zimmermann MB. Iron Fortification of foods for infants and children in Low-Income countries: Effects on the Gut Microbiome, Gut Inflammation, and Diarrhea. Nutrients. 2016;**8**(8):494

[62] Moreira-Araújo RSR. Utilização de snack com elevado conteúdo de ferro em pré-escolares para o controle da anemia ferropriva [Thesis]. São Paulo: Universidade de São Paulo (USP); 2000.

[63] Cardoso Santiago RA, Moreira-Araújo, RSR, Pinto e Silva MEM, Arêas JAG. The potential of extruded chickpea, corn and bovine lung for malfunction programs. Innovative Science and Emerging Technology. 2001;**2**:203-209

[64] Moreira-Araújo RSR, Araújo MAM, Silva AMSE, Carvalho CMR, Arêas JAG. Impacto de salgadinho de alto valor nutritivo na situação nutricional de crianças de creches municipais de Teresina-PI. Nutrire. 2002;**23**:7-21

[65] Carvalho RV. Formulações de snacks de terceira geração por extrusão: caracterização texturométrica e microestrutural [Thesis]. Lavras: Universidade Federal de Lavras; 2000

[66] Frota KMG, Morgano MA, Silva MG, Araújo MAM, Moreira-Araújo RSR. Utilização da farinha de feijão-caupi (*Vigna unguiculata* L. *Walp*) na elaboração de produtos de panificação. Ciência e Tecnologia de Alimentos. 2010;**30**:44-50

[67] Moreira-Araújo RSR, Barros NVA. Barra de cereais enriquecida com feijão-caupi, fibra de caju, mel e castanha de caju e o seu respectivo processo de obtenção. Brazil Patent: BR1020140169873. INPI deposit: June 17, 2014

[68] Moreira-Araújo RSR, Sousa IG. Barra de cereais enriquecida com feijão-caupi e o seu respectivo processo de obtenção. Brazil Patent: BR1020140169792. INPI deposit: June 17, 2014

[69] Landim LA, Pessoa ML, Brandão AC, Morgano MA, Araújo MAM, Rocha MM, Arêas JA, Moreira-Araújo RS. Impact of the two different iron fortified cookies on treatment of anemia in preschool children in Brazil. Nutricion Hospitalaria. 2016;**33**(5):579. DOI: 10.20960/nh.579